Trauma Systems Therapy
for Children and Teens

Trauma Systems Therapy for Children and Teens

SECOND EDITION

**Glenn N. Saxe
B. Heidi Ellis
Adam D. Brown**

THE GUILFORD PRESS
New York   London

© 2016 The Guilford Press
A Division of Guilford Publications, Inc.
370 Seventh Avenue, Suite 1200, New York, NY 10001
www.guilford.com

Printed in the United States of America

This book is printed on acid-free paper.

Last digit is print number: 9 8 7 6 5

The authors have checked with sources believed to be reliable in their efforts to provide information that is complete and generally in accord with the standards of practice that are accepted at the time of publication. However, in view of the possibility of human error or changes in behavioral, mental health, or medical sciences, neither the authors, nor the editors and publisher, nor any other party who has been involved in the preparation or publication of this work warrants that the information contained herein is in every respect accurate or complete, and they are not responsible for any errors or omissions or the results obtained from the use of such information. Readers are encouraged to confirm the information contained in this book with other sources.

Library of Congress Cataloging-in-Publication Data

Saxe, Glenn N.
  [Collaborative treatment of traumatized children and teens]
  Trauma systems therapy for children and teens / Glenn N. Saxe, B. Heidi Ellis, Adam D. Brown.—Second edition.
     pages cm
  Revision of: Collaborative treatment of traumatized children and teens. 2006.
  Includes bibliographical references and index.
  ISBN 978-1-4625-2145-6 (paperback : acid-free paper)—ISBN 978-1-4625-2150-0 (hardcover : acid-free paper)
  I. Ellis, Beverley Heidi, 1972– II. Brown, Adam D., 1965– III. Title.
  RJ506.P55S39 2016
  618.92′8521—dc23
                                                                            2015001486

The first edition of this book was published with the title *Collaborative Treatment of Traumatized Children and Teens: The Trauma Systems Therapy Approach.*

To the memory of Roslyn Sheps Saxe (1936–2005)
who, in her 69 years of life, blazed a path
from survival to transcendence, and in so doing,
inspired her son to develop an intervention for traumatized children,
so they could follow in her path

About the Authors

Glenn N. Saxe, MD, is the Arnold Simon Professor and Chair of the Department of Child and Adolescent Psychiatry at New York University (NYU) School of Medicine and Director of the NYU Child Study Center. He is a physician-scientist with a focus on the psychiatric consequences of traumatic events in children and on factors that contribute to children's risk and resilience in the face of adversity. Dr. Saxe is the principal developer of trauma systems therapy (TST), which is currently used to guide clinical care in 14 states. He is also Director of the Center for Coordinated Trauma Services in Child Welfare, a National Child Traumatic Stress Network academic center funded to improve trauma services for the nation's child welfare systems.

B. Heidi Ellis, PhD, is Assistant Professor of Psychiatry at Harvard Medical School and Boston Children's Hospital. She is also Director of the Refugee Trauma and Resilience Center at Boston Children's Hospital, a partner in the National Child Traumatic Stress Network. Dr. Ellis's primary focus is understanding how trauma and sociocultural contexts affect the mental health and development of youth, and translating this understanding into mental health and/or violence prevention intervention programs. She is the codeveloper of TST and oversees the adaptation and implementation of the model with refugee youth.

Adam D. Brown, PsyD, is Clinical Assistant Professor in the Department of Child and Adolescent Psychiatry at NYU School of Medicine. He is also the clinical coordinator of the trauma service at the NYU Child Study Center. At NYU, he directs training, consultation, and technical assistance in TST. Dr. Brown has overseen programs for youth in inpatient, day treatment, and residential settings, and has extensive training and expertise in the area of assessing and treating interpersonal trauma in children and adolescents. He has a focused interest in the complex interplay among traumatized youth and families, the people who provide care to these youth and families, and the systems that contain this care.

Preface

Welcome to the world of trauma systems therapy (TST). As you will read, TST is designed for children and families for whom trauma is not only part of the past, but also an ongoing part of present, everyday life. TST is designed for all children and families who are having difficulty related to a trauma. It has particular relevance for those facing such ongoing stress as family and community abuse and violence, child neglect, and parental mental illness and substance abuse. Frequently, these children receive care in services systems that are frayed and fragmented.

You will soon be introduced to such children as Gerald, Denise, Robert, and Tanisha and our approach to their treatment. As you read, you will learn that this treatment always addresses two things: (1) a traumatized child who is not able to regulate emotional states related to survival, and (2) a social environment and/or a service system that is not sufficiently able to help the child to regulate these survival states.

These two things define what we call a trauma system, and that is why we have called this treatment "trauma systems therapy." To address the trauma systems that Gerald, Denise, Robert, and Tanisha inhabit can require the engagement of a lot of people: parents, guardians, relatives, friends, teachers, social service workers, therapists, psychopharmacologists, advocates, and/or home- and community-based clinicians. TST offers these children a highly focused and integrative treatment approach to recovery.

This book, and TST, may be of particular interest to you if you are:

- A psychotherapist who wants to learn about the fundamentals of traumatic stress care and how to build integrated treatment approaches within the organization where you work.
- A psychopharmacologist who wants to learn how psychopharmacology fits synergistically with the other interventions that traumatized children receive, and have the tools to connect your practice with other elements of the services system.
- A social service worker who wants to build skills in safety assessment and learn how child protection work is a critical part of traumatic stress care.
- A home- or community-based clinician who wants to improve home-based interventions and connect these interventions to the other services traumatized children and families receive.
- An administrator of a mental health organization who wants to learn how services for traumatized children in your agency can be more focused, integrated, and effective.
- An administrator of any program in the child services system who wants to learn how your services can be better integrated with effective mental health services.
- A public policymaker who wants ideas about how to improve the services system for traumatized children.
- A student or trainee in social work, psychology, psychiatry, pediatrics, or law who wants to understand the fundamentals of traumatic stress and its treatment.

This book may also be of interest to parents, teenagers, teachers, and advocates of children who want to learn in straightforward language what trauma is and how it affects children and, most importantly, what can be done about it.

TST can involve such interventions as emotional regulation skill building, home- and community-based treatment, advocacy, and psychopharmacology. When these varied intervention approaches together address the trauma system, treatment becomes tightly focused, synergistic, and, most important, effective. As you will also read, the process of bringing together the people necessary to fix the trauma system (the people mentioned above) involves the critical process of collaboration. Often providers work in different agencies and have never talked to each other or have never sat down together with the child and family to really understand what is most important to them. Collaboration is critical, and doable.

We began developing TST in the late 1990s because we found that available treatments for traumatized children were not addressing the complexity of their problems, particularly related to ongoing stress and threat in their environments. Available treatments guided us to focus on the child's trauma history as if the traumatic experience was only part of the child's *history*. In reality, trauma was too often a part of a child's *everyday life*. Not only did existing treatments offer no guidance for handling this tragically ubiquitous problem, but we had a growing concern about the potential psychological and physical harm that might be caused when a child who faces ongoing threats and trauma receives intervention that hardly assesses his or her current reality nor prioritizes the imperative to address this reality in treatment. We designed TST to make sure this imperative is never missed. TST is designed for all children with traumatic stress problems—not only those with ongoing traumas—and it uniquely offers guidance to help children in such circumstances.

As you will read, we are very focused on understanding and orienting treatment to the practical realities of children's lives and the cost to the child—and everyone else—when treatment deviates from these practical realities.

From the beginning, we wanted the treatment we would develop to be practically implemented and to be useful for providers, administrators, children, and families. And, most important, we wanted our treatment to impact the problems for which children and families sought care. We also wanted—at all costs—to make sure that we did not oversimplify. Child traumatic stress is complex. What it takes to address this complexity requires a good-enough understanding of traumatized children's complex biobehavioral system, their complex social environment, and their complex services system—as well as the complexity of how all this fits together. As you will read, we turn from the ever-present temptation to accept easy answers or simple solutions that may look good on paper (including what we read in the clinical trials literature) but that we know will not work in the real world.

To make sure we properly addressed these complex realities, we designed TST to be *adapted*. What does this mean? We understand there are a great many variables at play within any given organization that will determine whether a new intervention can work within that setting. These variables include cost, access to services, administrative support, politics, and the reimbursement model within any given county or state. Every organization is different and contends with a unique array of these variables. Therefore, for any new treatment to be adapted, it must be flexible enough so that these unique organizational variables do not become insurmountable barriers to adaptation. As you will read, TST has a lot of structure and focus, but contains flexibility to make it work within a great many diverse organizations. The services contained within TST, for example, can usually be paid for by conventional funding vehicles available in most states and counties. The challenge is to form the right collaborations to make the treatment work.

TST is public property. It is designed to be used and is owned by its users. If you use TST, we consider you part of our innovation community and hope that you will use your skill and creativity to adapt it to best suit your needs and, more important, to the needs of the children and families whom you serve. If you make a useful adaptation to TST based on what will work in your organization, that is great and we hope you will share your innovation with us. It is our sincere hope that these innovations will continually work to create an ever-improved TST, and a model that users can feel they own. This process is called "lead-user innovation" and is introduced in Chapter 1 and detailed in Chapter 16. This means that the ideas contained in this book do not simply come from the minds of its three authors, but have been refined over time based on the experience and expertise of a great many practitioners who have delivered it to a much greater number of traumatized children and families in a wide variety of settings. TST has been used in mental health clinics, schools, child welfare prevention and foster care programs, residential programs, and pediatric intensive care units. It has been adapted for adolescents with substance abuse, for refugees, and for children with injuries and illnesses, in addition to its original development for children who have experienced maltreatment and family and community violence. TST is now being used successfully by many agencies across the nation.

We are tremendously grateful to the many members of our TST innovation community. You will find their experience and ideas reflected on every page of this book. There are far too many individuals to thank in these pages. There are several who deserve special thanks:

- Susan Hansen, Cheryl Qamar, Barbara Sorkin, and Lee Myer from the mental health and child welfare departments in Ulster County, New York, who were the first to disseminate TST and adapted it for children with mental health needs in child welfare prevention programs. (Susan and Cheryl now are part of our team at NYU.)
- Kelly McCauley of KVC Health Systems, Inc., in Kansas, who adapted TST for both residential care and child welfare.
- Bob Kilkenny and Lisa Baron from the Alliance for Inclusion and Prevention in Boston, who adapted TST for schools.
- Liza Suarez of the University of Illinois at Chicago, who adapted TST for children with substance abuse and traumatic stress and was instrumental in developing the Beyond Trauma phase of TST.
- Julie Kaplow of the University of Texas, who was closely involved in the early development of TST and was a coauthor of our first book.
- Bob Abramovitz of Hunter College and Virginia Strand of Fordham University, who integrated TST within the core curriculum of the National Child Traumatic Stress Network. (Bob also was instrumental in advancing TST for foster care at the Jewish Board for Family and Children's Services in New York.)

We are particularly grateful to members of our teams:

At New York University:

- Mary Dino, Susan Hansen, and Christina Laitner for review and suggestions of clinical content.
- Erika Tullberg for review and suggestions related to secondary traumatization and application to child welfare systems.
- Bonnie Kerker, Carol Quinlan, and Len Bickman (of Vanderbilt University and Florida State University) for evaluation of TST programs.
- Margo Fenner for her terrific work assisting in manuscript preparation.

At Boston Children's Hospital:

- Molly Benson and Saida Abdi for review and suggestions on the clinical content.
- Alisa Miller and Osob Issa for contributions to adapting TST for refugee populations.

We offer special thanks to our families for putting up with us and managing the many absences in the 2-year process of writing this book:

- Joanna Bures-Saxe, Ryan Saxe, and Benjamin Saxe.
- Chris Bogan, Eva, Ceci, and Jack (who thoughtfully made his appearance after the first drafts were in).
- Patty Goodman and Hannah Brown.

The process of treating children with traumatic stress, like the process of developing a treatment model for these children, is, in a way, never ending. What, really, is the finished product? The work of helping traumatized children requires, on the part of everyone, a continual struggle to make things better and better. This book is now the result of a 16-year effort to develop a treatment that will work. We hope, however, that this book is only the new version of a process that is continually improved in response to people's experiences. Similarly, when we leave a traumatized child at what we call the end of therapy, we do not really believe he or she is "better" or "cured" or whichever professional term is used to make us feel good. But we hope to leave the child and the family with tools they will use to meet their challenges throughout their lives.

So, welcome to the world of TST. You are now a member of a community of innovators. Use it. Change it. Make it better and do your best with the Geralds, Denises, Roberts, and Tanishas in your practice and in your lives.

Contents

PART III. DOING TRAUMA SYSTEMS THERAPY

PART IV. IMPROVING TRAUMA SYSTEMS THERAPY

Purchasers of this book can download and print larger versions
of the appendices from *www.guilford.com/saxe-forms*
for personal use or use with individual clients.

Introduction to Trauma Systems Therapy

Whatever It Takes to Help a Traumatized Child

LEARNING OBJECTIVES

- To introduce trauma systems therapy for child traumatic stress
- To describe the trauma system
- To outline the *whatever-it-takes* approach to providing care
- To provide a guide for the rest of this book

ICONS USED IN THIS CHAPTER

Essential Point	Academic Point	Danger	Quotation	Case Discussion

---

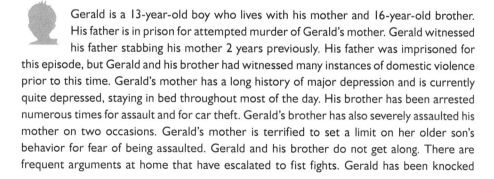

Gerald is a 13-year-old boy who lives with his mother and 16-year-old brother. His father is in prison for attempted murder of Gerald's mother. Gerald witnessed his father stabbing his mother 2 years previously. His father was imprisoned for this episode, but Gerald and his brother had witnessed many instances of domestic violence prior to this time. Gerald's mother has a long history of major depression and is currently quite depressed, staying in bed throughout most of the day. His brother has been arrested numerous times for assault and for car theft. Gerald's brother has also severely assaulted his mother on two occasions. Gerald's mother is terrified to set a limit on her older son's behavior for fear of being assaulted. Gerald and his brother do not get along. There are frequent arguments at home that have escalated to fist fights. Gerald has been knocked unconscious by his brother and is perpetually in fear that his brother will "lose it" again. Gerald has frequent intrusive memories of witnessing domestic violence, is vigilant about being assaulted, and has an exaggerated startle response. He has poor sleep with frequent nightmares and very poor concentration in his awake state; he failed the sixth grade because he found it hard to focus on school. He is at risk for failing the sixth grade again this year and has told his therapist that if he fails school again, he intends to kill himself.

What do you do? What do you say? Where do you begin? If you are like most providers* who work with traumatized children and families in the United States, you work out of your office or clinic. The story of Gerald is probably very familiar to you. You probably have five Geralds in your caseload. You see him for his first intake appointment. Perhaps you see him again for a follow-up visit. If you end up treating Gerald, his attendance is spotty. He is here for a few sessions, then gone for weeks or months at a time. If he attends regularly, you are faced with the real question: HOW CAN I HELP?! Does Gerald have cognitive distortions that need correcting? Does he have serotonin reuptake receptors that need blocking? Does he have conflicts that need interpreting? Does he have avoidance that needs exposing? Does he have eye movements that need desensitizing? Maybe . . . but . . . anything that you do; any distortion that you challenge; any interpretations that you make; any medication that you prescribe; any learning that you condition . . . is undermined as soon as Gerald leaves your office. What do you do?

Gerald travels through the system. He is seen in emergency rooms, residential programs, inpatient units, and outpatient clinics. His care involves mental health, education, social service, and soon the juvenile justice systems. If you are assigned to treat Gerald, then you know that sensible treatment requires a lot of integration with each of these systems. But who has time for that? He is hospitalized and you see him again. His medications are changed, but, for the life of you, you cannot figure out what "they" did in the hospital. He is failing school. You've gone to a few school meetings and explained about the stress and chaos in Gerald's life. The teachers are tired, and they have to think about the other kids in the class. They don't really know what to do. Gerald is missing school. He is missing appointments. You consider "closing the case" but just can't bear to do it. You've filed a couple of reports with your local child welfare agency, but they are "screened out." What do you do?

There Are No Easy Answers

We wish it were easy. We wish there was that one medication. We wish there was that 12-step, eight-session therapy that would make Gerald's nightmare go away.

---

*In this book we use the term "provider" to refer to any professional who provides services to traumatized children and families.

We know that you wish it, too. Sadly, what has created Gerald's nightmare is years of trauma, abuse, and neglect, some of which is ongoing. Real intervention will require rolling up your sleeves and helping to address the reality of Gerald's problems. But *how*?

This book is about an intervention model that attempts to address Gerald's needs and the tragic needs of children like him. Accordingly, intervention needs to be comprehensive, focused, and intensive. It must be in the home, in the school, and in the neighborhood. Interventions need to get to the essence of the problem and stick to it like a dog to a bone, never to let go until the work is done. Interventions must address the numerous barriers that get in the way of families accessing services. This work is not easy. It requires a lot of energy on the part of providers and a lot of support of providers from mental health agencies and service systems. Obviously, this type of work exists in a system that is far, far from perfect. There are enormous public policy concerns related to how services are delivered to traumatized children and how the service system is organized. Nevertheless, there are existing services in place in most states that can be maximized for effective treatment. This book is about using these existing services in a coherent treatment model aimed to maximize effectiveness.

> We wish it were easy. We wish there was that one medication. We wish there was that 12-step, eight-session therapy that would make Gerald's nightmare go away. We know that you wish it, too.

This book also tries to address the realities of a provider's practice. What are these realities?

- The average provider is busy, probably overworked, possibly "burning out," and has little "extra" time or resources to enhance treatment.
- The average agency that provides services is financially stretched and has few funds for the "extras" such as staff training, supervision, outcome monitoring, or home-based care.
- The average state service system is also stretched and fragmented, with insufficient communication between departments and inadequate cross-system service plans for children with traumatic stress.

We designed our intervention model with the needs of children with traumatic stress in mind, as well as the constraints of the realities of clinical practice in the United States at this particular time. Accordingly, we designed this intervention using services that are available in most states.

> We designed our intervention model with the needs of children with traumatic stress in mind, as well as the constraints of the realities of clinical practice in the United States at this particular time.

The answers we propose are not "easy"; how can they be? We offer a series of solutions that are in no way perfect. Service delivery takes place in a service system that is resource poor and problematic in many ways. Nevertheless, we believe that the solutions we propose will be very helpful for providers, agencies, and service systems as we all try to figure out what to do for children like Gerald.

Whatever It Takes

There are no half measures or tentative choices that are appropriate. It's "all in" or it's not; it's "whatever it takes" or it's not; it's about looking at the reality, or it's about averting our eyes.

Ultimately, the issue of addressing Gerald's needs—in all their complexity—boils down to the answer to a simple question: Do we look away, or not? Trauma is such a deep assault on the soul of a child—and on whom he or she might become—that our choice about how to help is not unlike what we must do when we walk along a riverbank and see a person drowning. There are no half measures or tentative choices that are appropriate. It's "all in" or it's not; it's "whatever it takes" or it's not; it's about looking at the reality, or it's about averting our eyes.

What do we think is in store for Gerald—and kids like him—if he doesn't get the help he needs? We know where far too many children like Gerald are going without treatments that will address their reality. They are going to our chronic psychiatric hospitals, our substance abuse programs, our homeless shelters, our prisons, and, far too often, prematurely to our morgues. We have to do *whatever it takes* to help. We know where these kids are going. The facts are clear. We know about the numbers of kids impacted by trauma. It's no longer good enough to say that our system is too limited and there are too many barriers in the way to provide help.

Regarding the great many of *our* Geralds left alone in that river: What do we tell ourselves that makes us not address their realities or that allows us to address them with half measures?

There are, of course, so many ways in which the system is limited—and so many barriers in the way of providing effective care. The question for us all is: How can we make it work, given these limitations? There may not be *easy* answers, but there *are* answers. It's not unlike the many things we might tell ourselves in an effort to feel OK about not jumping into the water to rescue the drowning person (e.g., "What drowning person?"; "He's going down anyway, not much I can do"; "I'll walk to town and call someone better equipped to help"; "What do you expect when you swim alone in a river?"). Regarding the great many of *our* Geralds left alone in that river: What do we tell ourselves that makes us not address their realities or that allows us to address them with half measures?

Judith Herman raised this very issue many years ago in her classic book on trauma, *Trauma and Recovery* (1997):

> It is very tempting to take the side of the perpetrator. All the perpetrator asks is that the bystander do nothing. He appeals to the universal desire to see, hear, speak no evil. The victim, on the contrary, asks the bystander to share the burden of pain. The victim demands action, engagement, and remembering. (pp. 7–8)

We cannot look away. We are called to act, to engage, to remember, to help, and to share the pain.

We cannot look away. We are called to act, to engage, to remember, to help, and to share the pain.

Is our perspective too harsh? A few facts to consider:

- From the general public, 52.1% of adults have reported having at least one adverse childhood experience, with 22% experiencing sexual abuse and 10.8% physical abuse (Felitti et al., 1998).
- In 2012, a nationally estimated 4.5 children died *every day* due to abuse and neglect (U.S. Department of Health and Human Services [HHS], Administration for Children and Families [ACF], Administration on Children, Youth, and Families [ACYF], Children's Bureau, 2013).
- 3.2 million children received a child protective services response in 2012 (HHS, ACF, ACYF, Children's Bureau, 2013).
- In a nationally representative sample, 60% of children were exposed to violence and 46% were assaulted within the past year (Finkelhor, Turner, Ormrod, Hamby, & Kracke, 2009).
- Among New York City families receiving child welfare services, 92% of children have been exposed to at least one traumatic event and *86% have experienced multiple traumatic events*. Among mothers, 92% have experienced a traumatic event, and *19% have experienced five or more* types of traumatic events (Chemtob, Griffing, Tullberg, Roberts, & Ellis, 2010).
- Childhood exposure to adverse experiences increases the risk for alcoholism, suicide attempts, depression, drug abuse, obesity, heart disease, and cancer (Felitti et al., 1998).

Our experience tells us that many of these children have problems as complex as Gerald's (would Gerald be the most complex kid in your practice?). These children need treatment. They need treatment that addresses trauma. And that trauma treatment must address the complex reality in which they live. One hundred percent of traumatized children deserve to have us do *whatever it takes* to help them.

We must not look away. We must be all in. We must figure out how to do whatever it takes. We know who bears the burden of our averted eyes.

We must not look away. We must be all in. We must figure out how to do whatever it takes. We know who bears the burden of our averted eyes.

Our Pledge: Offering a Treatment Approach That Helps You Do Whatever It Takes

We understand that there is a very tough reality ahead for those who will do whatever it takes. We join you in this spirit and are with you as you take this more courageous road. This book is written to help you to be as effective as possible. We start with a pledge to you.

- We write about the reality you face as you help with the reality your children face.
- We simplify this reality only to help us focus on what is most important. We do everything we can to *not* oversimplify.
- We offer practical solutions that will work in the world in which most people practice. In order for these solutions to work, clinical care must be embedded in the right type of organizational and systems-level approach and be financially viable within these organizations and systems. We address these areas methodically, practically, and clearly.
- We aim to provide an approach that offers value to whoever uses it, based on what is most important to them. The user may be a provider, an administrator, a parent, or a child. The only evidence base that matters to us is the accumulating evidence that our approach yields this type of value.
- We write to honor the courage of those who choose to do whatever it takes and to help with *your* very real needs as you take this difficult road.

Who Are We?

We are a child psychiatrist (Dr. Saxe) and a child psychologist (Dr. Ellis) who began to work together in the late 1990s with traumatized children and families at Boston Medical Center, Boston's inner-city hospital. We are also a child psychologist (Dr. Brown) who joined several years later and became the chief trauma systems therapy trainer. The children and families we worked with at Boston Medical Center continually faced considerable social problems such as poverty, community violence, parental mental illness and substance abuse, homelessness, and racism. Many of the families we served were highly traumatized. Ten percent of children seen in our primary care clinic reported seeing a shooting or stabbing before they were 6 years old (Taylor, Zuckerman, Harik, & Groves, 1994). Sixty-two percent of adolescents seen in our emergency room (for any reason) reported a history of experiencing or witnessing violent physical or sexual assault (Kassner & Kharasch, 1999).

We had been trying to do our best for these families with outpatient therapy, including what was considered "evidence-based" treatments and the highest-quality psychopharmacology. We directed a team of psychologists, psychiatrists, social workers, and many trainees, and were providing treatment to a great many traumatized children and families in Boston. At one point, faced with the frustration of the clinician assigned to Gerald (and a great many other children like him), we asked our team a very simple (but highly provocative) question: "Are we doing any good for the kids and families that come to us for treatment?" We saw the impulse on team members' faces to enthusiastically answer: *"Of course we are doing good!"* But people withstood the impulse and held their tongues for about 3 seconds—long enough to confirm our impressions—and then we were able to have an honest conversation.

> We began to ask a simple question: Are we helping? We were not able to provide a clear answer to that question.

The bottom line was this: Despite all our hard work, and the many hours we were putting in to try to help many people, we could not provide a clear answer to that question. There was simply no evidence to which we could appeal. Team members could describe families that did benefit from our work—but those were the families that returned to treatment. We knew that our "no-show" rate was about 50%. Furthermore, we were getting burned out. Our staff turnover rate was high. People were very frustrated. Frankly, it was feeling like we were banging our heads against the wall trying to help. We began to initiate a process of figuring out how we could do better. The first version of this book, published in 2007, was a result of that process. On the way, we investigated many different types of treatments and services for children. We also wanted our work to be helpful to others and so have worked with many people to try to operationalize our ideas into a useable format.

A huge catalyst for our efforts was our funding at the end of 2001 as an Intervention Development and Evaluation Center as part of the new National Child Traumatic Stress Network (NCTSN). This network is the nation's primary response to the problem of traumatic stress in children and provided the funding and infrastructure to help us develop this treatment that we began to call *trauma systems therapy* (TST).

The Never-Ending Story Based on a Community of Users

It is very important to understand that the ideas contained within the intervention model called TST come from an ever-widening community of users who have, over the years, agreed to work together to implement new interventions to help traumatized children and families, evaluate their utility, and then decide whether they should be integrated into the model. We began with a handful of clinicians who worked together on a clinical team in one clinical setting. Our team spent about 3 or 4 years tinkering with the model by slowly integrating and evaluating different approaches, until we felt we had a model that had a chance of helping us "do some good."

As soon as we arrived at the model we liked, we began writing the first version of our book and began to give presentations at local and national meetings about our work. Interest began to generate, primarily from providers and administrators who were asking themselves the same question we were asking: "Are we doing any good?" TST began to ride the wave of frustration such a question provokes.

Sometime in 2002 we received a call from three individuals—Susan Hansen, Cheryl Qamar, and Barbara Sorkin—who were administrators in the mental health and child welfare systems in Ulster County, New York. They had attended one of our lectures at a national meeting and thought our ideas for TST might be helpful for their work trying to provide integrated care between their county's mental health and child welfare systems. But there were several barriers in the way to our helping the Ulster County team:

- We had never even heard of Ulster County and had no idea how our intervention might be useful to them.
- We thought TST was an inner-city treatment model and had never even considered how it might be applied to a largely rural population.
- We designed TST as an outpatient mental health treatment and had no idea how it might help integrate services between county mental health and child welfare systems.

Fortunately, Susan, Cheryl, and Barbara are persistent people and convinced us to visit Ulster County and help them implement our treatment model there. Our visit surprised us on multiple counts, particularly how similar to our experience the clinical issues were in the families they were trying to help. Although figuring out how to adapt and implement TST in Ulster County was not easy, we helped them create a program that met their needs, helped a lot of children and families, and has been sustained for almost 12 years (at the time of this writing). Our first published outcome study was based on a cohort of children from Boston Medical Center and from Ulster County. Our experience in Ulster County taught us a number of very important things:

- Our ideas about trauma systems (described next) are quite useful outside the setting where they were developed.
- Our ideas could be extended and improved based on their use. By partnering with other agencies, we could create an ever-widening community of developers who could work with us to improve the TST model based on collective experience. At the time of this writing we have what we call a *TST Innovation Community* comprised of 25 agencies in 13 states and the District of Columbia, that continually work with us to improve TST based on this diverse experience (described in Chapter 16).
- Organizational issues are pivotal. TST is implemented within an organization or a group of collaborating organizations. Each organization has

its own human resource, financial, and political needs. Each organization has unique sets of stakeholders who must be mobilized for TST to be implemented and sustained. All of these issues required an organizational planning process. We describe this planning process in Chapter 8.

Whenever we implement TST, we learn how to make it more useful, and we now have access to an ever-widening community of TST innovators to help us adapt, evaluate, integrate, and implement. We feel very lucky to have such partners and, because of them, TST has been adapted for problems and for settings we had hardly considered: rural settings, residential care programs, crisis units, shelters for unaccompanied refugee minors, foster-care programs, child welfare prevention programs, school-based programs, refugee programs, and programs for children hospitalized with injuries and illnesses. Early partners such as Adam Brown at Children's Village in Dobbs Ferry, New York, helped work out the details of TST for residential care; Bob Abramovitz and Mary Dino at the Jewish Board for Family and Children's Services in Manhattan helped adapt TST for foster care; Kelly McCauley and Sherry Love of KVC Health Systems, Inc. in Kansas helped adapt TST for both residential care and child welfare; Bob Kilkenny and Lisa Baron from the Alliance for Inclusion and Prevention in Boston helped adapt TST for schools; and Liza Suarez of the University of Illinois at Chicago helped adapt TST for children with substance abuse and traumatic stress. Most recently, Erika Tullberg and Adam Brown worked out the details for how TST can best address the considerable problem of secondary traumatization.

TST started from a community of developers based at Boston Medical Center. Drs. Saxe and Ellis both left Boston Medical Center in 2007. Dr. Saxe now chairs the Department of Child and Adolescent Psychiatry at New York University School of Medicine and Directs the NYU Child Study Center. Dr. Ellis now directs the Center for Refugee Trauma and Resilience at Boston Children's Hospital. TST is now based in our new institutions and in institutions, agencies, homes, and schools around the United States.

TST has become a never-ending story based on an ever-widening community of users joined with a spirit to do *whatever it takes* to help traumatized children. We hope you will consider joining our community and contribute to the telling of our story.

What Is TST?

TST is both a clinical model for the treatment of children with traumatic stress (broadly defined) and an organizational model for the successful implementation of the TST clinical model based on the way organizations work. It has a defined position on the core clinical problems of traumatic stress in children and a defined position on how organizations can best support and sustain their TST program.

The Core Problem: The Trauma System

Traumatic stress occurs when a child is unable to regulate emotional states and in certain moments experiences his or her current environment as extremely threatening even when it is relatively safe. This happens when the child's brain regulation of emotional states is disturbed. In Chapters 2 and 3 we describe how this disturbed capacity to regulate emotional states leads to a child experiencing what we call a *survival-in-the-moment state.*

A survival-in-the-moment state is defined as:

an individual's experience of the present environment as threatening to his or her survival, with corresponding thoughts, emotions, behaviors, and neurochemical and neurophysiological responses.

A survival-in-the-moment state is defined as:

an individual's experience of the present environment as threatening to his or her survival, with corresponding thoughts, emotions, behaviors, and neurochemical and neurophysiological responses.

When there is a real threat to survival, then a survival-in-the-moment state is extremely adaptive. When there is not a clear threat to survival, then a survival-in-the-moment state can be extremely maladaptive. Here lies a very big problem for the child with traumatic stress:

1. He or she has a great propensity to shift into survival-in-the-moment states even when the present environment is relatively safe.

2. He or she also commonly lives in environments that can become truly unsafe and/or filled with reminders of past unsafe (traumatic) environments.

In order to effectively treat traumatized children, both of these problems must be addressed effectively.

system A group of interacting, interrelated, or interdependent elements forming a complex whole. (*American Heritage Dictionary, Fourth Edition*, 2000)

Accordingly, TST involves interventions that address what we call a *trauma system.* A trauma system emerges in response to disruption in the natural systemic balance between the developing child and his or her social environment. A trauma system is comprised of:

1. A traumatized child who experiences *survival-in-the-moment* states in specific, definable moments.

2. A social environment and/or system of care that is not able to help the child regulate these *survival-in-the-moment* states.

Our treatment explicitly addresses these two core problem domains. Because the social environment (e.g., family, school, peer group, neighborhood) ordinarily has a core function of helping a child to contain emotions or behavior, it is assumed that a child's inability to contain emotions or behavior means there is a diminished capacity of one or more levels of that social environment to help the child. Similarly, a child's inability to regulate emotional states also implies an inadequacy in the system of care to help the child contain emotions or behaviors. This failure has three possible sources: (1) The child has not yet accessed the system of care, (2) the child is "falling through the cracks," or (3) the services the child is receiving are insufficient in some way to help him or her contain those emotions or behavior.

TST includes an approach to assessing this "fit" between the child's regulation capacities and the adequacy of the social environment/system of care to help the child, and offers a variety of treatment modules based on the outcome of this assessment. We designed our intervention approach to help address the severe problems in children's environments and to do this work consistently holding in mind principles of child development and of systems of care. We designed our intervention approach with children like Gerald in mind.

Existing interventions do not offer clear approaches for addressing these severe social-environmental problems—approaches that are informed by theory about the way the social environment and the developing child interact. As is repeated throughout this book, our treatment addresses two core problem domains of the trauma system: (1) a child with dysregulated emotional states and (2) a social environment/system of care that is unable to help the child regulate these emotional states. Our intervention intensively targets the trauma system, which is why we call our intervention *trauma systems therapy.*

TST: Intervening with the Trauma System through Four Ecological Levels

In Chapters 2 and 3 we provide much detail about how survival-in-the-moment happens. We describe how specific signals in the child's present environment will evoke specific survival-laden responses in specific moments, based on a child's past history of specific traumas. You will learn how to identify the patterns by which a child transitions from his or her usual emotional state to these survival-in-the-moment states. The trauma system fits within a much broader social ecology comprised of family, school, neighborhood, and culture, and also includes the service system when problems need to be addressed. TST is an explicit social-ecological model of intervention (Bronfenbrenner, 1979) whose workings we describe in detail in Chapter 4. What does TST look like? Figure 1.1 provides this picture.

We first warn you: It's a complex picture! Please don't be daunted by it. We "unpack" these layers over the course of this book. For now, take a look at Figure 1.1 and then the outline of its various elements.

The Trauma System

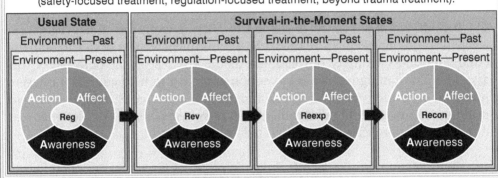

4. Capacity of the child service system to support the organization that houses the TST treatment team, to support the team's work supporting the child, and those around the child, for the child's regulation and growth.

3. Capacity of the organization that houses the TST treatment team to support their work supporting the child, and those around the child, for the child's regulation and growth.

2. Capacity of TST treatment team to support the child, and those around the child, for the child's regulation and growth.

1. Capacity of the child, and those around the child, for the child's regulation and growth (safety-focused treatment, regulation-focused treatment, beyond trauma treatment).

Usual State	Survival-in-the-Moment States		
Environment—Past	Environment—Past	Environment—Past	Environment—Past
Environment—Present	Environment—Present	Environment—Present	Environment—Present
Action Affect / Reg / Awareness	Action Affect / Rev / Awareness	Action Affect / Reexp / Awareness	Action Affect / Recon / Awareness

FIGURE 1.1. The TST picture.

Patterns of Survival-in-the-Moment

The boxes in Figure 1.1 labeled "Usual State" and "Survival-in-the-Moment States" describe the transition from the child's usual state to survival-in-the-moment. As we discuss in Chapter 3, these states are represented by four essential building blocks, each of which have a characteristic level of nervous system arousal: Regulating (Reg), Revving (Rev), Reexperiencing (Reexp), and Reconstituting (Recon). We call these the 4 R's and each are defined by three qualities of experience that we call the 3 A's—Affect, Action, and Awareness—all of which change based on what is going on in the child's environment at the time (environment—present). The way these shifts occur and, in particular, what causes the shifts can be understood through the child's experience of past environments, including traumatic environments (environment—past). What is critically important about all of this is the process by which a child transitions from her or his usual state (defined by the first R, regulating) to a survival-in-the-moment state (defined by the sequential transition through Revving, Reexperiencing, and Reconstituting). We return to this process, repeatedly throughout the book. The details of how the environment is arranged to support, or not support, the child's regulation and growth are described in Chapters 4 and 5, and the process for assessing this complex system is the focus of Chapter 9.

Four Levels of Ecological Intervention

1. **The capacity of the child, and those around him or her, to sustain, or fail to sustain, the child's regulation and growth.** The natural social environment is populated with people who ordinarily spend time with the child—parents, teachers, coaches, etc. Ordinarily, those around the child will be able to help him or her manage adversities, including trauma. Sometimes help beyond this naturalistic network is needed to support the child's regulation and growth, and this is when clinical intervention may be indicated. TST provides this clinical approach in three phases—safety-focused treatment, regulation-focused treatment, and beyond trauma treatment—discussed in detail in Chapters 12, 13, and 14, respectively.

2. **The capacity of the team supporting the child and those around him or her.** The child and those around him or her are supported by a multidisciplinary TST treatment team, with a defined approach to conducting the work (described in Chapter 7).

3. **The capacity of the organization supporting the team.** The TST treatment team is supported by an organization, or group of organizations. We have a very specific approach to ensure that the organizations in which this work is based can support and sustain their TST Program. The TST organizational approach is described in Chapter 8.

4. **The capacity of the service system supporting the organization.** Organizations that support TST treatment teams operate within a service system, the realities of which must be understood and well integrated so that the host organizations can fully support and sustain their teams. The realities of this service system are described in Chapter 4 and the integration of these realities within an overall organizational approach is described in Chapter 8.

Making It Work: The TST Organizational Model

We wrote our first edition of this book without a defined organizational model. We quickly learned, through our experience in Ulster County and in many of our early disseminations, that good clinical ideas only go so far. A clinical model such as TST is implemented in organizations with definable needs and reasons for supporting the implementation of a TST program in the organization. If the TST program is not developed with a good understanding of these needs and how the TST program will address them, then the program is unlikely to be properly implemented and sustained over time. As is described in Chapter 8, the implementation of TST requires an organizational plan struck in collaboration between TST developers and the right set of stakeholders from the organization. In particular, an organizational leader with sufficient authority must be included and the plan must be set to deliver on items the organization's leadership and staff identify as very important (whatever they may be).

Who Can Benefit from TST?

We've designed TST to address a very broad range of problems that traumatized children experience. It's not just for children with posttraumatic stress disorder (PTSD; more on the problems with PTSD in Chapter 3). It's for children who meet the following criteria:

1. A child with a plausible trauma history, and
2. A child who has difficulty regulating emotional states that are plausibly related to this trauma history.

Note the word *plausible*. We don't need to know all the details of the child's trauma history. We don't even need to know with 100% certainty that a child was exposed to a trauma. The most important thing to know, given the child's clinical presentation and what the child and others tell you, is that a trauma history is plausible. Similarly, you don't need to make a psychiatric diagnosis such as PTSD to offer TST. You need to see the child experiencing dysregulation of emotional states in certain moments and see that the way the child dysregulates in those moments may plausibly be related to his or her plausible history of trauma. We provide a lot more detail about what it means to meet the TST criteria in Chapters 3 and 7. What is most important for now is to know that TST can help a lot of traumatized children who need services. We are very proud of the fact that our model can help a broad range of children with issues ranging from the most straightforward to the most complex. One thing that we and others have observed: In most agencies that serve traumatized children, the great majority of providers' and administrators' time and attention is dedicated to a very small proportion of children served. These are the children with very severe and complex problems, including a high risk for harm. We are proudest of the fact that TST appears to provide agencies unique value for exactly these children and their families.

What Is Treatment?

Consistent with the theme of this book, we define treatment as whatever it takes to help a traumatized child. Accordingly, we don't ever predetermine what will help.

We know that, eventually, we'll have to get into this basic discussion, so we may as well dive in here. What do we mean by *treatment* or *therapy*? It's important to know that we take a very broad view here, perhaps broader than most other treatment models. Consistent with the theme of this book, we define treatment as *whatever it takes* to help a traumatized child. Accordingly, we don't ever predetermine what will help. Treatment is not necessarily something that is delivered by a clinician in a clinical setting according to well-defined psychotherapeutic or psychopharmacological protocols.

Treatment is *anything* that might be delivered by *anyone* who will help. Does this mean that anything goes? Well . . . yes and no. *Yes*: Just about anything could be considered a potential treatment or element of treatment. *No*: The only thing(s) that would be considered an actual treatment or element of treatment is that which we determine will specifically alleviate the child's well-defined trauma-related problem(s). Whatever it is and whatever it takes. As we detail in the assessment and treatment-planning chapters, there is a great deal of specificity to what we eventually decide should constitute the treatment for a particular child. It's highly strategic and highly specific. It's whatever it takes to help, given our well-defined understanding of the nature of the child's problem(s).

Five Goals of the Development of TST

We designed our intervention approach to help with the severe problems in children's environments, and do this work in a way that consistently incorporates principles of child development and of systems of care. We designed our intervention approach with children like Gerald in mind. Specifically, we set four goals for designing this intervention. As TST developed, we added a fifth goal that we see as critical for the success of any TST program.

1. Treatment must be developmentally informed.
2. Treatment must *directly* address the social ecology.
3. Treatment must be compatible with systems of care.
4. Treatment must be "disseminate-able" and sustainable.
5. Treatment must add value to users.

What Does Each Goal Mean?

1. Treatment Must Be Developmentally Informed

In order to treat Gerald, you need to know certain basic principles about child development. You need to know that the types of interventions effective for a 6-year-old are very different from those effective for a 16-year-old, and also that treatment of a child with developmental delays looks different from treatment of a child without them. You must consider how such areas as attachment, emotional regulation, identity, and cognition at different ages may be approached in treatment.

These ideas are very important for a child like Gerald. What type of attachment relationships might develop for a child with a depressed mother and a very violent father and brother? What does it do to the sense of identity of a 13-year-old boy to have a father in prison and to have witnessed this father beating up the boy's mother and brother? What does it do to his sense of identity, self-esteem, and feelings of control to have been beaten up by his father? How do these experiences, and their influence on attachments and identity formation, affect Gerald's ability to regulate his emotions? What type of peer groups is he likely to join? How does growing up in terror affect cognitive development and school performance? These types of questions need to be asked and answered in order to sensibly treat Gerald and all those like him. In Chapters 2, 3, and 4 we describe the developmental principles upon which our intervention approach is based.

> What does it do to the sense of identity of a 13-year-old boy to have a father in prison and to have witnessed this father beating up the boy's mother and brother?

2. Intervention Must Directly Address the Social Ecology

In order to treat Gerald and all those like him, you must be able to *directly* address the social ecology. If your treatment is conducted only in your office, you will be spinning your wheels for a very long time. If you try to approach Gerald's family problems by scheduling the occasional family meeting, you will probably not help anyone very much. Gerald's problems require on-site treatments that directly address the social-environmental contributors to the problem. Often families of children with traumatic stress experience significant barriers to receiving appropriate care. Intervention approaches, accordingly, must be flexible enough to surmount these barriers.

> If your treatment is conducted only in your office, you will be spinning your wheels for a very long time.

Perhaps the most successful intervention model to directly address the social ecology is multisystemic therapy (MST) for conduct disorder (Henggeler, Schoenwald, Borduin, Rowland, & Cunningham, 1998). MST uses community-based interventions to specifically target areas of a child's environment that are theoretically related to the development and maintenance of conduct problems. MST has demonstrated effectiveness for aggressive children by successfully targeting many fields in which the child interacts; "the child and family, school, work, peer, community, and cultural institutions are viewed as interconnected systems with dynamic and reciprocal influences on the behavior of family members," and are thus all engaged in the treatment process (Henggeler, Schoenwald, & Pickrel, 1995, p. 710). MST targets child and family problems in the multiple systems in which families are embedded and delivers treatments in the settings in which they are likely to have the highest impact. Services are delivered in a variety of settings, such as home, school, and the community.

> How could you approach Gerald's mental health problems from the distance of a clinic or office?

How could you approach Gerald's mental health problems from the distance of a clinic or office? His severe traumatic stress symptoms are highly reactive to conflicts and threats from his brother. His mother is too depressed and afraid to intervene or to reasonably engage in clinic- or office-based treatment. The consequences of these traumatic stress symptoms severely affect his school performance. Community-based interventions such as the following are essential for a child like Gerald:

- The provider must work in the home, helping Gerald's mother to protect him by engaging the police, social service agencies, relatives, or whoever is able and willing to help.
- The provider must actively work with Gerald's mother to help her understand her own traumatic stress symptoms and how they are impacting Gerald, and to ensure that she receives treatment and support so that she can better protect Gerald.
- The provider must work in the school, consulting teachers and other school staff about how to best teach him and help with the construction of an individualized education program (IEP).

The failure of two school years for a child like Gerald (who has normal intelligence) is a tragedy. Chapters 4, 11, and 12 offer details about the way in which the social environment can be engaged in the treatment of traumatic stress.

3. Treatment Must Be Compatible with Systems of Care

In order to treat Gerald, you must be able to clearly link his treatment with the wider system of care. This is not easy, given how fragmented this system has become. Nevertheless, as we describe in Chapters 4, 10, and 12, a number of tools can help. Gerald, like many children with traumatic stress, is seen in many different service systems. Within the mental health system, children like Gerald often drift between the inpatient, outpatient, residential, and emergency psychiatry systems. Gerald is currently treated in an outpatient setting. If his suicidal impulses increase, he may be seen in the emergency or inpatient psychiatry systems. If his mother continues to be too incapacitated to protect him, the social services and residential systems may become necessary. There is a clear and reciprocal relationship between his emotional symptoms and his school functioning. His traumatic stress-related anxiety and poor concentration have interfered with his performance at school. This poor school performance, in turn, has contributed to his low self-esteem and suicidal impulses. It is hard to imagine a sensible treatment plan that does not fully integrate the educational system.

> In order to treat Gerald, you must be able to clearly link his treatment with the wider system of care.

Clearly, there is a great need for service integration when treating traumatized children, and there is widespread acknowledgment of this need to create integrated systems of care for vulnerable, especially traumatized, children. The surgeon general's report on mental health specifically identifies the need for services integration:

> The organization of services . . . is the linchpin of effective treatment . . . it is not just services in isolation but the delivery system as a whole, that dictates the outcome of treatment. Among the fundamental elements of effective service delivery are integrated community-based services, continuity of providers and treatments, and culturally sensitive and high quality empowering services. (U.S. Department of Health and Human Services, 1999)

What would an integrated and highly coordinated array of community-based services look like for traumatized children? How might the specificity of trauma-related psychopathology guide the development of this array of services? What types of problems would be most likely to change as a result of these services? Our intervention model is designed toward such an integrated and highly coordinated system of services for an individual, traumatized child guided by the specific understandings of the nature of child traumatic stress. Our intervention approach can be seen as a guide for how services and interventions ought to be put together, given a child's emotional regulation capacities and the ability of the child's social environment and/or system of care to help him or her regulate emotion.

4. Treatment Must Be "Disseminate-able" and Sustainable

In order to treat Gerald, you must be able to work within an agency or service system that supports and pays for this treatment. It is critical that new interventions be developed with the financial and human realities of the clinicians, agencies, and service systems that will use them in mind. It is relatively easy to design a "pie-in-the-sky" intervention model that is prohibitively expensive to use. A new intervention must be "disseminate-able." It must be described in a clear way and address the clinical realities of practice in this time and place and also incorporate strategies for supporting clinicians and organizations in this difficult work. Chapters 9 and 10 review some of these strategies for supporting providers and the organizations for which they work.

We designed this intervention model with the needs of children with traumatic stress in mind, constrained by the realities of clinical practice in the United States at this particular time. Accordingly, we designed this intervention using services that are available in most states: a multidisciplinary team that assesses and treats all referred children. The TST team is typical of most multidisciplinary teams of psychiatrists, psychologists, and social workers, with three exceptions:

1. It has the capacity to deliver home- and community-based interventions in addition to clinic-based treatment.
2. It includes a child advocacy attorney who serves a key consultative role in the advocacy for services.
3. It functions from a very specific and operationalized model of assessment and treatment.

The enhancement of treatment with these "exceptions" to usual practice was chosen in a way that could be implemented with limited extra resources.

1. **Home- and community-based interventions.** Most states and counties fund short-term home-based intervention. We initially integrated a home-based team funded by the Commonwealth of Massachusetts Medicaid contract with a conventional multidisciplinary clinical team. This enhancement did not cost the agency implementing TST extra resources. When TST is being implemented with children receiving child welfare services, this service is often a standard part of care, provided by caseworkers who often play this role on the team. As is described in our organizational planning chapter (Chapter 8), an important part of the initial TST implementation plan is to identify the agency and providers who will offer the home- and community-based services.

2. **Child-advocacy attorney.** Finding an advocacy attorney who can consult with providers, the agency, and the team in certain key situations is very important. There are many types of partnerships that can be forged in a cost-effective way, including with legal aid clinics, pro bono services from law firms, law schools, and retired attorneys. If we embrace a whatever-it-takes spirit in this work, we must embrace partnerships with advocacy attorneys in these and other similar situations. We detail how legal consultation is used in Chapter 13 on safety-focused treatment. For now, here are some examples of how critical this consultation can be:

    a. The team is confident that the child is currently experiencing maltreatment and is similarly confident that treatment will make very little, if any, difference unless the maltreatment is sufficiently addressed. The child welfare agency has not sufficiently addressed the problem.
    b. The child is failing in school for the second consecutive year, has normal intelligence. An IEP is not in place, and the school does not believe an IEP is necessary.
    c. A refugee child is about to be deported back to the country where she witnessed her father's murder and is becoming suicidal.

3. **Model of assessment and treatment**. Most of the rest of this book is devoted to our description of our model of assessment and treatment. This model provides a blueprint for how services and interventions ought to be assembled. Our main aim in this regard is clinical utility.

THE TRAP OF GRANT FUNDING

Many of us have been here before. We win a federal, state, or foundation services grant to implement an intervention about which we are excited. We put everything we have into writing the proposal and celebrate when we are told the grant has been awarded. We use the grant to pay for the services that comprise this exciting program because the way services are paid for in our state and county cannot possibly cover the program. We have 4 or 5 years of funding. What can be better than this?

STOP! If this describes your current situation, please ask yourself a simple question: What will happen after the grant ends?

For almost all of us who have been in this situation, the program we have given our hearts and souls to implement disintegrates. It disintegrates because it was never designed to be funded through conventional means, and, in our experience, it is usually implemented based on wishful thinking: *If we achieve the outcomes we expect, the state, county, etc., will surely pay for this.*

We wish it were different, but this almost never happens. Most programs with services paid for through grant funds disintegrate when the funding is gone. One of our main objections to the evidence-based treatment (EBT) paradigm currently employed in our field is that most interventions evaluated through randomized clinical trials have not been designed to be delivered through conventional funding means, and the clinical trials that have "proven" their "evidence-based" status were based on treatment that was paid for by the grants that funded those clinical trials. It is therefore no surprise to us that in the real world, most EBT treatments are not sustainable after the funding period ends.

We designed TST to provide services that are largely paid for through conventional means, and we strongly discourage the use of grant funds to pay for services themselves so that the program will have the best chance of being sustained after the funding period ends. Grant funds do, occasionally, pay for elements within the implementation of a TST program. When grant funds are used within a TST program, we try to keep them as limited as possible and, within the organizational plan drafted, develop a vision for whether these funds will be necessary after the grant disappears or how the funds will be replaced when the grant ends. Expenses that are occasionally paid out of grant funds include:

1. The initial TST training and consultation
2. The evaluation of the TST program
3. The time for the TST attorney
4. The time for selected members of the team, particularly the psychiatrist/psychopharmacologist, to attend team meetings.

One more note about sustainability: If all the providers you have so diligently trained in the model burn out and quit, you are back to ground zero. TST is a model that is built around the idea that we must do whatever it takes to help kids. In order to sustain this kind of energy and focus in our providers, organizations must also commit to doing whatever it takes to sustain the well-being and commitment of its staff.

Providers and other individuals who are working with the child and family (e.g., foster parents, lawyers, advocates) may be impacted by trauma, either as a result of their personal experiences or through their work with trauma victims. Listening to stories of abuse, neglect, violence, and other types of trauma can cause people to develop vicarious trauma, compassion fatigue, or secondary traumatic stress. Although there are nuanced distinctions between these terms, for the most part they refer to the traumatic stress reactions one can develop as a result of working with trauma victims and the impact such symptoms can have on one's personal life and overall worldview. Throughout this book we refer to this as *secondary traumatic stress,* or STS.

In order to create stronger programs and ultimately to better serve children and families, organizations need to do whatever it takes to acknowledge and support the needs of staff and administrators. TST Treatment Principle 8, "Take care of yourself and your team," addresses this important reality.

5. Treatment Must Add Value to Users

The more we help organizations implement TST, the more we see that the idea of *value to users* is central. People have choices. They select solutions to the problems they face based on the plausibility that the selected solution will help with those problems, and they quickly revise their choice if the selected solution does not appear to help. There are many types of users of TST programs: children, parents, foster parents, clinicians, clinic administrators, child welfare workers, and child welfare administrators, to name a few. Each user has his or her own goals for engaging with TST, based on the problems he or she is facing.

> There is a universal truth: If a solution chosen for a given problem does not add value in a sufficiently compelling way to a person, based on that person's definition of the problem, then he or she will seek a different solution.

There is a universal truth: If a solution chosen for a given problem does not add value in a sufficiently compelling way to a person, based on that person's definition of the problem, then he or she will seek a different solution. With this universal truth in mind, we aim to provide value to the users of TST. This aim works at both the clinical and the organizational level in very similar ways. Our treatment engagement strategy, ready–set–go (described in Chapter 11), is based on this idea, as is a core part of our organizational engagement approach (described in Chapter 8).

Outline of the TST Manual

This book is to be read as a manual for implementing the TST intervention approach for children with traumatic stress. The book has four sections:

  I. Foundations
 II. Getting Started
III. Doing Trauma Systems Therapy
IV. Improving Trauma Systems Therapy

Part I (Chapters 2–5) describes the theoretical background necessary to implement TST. **Part II** (Chapters 6–8) describes the principles of TST and how the organizations and team that will implement TST get set up to apply these principles. **Part III** (Chapters 9–15) describes the activities providers and teams need to perform to "do" TST, and includes the practical elements of assessment, treatment planning, and treatment implementation. **Part IV** (Chapters 16–18) describes the process of improving TST through innovation by a community of individuals and agencies that use TST. In this section we also describe ideas for innovating the TST principles so that our treatment model can be used for problems other than traumatic stress.

Part I. Foundations

These chapters lay the foundation for understanding the trauma system, described previously. Starting with the biological processes underlying survival-in-the-moment and the way in which these processes influence regulation, we move up and down the layers of the trauma system to understand how a child's regulation and growth can be supported (or not supported) by the people, organizations, and service systems that surround him or her.

Chapter 2. Survival Circuits

The trauma system includes the basic biological processes that are evoked when a traumatized child experiences his or her survival to be at stake in definable moments. In those moments ancient systems of the brain and the body are engaged to help the child survive. These powerful systems are extremely adaptive, but they cause problems when they activate in situations when the child's survival is not actually at stake. We call this system the *survival circuit* and describe how it works in this chapter.

Chapter 3. The Regulation of Survival-in-the-Moment States

The trauma system also includes the process that occurs when a traumatized child shifts from his or her usual state of emotion to what we call *survival-in-the-moment* states. This shift relates to a bottom-line function of the survival circuit, described in Chapter 2: to recognize patterns related to information from the social environment and from the body to "decide" if there is sufficient threat in the environment. Once a threat pattern is recognized, thoughts, emotions, behaviors, and underlying chemical and physiological systems shift dramatically, and everything in the child is focused on maintaining survival; that's what we mean by *survival-in-the-moment*, and a core part of treatment is to help the child to regulate these states so they are not expressed in situations that are not truly threatening. This chapter details these survival-in-the-moment states and the importance of regulating them.

Chapter 4. The Social Environment and the Services System

Survival-in-the-moment states are expressed in specific contexts that are either truly threatening or are safe enough but remind the child (consciously or unconsciously) of his or her trauma experience. This chapter offers an account of the various interacting components of the social environment, including the family, school, peer group, neighborhood, and culture. These components of the child's natural social environment are understood in relation to the first level of the trauma system: That is, we focus on how these areas of the social environment can serve to promote or diminish the self-regulation capacities of the child. We also examine how elements of the services system may impact this work.

Chapter 5. Safety Signals

The traumatized child's main source of hope is related to the type of relationships to which he or she has access. Are there people in his or her life who the child perceives to be in his or her corner? Are there people whom the child can trust? Such people emit what are called "safety signals," and if there are enough of these signals, the traumatized child can be helped to regulate emotion in a host of environments. The parent–child relationship and the therapeutic relationship are two critical relationships through which safety signals, and the child's ability to recognize them, can be leveraged. This chapter discusses the importance of those safety signals in promoting the child's regulation and growth.

Part II. Getting Started

Once the foundations are well understood, it's time to get ready to help. Where to start? First we review the 10 principles of intervention that ground all the work in TST. We then describe how these principles are delivered by a team of providers, and how this team needs to be supported by the agency in which it works. As described, TST is always delivered by a team of providers that operates—together—in specific ways. In order to be able to do this work, organizations need to support their providers and teams in specific ways. All of these needs and requirements are described in the chapters of Part II.

Chapter 6. Ten Treatment Principles

This chapter outlines the 10 principles that anchor TST treatment. These principles are:

1. Fix a broken system.
2. Safety first.
3. Create clear, focused plans that are based on facts.
4. Don't "go" before you are "ready."
5. Put scarce resources where they'll work.
6. Insist on accountability, particularly your own.
7. Align with reality.
8. Take care of yourself and your team.
9. Build from strength.
10. Leave a better system.

Chapter 7. The Treatment Team

The treatment team is an essential component of TST. This chapter describes the importance of having a multidisciplinary treatment team for conducting the work that needs to be done, including the strategies needed for creating a supportive team environment. The chapter suggests how the team should operate to guide treatment toward achieving fidelity to the TST principles.

Chapter 8. Organizing Your Program

The TST treatment team operates within an organization or several organizations that have agreed to collaborate with each other. How will this team be supported to do this difficult work? What does the organization or organizations need to know about TST so they may help it fit and stick? How can TST be adjusted to best fit within the needs of the organization or organizations that use it? How can TST help address secondary traumatic stress experienced by those working within the organization and by the organization itself? TST is only implemented when there is a defined organizational plan that works out these issues. This chapter describes the process of getting to this organizational plan.

Part III. Doing Trauma Systems Therapy

Once a team is set to implement TST and an organization is set to support that team, the team and its providers work with children and families to deliver TST in a set of defined steps. Fidelity to TST is defined by how closely the implementation of these steps follows the TST model. What are these steps? Each is detailed in a separate chapter in this part.

Chapter 9. Assessment

To deliver an intervention that will truly address the complexity of a traumatized child's problems, the right type of information must be gathered to know what to do. This chapter offers a clear approach to gathering information to answer five questions that will form the child's treatment plan. The five questions are:

1. What problem(s) should be the focus of the child's treatment?
2. Why are these problems important, and to whom?
3. What interventions will be used to address the child's problems?
4. What strengths can be used to address the child's problems?
5. What can interfere with addressing the child's problems?

Chapter 10. Treatment Planning

Once the information is gathered from our TST assessment, we are ready to answer those five questions that will form the basis of our treatment plan. This chapter offers guidelines for using the information gathered in Chapter 9 to answer these questions and to arrive at these decisions.

Chapter 11. Ready–Set–Go

Providers and their teams may feel they are close to making decisions on what to do in treatment based on what they have learned in Chapters 9 and 10, but their decision can never be made without the right type of partnership with the family. How much does the problem the team wants to address relate to the problems the child and family see as most important? How much does the team understand the practical barriers to successful implementation of treatment? This chapter discusses the potential difficulties of engaging families in treatment, and reviews an approach to partnering with families to make the best decisions about what to do in treatment.

Chapters 12–15. Treatment Implementation

Once the right type of information has been gathered, and the team uses that information to develop preliminary ideas on how treatment will be conducted and partners with the family to finalize these decisions, everything is lined up for success. Now: What do you do to achieve success? These next four chapters are designed to answer this question. TST is "done" in three sequential phases of implementation based on what is needed. Each phase defines a specific theme of trauma treatment and includes a set of specific treatment activities that are initiated and/or delivered within the given phase. Through learning how to implement the activities described in Chapters 9–11, you will know which TST phase is the best place to start. Chapters 12–14 will tell you what to do in each phase. The phase in which you start is based on what is needed. Chapter 15 provides the approach to psychopharmacology within TST, how psychotropic agents may be used to support the work (and the child) in each of the three treatment phases, and the role of the psychiatric consultant on the TST team.

Chapter 12. Safety-Focused Treatment

The primary goal of the safety-focused phase of TST is to establish and maintain the safety and stability of the child's social environment and to minimize risk to the child and others based on the child's difficulty regulating emotional and behavioral states. This intensive home-/community-based phase of treatment is always offered if the child is at risk to be harmed or is at risk to harm him- or herself or others. This phase of treatment is organized around the following set of activities: *Establish Safety, Maintain Safety*, and *Care for Caregivers. Establish Safety* is designed to make sure the child's environment is safe enough. *Maintain Safety* is designed to make sure that the level of safety that has been established is real and will last. *Care for Caregivers* is designed to provide the right type of support for caregivers to make the needed changes. Two guides, the Safety-Focused Guide (for clinicians; see Appendix 7) and the HELPers Guide (for caregivers; see Appendix 8), structure the treatment in this phase.

Chapter 13. Regulation-Focused Treatment

The primary goal of the regulation-focused phase is to give the child sufficient skills to manage emotional states when triggered by stimuli from his or her social environment. Unlike treatment delivered in the safety-focused phase, treatment delivered in the regulation-focused phase may occur in the clinic or office. Regulation-focused treatment is offered when the child continues to have difficulties regulating emotional states even when the environment is safe enough. This phase of treatment is focused on developing the child's emotional regulation skills and is organized by the following set of activities: *Build Awareness, Apply Awareness*, and *Spread Awareness*. The *awareness* we seek to *build, apply*, and *spread* is about what stimuli leads to the dysregulation and about what strategy the child—and those around him or her—may use to achieve regulation once the child is stimulated. This phase is organized by two guides: the Regulation-Focused Guide (for clinicians; see Appendix 9) and the Managing Emotions Guide (for children and families; see Appendix 10).

Chapter 14. Beyond Trauma Treatment

The primary goal of the beyond trauma phase is to work with the child and family to gain sufficient perspective on the trauma experience so that the trauma no longer defines the child's view of the self, world, and future. The phase is comprised of learning cognitive skills and processing the trauma. This phase of treatment is typically offered when the social environment is stable and the child is sufficiently able to regulate emotional states. The goals of this phase of treatment are guided by the mnemonic STRONG: **S**trengthening cognitive skills, **T**elling your story, **R**eevaluating needs, **O**rienting toward the future, **N**urturing caregiving, **G**oing forward. This phase is structured by two guides: the Beyond Trauma Guide (for providers; see Appendix 12) and the Cognitive Awareness Log (for children and families; see Appendix 13).

Chapter 15. Psychopharmacology

Psychotropic agents are occasionally helpful for supporting the work conducted in each of the treatment phases. This chapter details the indications for these agents within TST, how they may be used in each phase, and the principles and practice of psychopharmacology within TST.

Part IV. Improving Trauma Systems Therapy

As we've discussed previously in this chapter, TST is a never-ending story based on a community of users who are continually tinkering with the model to make it better able to address their needs. The contributing members of this community share the information they discover about improvements to TST with anyone who may benefit. Over time this collaborative process has created a powerful process of continually improving TST so that it may benefit a wide and diverse community of users. Our approach to improving TST is based on a lead-user model of innovation described by Eric von Hippel in his book Democratizing Innovation *(2005). Accordingly, Chapter 16 is called "Democratizing Trauma Systems Therapy," and in it we describe this process and provide examples of TST innovations and adaptations based on this approach. Chapter 17 provides ideas for the most radical innovation yet: using the TST approach for intervening with disorders that don't involve trauma.*

Chapter 16. Democratizing Trauma Systems Therapy

In this chapter we describe how TST has been used in a variety of settings and how we work with a growing community of users. We use this chapter to explore how the process of innovation works within TST, such that the innovations of users are continually integrated into our model and TST becomes this never-ending story that helps people do *whatever it takes* to help traumatized children. In this chapter we highlight some of these innovations and adaptations in real-world settings.

Chapter 17. Extending Trauma Systems Therapy Beyond Trauma

Children with many emotional, behavioral, and developmental disorders have difficulty regulating emotional states in certain definable moments. Children with autism, for example, may become dysregulated when required to manage social information that is too much for them. Children with attention deficit hyperactivity disorder may become dysregulated when they are expected to organize their lives in a way in which they are not capable. Children with depression may become dysregulated when they need to manage situations in which loss occurs. In this chapter we describe how ideas related to TST for traumatized children may be relevant to the treatment of problems beyond trauma.

Chapter 18. Conclusions

The book ends with a concluding chapter that highlights the possible roles that TST can play in the system of care and the public policy concerns relevant to creating an effective and integrated system of care for traumatized children.

Use of Icons

Throughout this manual we use icons to guide you through the elements of our interventions. The icons should be read as symbols that provide "at-a-glance" ideas concerning what a given section is about. The following table describes the six icons that are used in this manual. Each chapter begins with a table indicating the icons that are used in that chapter.

	ICON KEY	
	Essential Point	An *essential point* indicates a section that contains information that **must** be understood to master the TST treatment approach.
	Academic Point	An *academic point* indicates a section that contains information that is interesting or academically important but is not absolutely necessary for mastering the TST approach.
	Quotation	A *quotation* is a piece of writing taken from others that we believe is very important to illuminate the TST treatment approach.
	Case Discussion	*Case discussions* are used liberally throughout this manual to illustrate our treatment approach. We believe case discussions are particularly important to understand the concepts described in the manual.
	Useful Tool	A *useful tool* is used in our treatment sections to highlight an intervention technique that is highly useful.
	Danger	A *danger icon* indicates a potential pitfall of practice. This icon should serve as a warning to pay attention to the section (or skip at your own peril!).

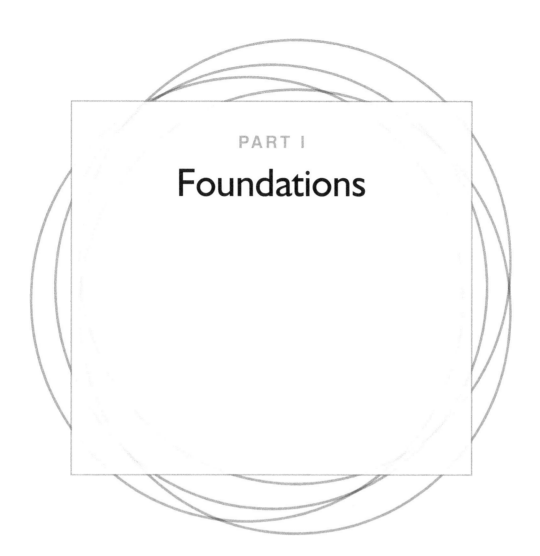

PART I

Foundations

Survival Circuits

The Way the Brain Processes Information Related to Threat Helps Us Understand Traumatic Stress

---

LEARNING OBJECTIVES

- To understand how traumatic stress responses relate to systems of the brain evolved for survival
- To understand how trauma affects threat pattern recognition
- To learn about key brain structures involved in traumatic stress responses

---

ICONS USED IN THIS CHAPTER

Essential Point	Academic Point	Quotation	Case Discussion

Traumatic stress is about *survival-in-the-moment,* a state that is controlled by ancient systems of the brain and body that we call the *survival circuits.* These survival circuits control the way we process traumatic events and the hold that these events may have on us throughout our lives. We begin our discussion of the foundations of TST with a review of these survival circuits and their implications for treating traumatic stress. First, let us briefly think about the word *survival.* Any discussion of survival must begin with the amazing work of the 19th-century British naturalist, Charles Darwin (1809–1882). As most of us know, Darwin proposed his theory of evolution to explain the natural origins of human beings. Through his observations of animals on the Galapagos Islands, he noted that those animals who were best equipped to survive were the most likely to live long enough to pass on their survival-enhancing traits to their offspring. Traits that help to promote survival continue and those that do not promote survival die out. This is a process called *adaptation*. New traits can suddenly develop in a given organism out of what is called "chance mutation." Those new traits that give their owner enough of an advantage to reproduce become integrated into the biology of the species. Over many millions of years, this process creates species with ever-increasing advantages for survival.

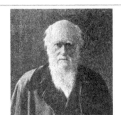

Charles Darwin (1809–1882)

Although Darwin's revolutionary proposal, *The Origin of Species* (1859), was published more than 150 years ago, it anticipated and is supported by groundbreaking work in genetics, molecular biology, and developmental neuroscience that has been published in the last 10 years. The need to survive has sculpted our biology. This sculpture has occurred over many millions of years and has given us, in our genes, our cells, our brains, and our bodies, powerful mechanisms that foster survival. Survival behavior is at the core of traumatic stress. It is enacted in the moment that we perceive our life to be in danger, and the *survival circuits* control it.

Survival Circuits

We human beings are at the top of the evolutionary ladder. What puts us up there? We have a biology that has been refined over millions of years, giving us the remarkable capacity to have some control over our environments. We have biologies that give us the potential to create great works of art, science, mathematics, technology, and culture. Our ability to master our environments and to achieve the enormous advances in diverse areas of pursuit, requires our evolutionarily advanced neurobiological systems to be working properly. The main part of our biology that has allowed us such powerful and flexible adaptive capacities is the human brain, particularly the higher-order systems of the brain located in the *cerebral cortex*.

One of the primary ways that these advanced, higher order brain systems become unable to do their great work is if there is a perceived threat to survival in the environment.

Lower-order systems of the brain, such as those that control basic emotionality, physiology, and survival-motivated behaviors, are also found in the brains of lower animal species. These lower neurobiological systems are largely responsible for maintaining our survival so that our higher-order brain systems can do their great work. One of the primary ways that these advanced, higher-order brain systems become unable to do their great work is if there is a perceived threat to survival in the environment. When this threat occurs, all neurobiological systems work at only one goal, by virtue of millions of years of evolution and adaptation: to foster *survival-in-the-moment*. As described, the survival circuits are responsible for *survival-in-the-moment* responses. It is the engagement of these survival circuits in situations where there actually is no threat that causes the problem of traumatic stress.

Once these powerful and ancient systems are triggered, the brain and the body enter a state of processing in order to survive in the face of life-threatening events. But most of the time there *is* no current and immediate life threat. Individuals with traumatic stress, however, have brains and bodies that are responding to a past life threat in the present. Almost all traumatic stress problems relate to these powerful survival circuits. It is therefore extremely important to understand how seemingly innocuous *stimuli* can create extreme, survival-motivated *responses* in order to help traumatized children respond in more adaptive ways.

Survival-in-the-Moment

As we describe in this book, there is a great deal of focus in TST on understanding specific moments in the traumatized child's life. In essence, these are the

TST is about preventing survival-in-the-moment responses.

moments when the survival circuits get engaged. These are the moments when children feel and do things that become very problematic for themselves and/or others and lead to the need for mental health intervention. If these moments were somehow magically removed from a traumatized child's life, there would be no need for mental health intervention. As we introduced in Chapter 1, traumatic stress is about survival-in-the-moment, defined as follows:

> *an individual's experience of the present environment as threatening to his or her survival, with corresponding thoughts, emotions, behaviors, and neurochemical and neurophysiological responses.*

In children who have experienced traumatic stress, there are fundamental problems with the way in which the brain processes potentially life-threatening stimuli.

TST is about preventing these survival-in-the-moment responses. Our TST picture, shown in Figure 1.1 (p. 12), puts survival-in-the-moment in the center of everything.

What goes on within the brain and body between the potentially life-threatening stimulus and the potentially life-preserving response? We begin the discussion of this fundamental process with a description of a moment in the life of a child with traumatic stress. Consider what happens to Denise in the moment:

Denise is a 16-year-old girl with a history of sexual abuse from her mother's ex-boyfriend. While at a local mall with friends, she saw a man who frightened her. She later reported that this man reminded her of her mother's ex-boyfriend. Denise remembers becoming extremely anxious and flooded with memories of sexual abuse. She does not remember walking away. Her friends found her curled up in a bathroom stall, unresponsive.

States of extreme fear and dissociation are entirely motivated by survival.

This is the case of an adolescent with a history of sexual abuse who was functioning well until she saw a man who reminded her of the man who had abused her. When she saw this man, her brain rapidly shifted to a survival-in-the-moment state. It is exactly this moment that must be understood and changed within TST.

Denise generally functions well. Most of the time, her higher-order brain systems are engaged and doing their great work. Denise was at the mall having fun with friends. She was happy, socializing, and calm. At the moment she saw this man, she entered a state of extreme fear and then dissociation. These states of extreme fear and dissociation are entirely motivated by survival. Traumatized children go from the stimulus (a traumatic reminder) to the response (an extreme emotional state) without the ability to think, calm, and self-soothe. This stress response can be immediate, extreme, and outside of conscious control. An essential part of intervention is to help children to calm themselves when confronted by a traumatic reminder so that they do not enter these extreme, survival-in-the-moment states.

One of the main goals of intervention is to prevent children from going from stimulus to immediate extreme response. A critical problem for traumatized children is that they frequently live in environments riddled with traumatic reminders. The stresses of ongoing family violence, community violence, parental substance abuse and mental illness, for example, are frequently part of the everyday life of a traumatized child. All children must learn to identify, manage, and reasonably respond to signals from their social environment. How does a child with traumatic stress learn to differentiate between real and perceived threats? How can such a child do this when he or she hears any loud voice as angry, or misinterprets a classmate's playful nudge as aggressive? How much more difficult is this task when the child is exposed to ongoing domestic or community violence, endures parental substance abuse, or fears impending homelessness? This is the core problem that our intervention model is designed to address.

If Denise does not immediately respond with extreme emotional or behavioral changes and instead can *think* about the stimuli of a man who reminds her of her mother's ex-boyfriend in the moment, she could perhaps understand that the man is *not* her mother's ex-boyfriend. Once Denise has the ability to think in this way, a lot of good things can happen for her. The ability to think in this way requires the engagement of the higher-order brain systems that we mentioned. Again: These higher-order systems are trumped by the lower-order systems in situations that evoke survival-in-the-moment responses. How can higher-order brain systems *stay* engaged in situations that are not truly threatening, but in which a traumatized child perceives threat? TST is designed to help traumatized children's brains do just this.

> How can higher-order brain systems *stay* engaged in situations that are not truly threatening, but in which a traumatized child perceives threat? TST is designed to help traumatized children's brains do just this.

Your Moment in the Zoo

In order to best understand how this stress response works, we will take an imagined walk through your brain in a given moment between a stressful stimulus and a response. Please imagine yourself in the following situation:

> You are walking down a path in your own thoughts. It is a nice, sunny day. You feel calm. Suddenly, you notice an object coming at you from the right. You freeze. Your feet are planted in the ground. Your heart is pounding. You are sweating . . . you then recognize that the object walking toward you is a *lion* . . . but that it is in a cage . . . and that you are in the zoo. . . . You continue walking and continue to enjoy your pleasant day at the zoo.

The moment described in the above scenario probably would take under 2 seconds. Within that brief span of time, a lot of activity occurred in your brain that illustrates very important ideas about the nature of traumatic stress, the emotional nervous system, and its integral role in survival. This example of the moment and the following discussion is adapted from the work of one of our colleagues at New York University, Joseph LeDoux, a neuroscientist who has conducted some of the pioneering work that has illuminated our understanding of the specific brain processes involved in emotional experiences, particularly related to fear. His books *The Emotional Brain* (1998) and *Synaptic Self* (2002) are central to understanding how the brain processes threatening stimuli and for understanding survival-in-the-moment responses. We also rely on Antonio Damasio's *The Feeling of What Happens* (1999) in our discussion of how emotion, memory, and consciousness interact. In this brief chapter, it is hard to truly do justice to these great areas of research, and even though we oversimplify our discussion, we retain the salient points that are necessary to understand the TST intervention components and their rationale.

According to LeDoux (1998, 2002), there are two emotional processing systems of the brain. These two systems work closely together such that we are usually unaware that there are these discrete systems. Both systems are critical for our survival and, more or less, distinguish between the higher-order and lower-order systems of the brain we've already mentioned. LeDoux refers to these two systems as the "low road" and "high road" of emotional processing. We call these systems, considered together, the *survival circuits*.

The Survival Circuits in Four Steps

 Let's walk along these two critical roads to see if we can understand what is going on when children experience traumatic stress. We will walk these roads in four steps, as shown in Figure 2.1.

Step I: Picking Up Threat Information

People's responses to the external world are based on how they appraise external stimuli and integrate those bits of information with the internal state of their bodies.

People's responses to the external world are based on how they appraise external stimuli and integrate those bits of information with the internal state of their bodies. Humans have incredibly sophisticated ways of picking up information about the external world through the five senses. This information is

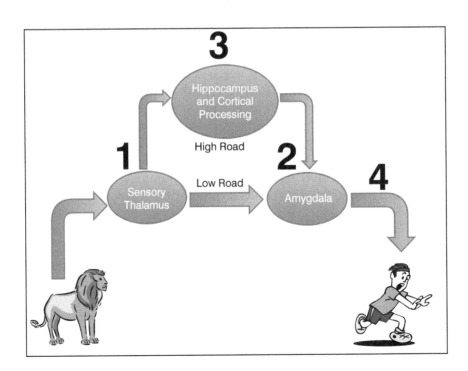

FIGURE 2.1. Four steps from threat to response.

transmitted from the respective perceptual system (vision, sound, etc.) to the sensory thalamus for more detailed processing. The sensory thalamus is located about midway between the frontal cortex and the midbrain. In this step we are talking about information passing through any of the five senses that *may* indicate threat. Most stimuli that are processed do not signal a threat to life and limb. Some stimuli, however, indicate such a threat. The way in which people make this distinction is critical for survival and for adaptive responding. At the zoo, you were confronted with a stimulus that you *eventually* recognized as a lion in a cage. How did you decide you were safe? How much did you need to think about the lion walking toward you before you knew that you were (very) unlikely to be attacked? What about Denise in the mall? How did she decide that the stimulus of a man walking toward her indicated that her life could be threatened? How did that appraisal determine a response? Much of this appraisal is done unconsciously, such that we are completely unaware of the information that bears on survival-laden responses in the moment. It is very fortunate that these responses can be processed outside of conscious awareness for the simple reason that conscious processing takes time. As we discuss next, once potentially threatening information is picked up by the sensory thalamus, it is then transmitted along two routes: a very fast low road and a slower high road. Without these two roads, we would be in very big trouble.

Step 2: Reacting to Information Related to Survival (So That We Will Not Be Eaten)

Survival and speed are related. Over the course of evolution, animals (including humans) had to act quickly on information from the environment indicating a possible threat to survival because to hesitate might well mean that the animal (including a human) would be the predator's next meal. Fortunately, evolution has given animals with central nervous systems a means of acting very quickly when threat in the environment is detected. This system is what LeDoux (1998, 2002) calls the "low road" of emotional processing. This low road is extremely fast and unconscious. Low-road brain processing transmits bits of threat-related information very quickly to the amygdala, in the center of the brain. The amygdala's job is to initiate emergency responses, if indicated. This type of information does not include the contextual details; these details are sacrificed in the service of speed so that you can respond to maximize your chance of survival.

Step 3: Making a More Accurate Appraisal of the Threat Information

LeDoux's (1998, 2002) high road of emotional processing includes the sensory cortex, the medial temporal lobe memory system (especially the hippocampus), and the prefrontal cortex. These brain regions are all engaged to perceive the details of the situation and to compare them to the person's (or animal's) memory of prior experience so that the most adaptive response is possible, given the nature of the stimuli. It is these systems, working together, that help an individual know just how threatening the stimuli are. A balance must be struck between accuracy and speed. If you are walking down a path in the African savanna and a lion happens to be ambling toward you, the initiation of immediate behavioral responses to maximize your chance of survival is extremely important. Because the vast majority of signals we process do not connote extreme threat, it is very important to have brain systems that provide a more nuanced and accurate appraisal of signals. These systems must work quickly enough to shut down the emergency response from the low road/amygdala system so that such responses do not continually overappraise the threat in signals that are not truly threatening. As described, the low road/amygdala system does its work in a decontextualized way. It is concerned *only* with survival. The high-road system that processes information transmitted from the sensory thalamus is meant to provide this context. The memory system in the medial temporal lobe, particularly the hippocampus, provides the contextual details. This is the system that works with the sensory cortex and other areas of the higher-order cerebral cortex to bring accurate, context-laden details provided by the long-term memory systems of the cerebral cortex to help an individual accurately understand the proper time and place of the stimulus.

The ability to accurately place a given stimulus in proper time and place is extremely important. What let you know that the stimulus of the lion was not life-threatening? You could correctly place it in the zoo and connect it with your long-term memory stores of your experiences in zoos. To the degree that none of these memories includes being attacked by a lion in a zoo, but rather pleasant times and the safety of lions in zoos, you will feel safe and continue to have your current pleasant day at the zoo. In fact, your initial response (heart pounding, sweating, feet planted, etc.) was mediated by the low road/amygdala but terminated so quickly and unconsciously that you could have continued completely unaware that it had occurred. What terminated this immediate, low-road response? The high-road medial temporal memory system, indicating you were safe by allowing you access to information so that you could correctly recognize the context you were in. This information would include that you have been to the zoo many times before, that you have never been attacked by a lion, that you have never before seen anyone attacked by a lion, and that lions in zoos, generally, do not leave their cages. Access to this information diminishes the body's emergency responses and leads to the sense of calmness that you felt only moments after you were alarmed.

Step 4: Doing Something about the Threat Information

Ultimately, the survival circuit is about what you will do and how quickly you will do it. If the amygdala, via its low-road pathway, is engaged, it will fire to initiate highly adaptive emotional and behavioral response systems in the body to maintain survival. If the amygdala is not engaged, either because the low-road signal is not strong enough or because the high-road system indicates it's a false alarm, then usual emotion and behavior continues and you go about your day hardly conscious that your brain had a false alarm at the zoo. The reason it is important to know about these systems is that, as we discuss in the next chapter, they more or less define traumatic stress reactions. These reactions relate to a person's emotional experience and the behaviors exerted to manage the perceived threat in the environment. How do these emotional and behavioral reactions work? The lateral nucleus of the amygdala integrates the information about the threat, and if the information is determined to be an actual threat, then signals passed to the central nucleus of the amygdala engage powerful, evolutionarily driven, bodily responses to manage the threat. These responses include activation of the hormonal systems via the hypothalamic–pituitary–adrenal (HPA) axis, which releases energy stores using the stress hormone cortisol; the locus coeruleus/norepinepherine system that activates the heart and focuses attention on the threat; and the polyvagal system, which increases social engagement via the myelinated vagus nerve or initiates immobilization or freezing via the unmyelinated vagus nerve. These systems also feed back to the amygdala and to the higher-order cortical systems and result in an awareness of the feeling state of our body. This process of self-awareness is extremely adaptive. It allows an individual to use emotions as signals for effective action and underlies the critical process of emotional regulation that is detailed in the next chapter. In fact, the engagement of these emotional and behavioral response systems is the basis for the regulation of survival-in-the-moment states, as described in Chapter 3.

What about You and Denise?

In the first moments after seeing the object moving toward you at the zoo (before you were even aware that it was a lion), the amygdala's lateral nucleus alarmed its central nucleus, which initiated systems that resulted in cortisol surges (HPA axis), rapid heart rate and increased attention (norepinepherine and autonomic nervous system), and sweating (autonomic nervous system). Fortunately, this low-road cascade became inhibited almost immediately by the high-road response, and you continued to have your nice day at the zoo. Denise, in contrast, does not have access to a high-road system that could have helped her correctly identify the stimulus and bring the context of the mall into her awareness in the moment. Her response is thus primarily mediated by the very quick pathway from the sensory thalamus to the lateral nucleus of the amygdala. Although it is hard to tell exactly what emotions she was experiencing after she saw the man in the mall, it is likely that extreme fear was a part of her response; as she was curled up on the floor of the bathroom, unresponsive, she was likely experiencing a significant dissociative state. For Denise, this emotional roller coaster from extreme fear to an unresponsive dissociation constituted her survival-in-the-moment response.

Stepping into the Light: The Importance of Conscious Experience

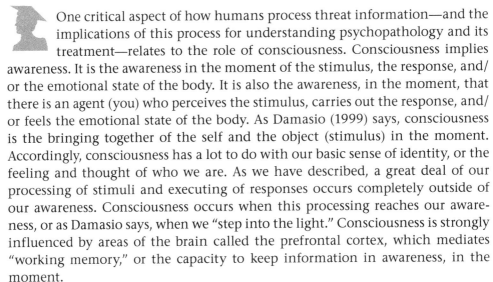 One critical aspect of how humans process threat information—and the implications of this process for understanding psychopathology and its treatment—relates to the role of consciousness. Consciousness implies awareness. It is the awareness in the moment of the stimulus, the response, and/ or the emotional state of the body. It is also the awareness, in the moment, that there is an agent (you) who perceives the stimulus, carries out the response, and/ or feels the emotional state of the body. As Damasio (1999) says, consciousness is the bringing together of the self and the object (stimulus) in the moment. Accordingly, consciousness has a lot to do with our basic sense of identity, or the feeling and thought of who we are. As we have described, a great deal of our processing of stimuli and executing of responses occurs completely outside of our awareness. Consciousness occurs when this processing reaches our awareness, or as Damasio says, when we "step into the light." Consciousness is strongly influenced by areas of the brain called the prefrontal cortex, which mediates "working memory," or the capacity to keep information in awareness, in the moment.

> Conscious thought is experimental action. It allows us to carefully consider our responses before acting. Consciousness involves the ability to shift attention to the things on which we want to focus.

Consciousness is a very important component for treating traumatic stress. When you were walking in the zoo, you were initially lost in your thoughts and momentarily not really conscious about being in the zoo. At any moment you could have easily shifted your attention from your thoughts to what you were doing (walking in the zoo), but it is a good thing that you did not need to be completely conscious of the zoo if you did not need to be. If we do not always need to be conscious of the context we are in, then we can shift our attention to other things and let our higher-order brain systems do their great work (perhaps while you were walking in the zoo you were composing a symphony, solving a scientific problem, or trying to solve an interpersonal conflict). Conscious thought is experimental action. It allows us to carefully consider our responses before acting. Consciousness involves the ability to shift attention to the things on which we want to focus. When we perceive stimuli suggesting that our life is in danger, however, it is very hard to attend to anything else. How might this work for you and for Denise?

You were "in your thoughts" on your walk in the zoo. At some point, the context of the zoo intruded on your consciousness in the form of a lion walking toward you. Just prior to this awareness, your low-road system briefly engaged. Momentarily after your low-road system engaged, your high-road system processed the sensation of the lion, compared it with previous memories of lions in zoos, accurately brought your current context (the zoo) to your moment, and brought some of that information into your consciousness. Each of the high-road systems—the sensory cortex (accurate perception), medial temporal lobe memory system (context), and prefrontal cortex (consciousness)—sent safe signals to the amygdala, allowing you to continue to enjoy your day. In Denise's case, once she was stimulated, she was, sadly, far less able to shift her attention back to her good time at the mall. The stimulus of the man who reminded her of her mother's ex-boyfriend signaled danger, and her low-road amygdala system responded rapidly and extremely. Her higher-road systems were not able to accurately perceive the stimulus to tell her that the man was not her mother's ex-boyfriend and to keep her in the safer context of the mall. Accordingly, what entered her consciousness was only the context of past abuse. Consciousness involves orientation to time, place, and person. In the moment, she was disoriented to when this was, where she was, and who she was. She was a little girl, in her bedroom, being abused.

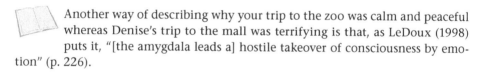 Another way of describing why your trip to the zoo was calm and peaceful whereas Denise's trip to the mall was terrifying is that, as LeDoux (1998) puts it, "[the amygdala leads a] hostile takeover of consciousness by emotion" (p. 226).

When presented with a stressful stimulus, the emotional nervous system becomes so overwhelmed that what enters an individual's awareness is dominated by low-road amygdala processing (i.e., fast, fragmented, decontextualized, aroused), rather than high-road processing (i.e., slower, calm, linear, contextual, and more conscious). When Denise saw the man at the mall, the amygdala succeeded in its hostile takeover. When you saw the lion, your higher-order systems fought it back (the amygdala . . . not the lion).

What's It All About?: Pattern Recognition of Threat Information and Shifting the State of the Body Based on Recognized Patterns

Recently, a great deal of attention has been devoted to understanding the logical structure and function of the brain. How does it work? Can its functioning be boiled down to its logical essence? In his recent book *How to Create a Mind: The Secret of Human Thought Revealed* (2012), Ray Kurzweil proposes that the central organizing unit of the brain is comprised of groups of neurons that work together to recognize patterns. These pattern recognition units are organized hierarchically, in increasing levels of abstraction, ranging from the basic elements of sensation to highly abstract mathematical and linguistic concepts.

From this perspective, the survival circuit we described above is a midlevel pattern recognition unit that is designed to recognize and integrate patterns relating to:

1. Information from the external world related to threat and safety.
2. Information from the body related to threat and safety.
3. Information about past experience related to threat and safety stored in memory.

As described, the survival circuit brings this converging information to the amygdala, which then responds if a threat pattern is recognized and leads the body's adaptive response to that threat.

The bottom line for individuals with traumatic stress:

Their survival circuit, a pattern recognition unit, has a much greater propensity to "see" threat patterns in signals from the external and internal worlds than the survival circuits of those who do not have traumatic stress. As we discuss in Chapter 3, the result of the survival circuit "deciding" that a threat pattern is present leads to response patterns involving thoughts, emotions, and behaviors as well as specific neurochemical and neurophysiological actions. We call these response patterns *survival-in-the-moment states* and detail the regulation of them in the next chapter.

The survival circuit is a pattern recognition unit for detecting threat information and functions by shifting the state of the body based on the recognition of threat patterns.

From this perspective, the amygdala integrates all this information and acts as a switch. When switched "on," the chemical and physiological state of the body, with corresponding conscious and unconscious emotional and behavioral responses, are all interrelated and dedicated to a singular focus: managing a perceived, impending threat to survival. When switched "off," these systems are not engaged and humans and animals feel and do whatever else they might feel and do when they don't perceive immediate threat to their survival. There are only two choices: "on" or "off." That's it. Threat pattern or not: survival-in-the-moment state or not. The overt

That's it. Threat pattern or not: survival-in-the-moment state or not. The overt expressions of a survival-in-the-moment state in threat-related emotional and behavioral response systems are what we call *traumatic stress*.

expressions of a survival-in-the-moment state in threat-related emotional and behavioral response systems are what we call *traumatic stress.*

Here's a peek ahead in this book:

If we see the central problem related to traumatic stress as a problem with the way an individual responds to patterns of signals related to survival, then it will be critically important to help him or her perceive and integrate these patterns of signals in a way that is more adaptive in a given moment. Clinical pattern recognition is a key part of our approach to helping children. As is detailed in Chapter 7, the definition of a clinical problem in TST is

> *patterns of links between potentially threatening signals and the expression of survival-in-the-moment states.*

The assessment process in TST is heavily based on pattern recognition. It is the pattern recognition of an observer (you) who notes the regularities in the expression of these survival-in-the-moment states within their social contexts and then decides how to break that pattern. That breaking of the pattern, in essence, is the focus of the TST Treatment Plan.

At this point it may be helpful to think about how this type of pattern recognition may work for Gerald and Denise. Think about how their survival circuit pattern recognition may be working and how your clinical pattern recognition may be able to help.

Helping Children Step into the Light

Our most important aim in developing TST is to help children and their families to move beyond the haunting influence of their pasts so that they have a chance at a happy, healthy, and successful future. If children are perpetually responding to potential threats from their environment by entering survival-in-the-moment states, then it is very hard to move into such a future. Their *present* is full of survival-in-the-moment states based on their *past* experience. This effect can be seen in the brain: When threat in the environment is recognized, higher-order systems of the brain responsible for anticipating, planning, and strategizing go offline. That is, the future-oriented brain is undermined by the survival-oriented brain. This makes sense from an evolutionary perspective. It's not terribly relevant to plan for the future when there is an impending risk of being eaten in the present. We have to help get traumatized children beyond this state because, in most cases, there is not an immediate risk of harm in the present (and if there is such risk, we respond by getting the child to a safer place).

Again: One of the most devastating effects of traumatic stress is that it robs children of the ability to think into the future. If consciousness is about the present and memory is about the past, then planning and anticipation are about the future. The TST approach focuses on the use of present consciousness and long-term memory stores to anticipate the risk and reward of future events and to plan so that ones' needs are met into the future.

The silver lining in the cloud of trauma is that just as bad events can change the brain in deleterious ways, good events can change the brain in beneficial ways. We designed TST to help retrain the brain, and the child who owns it, to have experiences that will help him or her have the future he or she deserves.

In children with traumatic stress these calculations can be skewed, causing great problems. An overestimate of the likely risk in events leads to the serious problem of avoidance of people, places, and things that might remind the child of his or her past trauma. As a result, traumatized children can lead overly restrictive lives. Traumatized children can also underestimate the risk of danger and put themselves in highly dangerous situations. This can happen when the child is not able to act on interpersonal warning signs and therefore forms relationships with individuals who repeat the trauma. Traumatized children also have trouble calculating the likely reward inherent in future events. They underestimate the pleasure that they might experience in relationships and activities. The calculation of the probability of risk and reward of future events is a part of an individual's ability to visualize him- or herself in the future. One of the tragic consequences of traumatic stress is this lack of ability to see oneself into the future. Lenore Terr (1990) has described this as a sense of a "foreshortened future." Traumatized children will not be able to see their futures if they are fighting for their lives in the present and if they have trouble seeing any likelihood of rewards or pleasure in future events.

The silver lining in the cloud of trauma is that just as bad events can change the brain in deleterious ways, good events can change the brain in beneficial ways. We designed TST to help retrain the brain, and the child who owns it, to have experiences that will help him or her have the future he or she deserves.

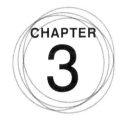

CHAPTER

3

The Regulation of Survival-in-the-Moment States

How Child Traumatic Stress Is a Disorder of the Regulation of Survival-in-the-Moment States

---

LEARNING OBJECTIVES

- To understand how traumatized children shift into survival-in-the-moment states in specific moments
- To learn about the survival-in-the-moment state building blocks
- To understand the importance of this survival-in-the-moment state process for organizing treatment

---

ICONS USED IN THIS CHAPTER

Essential Point	Academic Point	Quotation	Case Discussion

We described the survival circuit as a pattern recognition unit whose entire purpose is to maintain the survival of the individual. When this unit "decides" that the individual's survival is at stake, the individual quickly transitions into a survival-in-the-moment state* to effectively manage this threat. In Chapter 1,

---

A word about language: The term *survival-in-the-moment* accurately describes what we mean by a child's switch to a survival-laden emotional state the moment a threat is perceived in the present environment. The term can also sound awkward in some contexts. Accordingly, we sometimes refer to this same process as *survival states*. The terms are interchangeable.

we defined a survival-in-the-moment state and introduced the idea of survival-in-the-moment building blocks to set the stage for a detailed description of how a child transitions from his or her usual state to a survival-in-the-moment state (Figure 1.1, p. 12). In this chapter we describe how this works. First, we repeat the definition of a survival-in-the-moment state (or survival state):

> *an individual's experience of the present environment as threatening to his or her survival, with corresponding thoughts, emotions, behaviors, and neurochemical and neurophysiological responses.*

We define the survival-in-the-moment state as a critical part of the trauma system upon which TST is entirely based. This trauma system has two components:

1. A traumatized child who experiences survival states in specific, definable moments.
2. A social environment and/or system of care that is not able to help the child regulate these survival states.

This chapter addresses the first part of the trauma system: the traumatized child. The next chapter is about the second part of the trauma system, the system of care. In this chapter, we detail the process by which traumatized individuals shift into survival-in-the-moment states in specific moments and the importance of understanding this process for organizing treatment. This idea has very important implications in relation to the nature of psychiatric diagnosis. As is discussed, we see significant limitations to the usefulness of the information that comes from a psychiatric diagnosis—based on the DSM approach—for clinical decision making, and believe that the process we describe yields much more useful information for this purpose. In Chapter 9 we explain how the assessment of survival-in-the-moment states fits into the overall assessment of traumatized children. Our treatment chapters detail how to help children with these states.

To start this discussion, let's introduce a new child:

Consider Robert . . .

> Robert is a 10-year-old boy with a history of severe physical abuse from his stepfather. He has a long history of extreme and impulsive aggressive behavior. While on the playground at recess, another child made a demeaning comment about Robert. Without thinking, Robert lunged at him and continued to pound him in the face with his fists until the school monitors pulled him off.

Robert and Denise (from Chapters 1 and 2) each enter survival-in-the-moment states when reminded of prior traumatic events. As described in Chapter 2, the reactions of Denise and Robert can be understood in terms of the functioning of deeply ingrained neurobiological systems that we have called the *survival circuit*.

The survival circuit recognizes patterns of stimuli that indicate threat and activates emotional and behavioral responses to help individuals manage this threat. Recall our discussion of the survival circuit as a pattern recognition unit in which the lateral nucleus of the amygdala acts as an on–off switch related to perceived threat. Survival-in-the-moment states occur if (and only if) this switch turns on. This chapter is about what happens when the switch turns from off to on.

Think about what is going on inside Denise as she is curled up on the bathroom floor. Think about what is going on inside Robert as he lunges after the boy on the playground. Think about both these children in the instant before they behaved in these extreme

> The survival circuit recognizes patterns of stimuli that indicate threat and activates emotional and behavioral responses to help individuals manage this threat.

ways. In that instant the survival circuit switch was turned off. Now think about what changed after both these children were reminded of a traumatic event, which flipped the switch to *on*. If you have a good sense of what changed for them between the off and on points, then you know what survival-in-the-moment states are.

In truth, it's a little more complicated than simply an on–off switch. Just as a lot goes on "behind the walls" that determines whether the switch in your living room will turn your lights on or off, there's a lot that goes on inside a traumatized child's brain and body that will determine whether the switch to survival-in-the-moment state turns on or not. Chapter 2 reviewed some of the brain and body mechanisms involved. In this chapter, we add the necessary complexity (and only what is necessary) for you to help the children with whom you work. To do this, we must introduce a building block.

Survival State Building Blocks

What is a state? A *state* is a configuration of specific elements that come together in certain specific moments. There is usually a context to those moments that cause the elements that constitute a state to come together. In the case of traumatic stress, the context is information in the present environment that reminds the child (consciously or unconsciously) about a past environment of trauma. We call these two related contexts (or environments) the two E's: environment-past and environment-present. What elements come together? These are elements of experience, driven by biology, that prepare an individual to survive. The three elements on which we focus are *awareness*, *affect*, and *action*: We call these the three A's. These are not the only elements to come together in certain moments: There are chemical, physiological, and neurological elements as well. The three A's are closest to the surface and therefore most accessible to providers and the people with whom we work. There is one more aspect of a state to consider: It shifts in predictable ways based on the context.

We describe four specific states that shift based on context and call these the four R's: regulating, revving, reexperiencing, and reconstituting. Two E's, three A's, four R's comprise the building blocks of survival-in-the-moment states. Figure 3.1 shows what such a building block looks like.

Children's extreme reactions in their present environment are often not understandable to those around them because they cannot see how the environment-present evokes memories (consciously or unconsciously) about the children's environment-past.

As can be seen, the outermost component of our building block is the *environment-past*. This component provides the frame within which we can understand the child's experience in specific moments based on the second E: *environment-present*. Children's extreme reactions in their present environment are often not understandable to those around them because they cannot see how the environment-present evokes memories (consciously or unconsciously) about the children's environment-past. Therefore, to understand everything else, we must understand the two E's. The next chapter focuses on the two E's, so we spend the least time with these components in this chapter. For now we provide the following definitions of the two E's. We then devote the rest of this chapter to the three A's and the four R's of our building blocks.

The Two E's

Environment-Past

Information about a child's past environment, related to trauma, which may inform how the child experiences his or her present environment as threatening.

Environment-Present

Information about a child's present environment, at a specific moment, to inform how it is experienced as threatening.

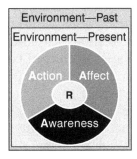

FIGURE 3.1. One building block of a survival-in-the-moment state.

The Three A's

Once we have framed a child's reaction within the social environment, past and present, we need to define his or her reactions with as much specificity and accuracy as possible. This is how the three A's come together in specific moments and contexts. Let's describe the three A's of our building block next. As you consider the three A's, think about Denise and Robert in the moment just before and just after their present environment changed such that they were reminded of their past trauma. Think about how they change when the survival circuit switch turns on.

Awareness

In the moment just before and after a traumatized child is reminded of the trauma, there are significant shifts in the child's awareness of what is going on. Before a traumatized child experiences threat in the environment, the child is most likely aware of and engaged in the external world in relation to the tasks at hand. After threat is experienced, the child is usually aware of only very specific features in the environment that are important for survival. The child also may be more focused on his or her internal world of strong reactions than on the external environment as old traumatic memories begin to dominate consciousness. In other words, there are dramatic shifts in the focus of attention the moment the survival circuit switch turns on.

Awareness, or consciousness, also implies a sense of self: the subject who is aware or is conscious. Damasio (1999) defines consciousness as "...the unified mental pattern that brings together the object and the self" (p. 11). According to Damasio, consciousness is a critical evolutionary advance that allows an individual to be aware of the environment and of his or her internal states in order to decide on the most adaptive response for a given stimulus (or object). As we describe, it is the awareness element of the three A's, rather than affect or action, that we work to engage in treatment. Awareness is primarily controlled by the higher-order brain systems, referred to as the *high road* in Chapter 2, whereas affect and action stem from lower-order (*low road*) brain systems. It is through awareness that affect and action will become regulated.

> Consciousness is a critical evolutionary advance that allows an individual to be aware of the environment and of his or her internal states in order to decide on the most adaptive response for a given stimulus (or object).

At its simplest and most basic level, consciousness lets us recognize an irresistible urge to stay alive and develop a concern for self. At its most complex and elaborate level, consciousness helps us develop a concern for other selves and improve the art of life. (Damasio, 1999, p. 5)

There are three main components of awareness (or consciousness) that must be assessed:

1. **Attention**. Concerns the degree to which the child changes awareness of what is going on around him or her after experiencing threat.
2. **Orientation**. Refers to how the child's experience of place and time can change after experiencing threat.
3. **Sense of self**. Refers to how a child's experience of who he or she is can change after experiencing threat.

Affect (or Emotion)

Emotions have evolved to be highly adaptive. Unfortunately, in response to traumatic stress, these emotions can be highly maladaptive.

A child's emotions can shift dramatically after experiencing a threat in the environment. Affect, or emotion, has two key biological functions: (1) to produce a specific reaction to a stimulus (e.g., fight–flight–freeze) and (2) to help regulate the internal state of the individual so he or she can be prepared to react to that stimulus. Emotions have evolved to be highly adaptive. Unfortunately, in response to traumatic stress, these emotions can become highly maladaptive, leaving the individual feeling extremely disoriented. Robert entered a state of anger when he punched his classmate. Denise experienced a state of intense anxiety when she saw a man at the mall who reminded her of her mother's ex-boyfriend. These affects, or emotions, are experienced because in the context of trauma, they may have facilitated survival. The problem is that the child is unable to see that the context has changed.

Action (or Behavior)

A child's behavior can change dramatically after perceiving a threat. Sometimes these dramatic changes are motivated by efforts to diminish the intense and painful emotions elicited. Behaviors such as running away, self-destructive actions, suicide attempts, aggression, substance abuse, binge eating and purging, fire setting, and compulsive sexual engagement can all be behavioral efforts to manage posttraumatic emotion. Robert, for example, discharges rageful emotions through aggressive behaviors. Again, as in the case of awareness and affect, action has developed to facilitate survival. *From the child's point of view, this behavior is a matter of life or death.* The behavior of a traumatized child in this type of state, no matter how extreme, dangerous, or destructive, is the child's way of surviving. As we discuss in other sections, if we expect children to stop doing what they do in order to survive, we better have something effective with which to replace it.

The Four R's

If you noticed, there is a big letter *R* in the middle of our building block. This letter is the "address label" for four different states that define survival responses in the moment: regulating, revving, reexperiencing, and reconstituting. Accordingly, there are four different building blocks, each defined by its own *R*, which comprise survival-in-the-moment reactions. Knowledge about each of these building blocks is important because each points to different approaches for helping a child.

Regulating

Traumatized children spend most of their time in the first R: *regulating*. These regulating states are characterized by their calmness, continuity of experience, control over emotions and behavior, and engagement in the environment. During regulating *states* children are learning, playing, working, talking, and otherwise fully engaged in and responsive to their social environment. Robert was in a regulating state prior to hearing the demeaning comment. Similarly, Denise was in this regulating state while at the mall before seeing a man who reminded her of her rapist. When a child is in a regulating state, higher-order brain systems are working. The amygdala has not yet made its switch. The three A's are consistent with an environment that is not perceived as threatening.

Revving

During a *revving state*, children with traumatic stress have experienced (consciously or unconsciously) that the environment has changed and threat is present. During this state, their coping skills are challenged. They may attempt to utilize existing coping skills to calm and self-soothe. They may seek out others whom they expect will help them to manage emotion. The three A's are beginning to change in a revving state. Children may begin to feel disoriented and their focus of attention is shifting (awareness), affect is changing, as are their actions, which are shifting into defensive behaviors. When Denise was becoming anxious after seeing a man who reminded her of her mother's ex-boyfriend (who raped her), and as she began to have memories of the assault, she was in a revving emotional state. This state is a critical point for intervention. Children send out signals of distress in this phase. If intervention does not happen, it is very easy for children to enter the *reexperiencing* state. In a revving state the switch is on, but it is very easy to turn it off. It becomes a question whether a particular child has the capacity to become *aware* that his or survival circuit switch is on and to turn it off before it is too late. As we describe in Chapter 13 on regulation-focused

It becomes a question whether a particular child has the capacity to become *aware* that his or her survival circuit switch is on and to turn it off before it is too late.

treatment, an important part of intervention is helping a child to become *aware* that the switch is on (while still in the revving state).

Reexperiencing

During *reexperiencing* states children are often flooded with feelings that remind them of their trauma. The three A's have shifted dramatically at this point. The child's awareness and engagement in the environment are markedly changed. Attention is focused on basic facts of survival. As the child is reexperiencing the trauma, he or she becomes disoriented to time and place, feeling as if he or she were "back then" and "back there." The way that children feel about themselves is very different in a reexperiencing state, and at the extreme, they may become disoriented to *who* they are (dissociative identity disorder). Similarly, emotions and behaviors activated to manage these emotions also change dramatically. In reexperiencing, the switch is fully on; survival-in-the-moment responses are in full swing. Again, this system is built for managing threats to survival and gives the individual only the survival-essential fragments of information at the expense of the contextual details. Amygdala-mediated information processing prepares the body to fight, flee, or freeze in order to maximize the chance of survival. The speed of information processing necessary for survival sacrifices the details of the context. As contextual processing diminishes, the child becomes disoriented. Accordingly, when a child is in a reexperiencing emotional state he or she experiences flashes and bits and pieces of highly threatening information. Our ability to help a child in a reexperiencing state is dramatically limited. Our focus is always to prevent such states. When it is too late, our main aim is to do whatever we can to make the environment safe enough, from the child's perspective, and to keep the child and others as safe as possible.

Reconstituting

> This period of reconstitution is very important because the child is particularly vulnerable to being triggered and to reentering the reexperiencing state.

As described, reexperiencing states are marked by extreme emotion and behavior with changes in awareness or consciousness (attention, orientation, sense of self). Once these states are terminated via therapeutic means or otherwise, the child transitions back to the regulating emotional state. This transition requires a period of time during which the child reorients to his or her surroundings and tries to calm and soothe him- or herself. Some reparation for the damage done during reexperiencing states (to the child's sense of self, to relationships with others, to physical objects) may be needed to help the child and the environment to return to a calm and stable state. This period of reconstitution is very important because the child is particularly vulnerable to being triggered and to reentering the reexperiencing state. It's important not to confuse a reconstituting state for a regulating state, even though they may overtly look the same. A child in a reconstituting state may be much quieter and appear much calmer, but he or she is at very high risk of slipping back into a reexperiencing state if he or she perceives any signal of threat.

Putting It All Together: Four Building Blocks That Define Survival-in-the-Moment

We started with one building block that defined the elements of a state that becomes survival-in-the-moment. With the four R's, we described how survival-in-the-moment is the process of transition between four state building blocks, each defined by its own *R*. Figure 3.2 puts this all together. As you will recognize, Figure 3.2 reproduces the innermost section of the TST picture shown in Figure 1.1 (p. 12).

As described, children spend most of their time in the regulating state as their usual state of being. Survival-in-the-moment, itself, can be described as three interrelated states (i.e., revving, reexperiencing, reconstituting) that begin when *environment-present* changes from one the child perceives as safe to one the child perceives as threatening. The way we can best understand why the child, and perhaps no one else in that environment-present, perceives a threat is through our knowledge of the child's *environment-past*. We began this chapter by saying that traumatic stress is a little more complex than an on–off switch. Figure 3.2 illustrates this complexity. The core of Figure 3.2, however, maintains that simplicity. A child's survival circuit, in his or her usual, regulating state, is off. It switches on with the transition to the three interrelated survival-in-the-moment states. And that's it.

What does all this mean for intervention?

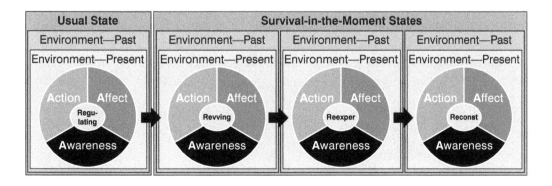

FIGURE 3.2. The four building blocks of survival-in-the-moment.

The information contained in Figure 3.2 also makes it clear where intervention fits in this picture. What components of the building blocks shown in Figure 3.2 might we have any influence over? Only two: the (1) environment-present and (2) awareness. Obviously, we cannot change the past environment, but we can help the child to be aware of the differences between the present and the past environments, even though this may be hard to see, given the child's history. We can help the child to be aware of alternative responses to the present environment and to learn, through this awareness, skills to manage his or her affects and actions. In the traumatized child both affect and action are wired to maintain survival in the face of threat, and both are fully mediated by low-road brain processes. The only hope of rewiring them to the high road is through awareness. Our intervention chapters will help you do this. The other point of intervention is the present environment. Once we learn how the present environment may be perceived by the child as threatening, there are ways we can intervene within the environment to address this problem. Obviously, if the present environment is truly threatening, we would need to definitively address this danger. These issues are fully explored in our assessment and intervention chapters.

We cannot change the past environment: but we can help the child to be Aware of the differences between the present and the past environment.

What about Denise and Robert?

How, exactly, can we use this information to understand and help Denise and Robert? In Chapter 9, we introduce a process called the Moment-by-Moment Assessment to gather the information we need in order to know how to help traumatized children. The Moment-by-Moment Assessment gathers the information on the two E's, three A's, and four R's described in this chapter. In Chapter 9, we provide the details on how this is done. For now, to illustrate the importance of this information for understanding how to help a traumatized child, we show Robert and Denise's Moment-by-Moment information as they leave their usual, regulating state and switch to survival-in-the-moment.

Figures 3.3 and 3.4 show this process with Robert and Denise.

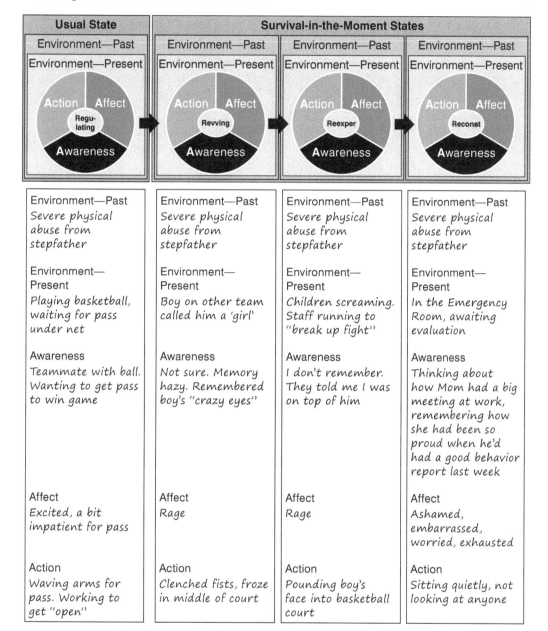

Usual State	Survival-in-the-Moment States		
Environment—Past	Environment—Past	Environment—Past	Environment—Past
Environment—Present	Environment—Present	Environment—Present	Environment—Present
Action / Affect / **Regulating** / **Awareness**	Action / Affect / **Revving** / **Awareness**	Action / Affect / **Reexper** / **Awareness**	Action / Affect / **Reconst** / **Awareness**

Environment—Past	Environment—Past	Environment—Past	Environment—Past
Severe physical abuse from stepfather	*Severe physical abuse from stepfather*	*Severe physical abuse from stepfather*	*Severe physical abuse from stepfather*
Environment—Present	Environment—Present	Environment—Present	Environment—Present
Playing basketball, waiting for pass under net	*Boy on other team called him a 'girl'*	*Children screaming. Staff running to "break up fight"*	*In the Emergency Room, awaiting evaluation*
Awareness	Awareness	Awareness	Awareness
Teammate with ball. Wanting to get pass to win game	*Not sure. Memory hazy. Remembered boy's "crazy eyes"*	*I don't remember. They told me I was on top of him*	*Thinking about how Mom had a big meeting at work, remembering how she had been so proud when he'd had a good behavior report last week*
Affect	Affect	Affect	Affect
Excited, a bit impatient for pass	*Rage*	*Rage*	*Ashamed, embarrassed, worried, exhausted*
Action	Action	Action	Action
Waving arms for pass. Working to get "open"	*Clenched fists, froze in middle of court*	*Pounding boy's face into basketball court*	*Sitting quietly, not looking at anyone*

FIGURE 3.3. Robert's survival-in-the-moment episode.

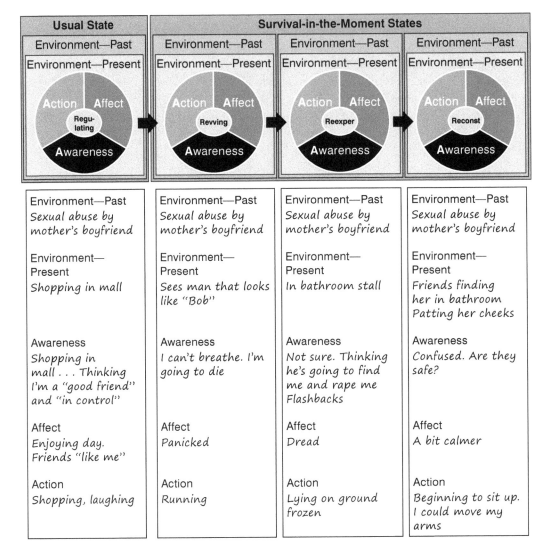

Usual State	Survival-in-the-Moment States		
Environment—Past	Environment—Past	Environment—Past	Environment—Past
Environment—Present	Environment—Present	Environment—Present	Environment—Present
Action / Affect / Regulating / Awareness	Action / Affect / Revving / Awareness	Action / Affect / Reexper / Awareness	Action / Affect / Reconst / Awareness
Environment—Past *Sexual abuse by mother's boyfriend*	Environment—Past *Sexual abuse by mother's boyfriend*	Environment—Past *Sexual abuse by mother's boyfriend*	Environment—Past *Sexual abuse by mother's boyfriend*
Environment— Present *Shopping in mall*	Environment— Present *Sees man that looks like "Bob"*	Environment— Present *In bathroom stall*	Environment— Present *Friends finding her in bathroom Patting her cheeks*
Awareness *Shopping in mall . . . Thinking I'm a "good friend" and "in control"*	Awareness *I can't breathe. I'm going to die*	Awareness *Not sure. Thinking he's going to find me and rape me Flashbacks*	Awareness *Confused. Are they safe?*
Affect *Enjoying day. Friends "like me"*	Affect *Panicked*	Affect *Dread*	Affect *A bit calmer*
Action *Shopping, laughing*	Action *Running*	Action *Lying on ground frozen*	Action *Beginning to sit up. I could move my arms*

FIGURE 3.4. Denise's survival-in-the-moment episode.

States and Traits

We have described child traumatic stress as a disorder of survival states. This wording implies a continually changing clinical picture depending on what is going on with the child. Although states are changing, they change in regular and predictable ways. What about "traits"? Traits imply relatively enduring patterns of thinking, feeling, behaving, and relating and are important for a child's developing personality. The way that "states" can become "traits" in traumatized children is very important to understand. Perry, Pollard, Blakley, Baker, and Vigilante (1995) wrote an influential paper on how states turn into traits in the context of child traumatic stress. In essence, this process involves how the child adapts over time to being overwhelmed by extreme emotion.

The tragic and complex process by which survival-in-the-moment states become embedded into enduring components of a child's personality can be approached through considering the following questions:

- What does it do to a child's sense of self-esteem and self-control to grow up continually having difficulty controlling affect, awareness, and actions? How much worse is the impact of this state of dysregulation if the child has difficulty remembering what he or she said or did in a given emotional state?
- What does it do to a child's sense of identity to grow up having a dramatically different feeling about him- or herself in different emotional states? What does it do to a child's sense of identity over time when the sense of self is dependent on the state the child happens to be in?
- What does it do to a child's capacity to learn when he or she is regularly overwhelmed with emotion and the consequential changes in attention and information processing?
- How does the experience of the trauma and the child's continuing state regulation problems affect the way the child thinks about him- or herself in relation to other people, to the world, and to the future?
- How do these changes in affect, awareness, and actions influence the child's relationships over time?

We do not have clear answers to all these questions. Nevertheless, traumatic stress in children is more than a disorder of extreme emotional states. It is also a disorder of children's adaptations to these states as reflected in how they think about themselves, their world, and their future. These adaptations can be thought of as *enduring negative cognitions* and are

> Traumatic stress in children is more than a disorder of extreme emotional states. It is also a disorder of children's adaptations to these states as reflected in how they think about themselves, their world, and their future.

best seen in what Aaron Beck, the father of cognitive-behavioral therapy (CBT), called the *cognitive triad*: relatively stable ways of thinking that serve to maintain psychopathology, particularly depression and anxiety (Beck, Rush, Shaw, & Emery, 1979). According to Beck and colleagues (1979), treatment aims to address cognitive distortions related to:

- The self
- The world
- The future

These ideas have been applied to traumatic stress in children and adults and form the basis of CBT as applied to traumatic stress. We integrate this approach in TST, but only after children are good enough at regulating their emotional states and the social environment is stable enough so that it is not provoking dysregulation. This work is detailed in Chapter 14, "Beyond Trauma Treatment."

Impact on Others

Just as a child's experience of survival states can, over time, shape more enduring traits, the *impact* of these survival states can affect both immediate interactions with others as well as enduring patterns of relationships. Imagine for a moment that you are an employee at Robert's school and are assigned to monitor the children on the playground. You are enjoying the spring day, watching the children play, and feeling good about your job and the world. Suddenly a fight breaks out, and you spot Robert pounding another child to the ground. You will likely quickly shift your attention (awareness), may feel a surge of anxiety and concern (affect), and may move forward to put a quick end to the physical altercation (action). Later that night, over dinner, you might mention the incident (rather than sharing how nice the weather was as you watched the children play). Robert's dysregulation clearly has an impact on how those around him feel, think, and react in the moment.

But Robert's dysregulation may, over time, impact not only those moments but all the many moments to follow. Imagine over the next several months that you continue to be assigned the job of playground monitor, and you have now pulled Robert out of countless fights. You walk out on the playground on another sunny day, but instead of optimistically and bemusedly watching the children play, you feel keyed up—your muscles are tense, your brow furrowed; this is the time of day when Robert's class comes out to play. As Robert emerges from the classroom, you watch him suspiciously. How soon will he blow up? How will yet another playground fight on your watch be perceived by the principal? Why did you get saddled with dealing with this obstreperous youngster? And isn't it about time someone taught him some respect and discipline?

The problems depicted in the above scenario are manifold. The playground monitor has been affected in an enduring way by Robert, and is now less able to do well in the very important job he has—to fairly and respectfully help the children learn to play. Robert may (rightly) pick up on signals of hostility from the playground monitor, and rather than learning to turn to an ally for help, instead perceives an enemy. The monitor, in a heightened physiological state, may respond too quickly and harshly. And so a downward spiral begins.

In TST a child's survival states, the enduring traits, and the ways in which these impact others around him or her must all be considered and addressed; trauma *systems* therapy acknowledges and addresses these very important interrelationships.

What about Psychiatric Diagnoses?

What about posttraumatic stress disorder (PTSD) and other psychiatric disorders that have been associated with trauma (e.g., depression, dissociative disorders, substance abuse)? Why have we not even mentioned PTSD or those other disorders in this manual on the treatment of trauma? We mentioned earlier that we are not big fans of psychiatric diagnosis. Here's why:

Knowing the diagnosis is not clearly related to knowing what to do.

Another way of stating this perspective is simply to ask how much any diagnosis communicates information that tells you how you can help Robert or Denise. Let's say that you knew that Robert and Denise have PTSD. How much would that guide you in formulating what is needed to reduce the likelihood of Denise curling into a ball in the bathroom in specific moments or Robert punching someone in specific moments? Those are the reasons kids like Denise and Robert come to treatment. They don't seek our help to cure their PTSD; they seek our help to stop having definable episodes that lead to their undoing. How much information is contained in the diagnosis of PTSD that would be helpful for Denise or Robert to prevent these moments? How much information is contained in the diagnosis of PTSD that would help you predict these moments? Is it only PTSD? What if you knew that Denise also had a diagnosis of depression and that Robert had conduct disorder? How much would these additional diagnoses add to your knowledge of what to do to help Denise and Robert prevent their moments of undoing? We are not saying that these diagnoses are irrelevant; we simply believe the information they reveal about what to do is very limited. What is the missing information that can tell you what to do? We believe that psychiatric diagnosis misses two categories of information critical to formulating what to do to help children like Denise and Robert:

> They don't seek our help to cure their PTSD; they seek our help to stop having definable episodes that lead to their undoing.

1. Psychiatric diagnoses related to trauma do not contain sufficient *information about the process of how children shift into specific survival-related states* in specific moments.

2. Psychiatric diagnoses related to trauma do not contain sufficient *information about how symptoms and the social environment fit together.*

Let's take these problems one at a time.

1. **Information about the process of how children shift into specific survival-related states.** Our main concern about the diagnosis of PTSD is that it obscures the primary developmental pathology of traumatized children: the dysregulation of emotional states when threat is perceived in the present environment. The understanding of this critical process—and in particular, how awareness, affect, and action can dramatically change in the context of perceived threat—gives providers actionable information that can guide how to intervene.

> Our main concern about the diagnosis of PTSD is that it obscures the primary developmental pathology of traumatized children: the dysregulation of emotional states when confronted by a stressor.

2. **Information about how symptoms and the social environment fit together.** We have described repeatedly that the core problem of traumatized children involves the "fit" between the social environment or system of care and the children's capacity to regulate emotional states (further described in Chapter 4). There is no mention of the social environment within the definition of PTSD. We have aimed our assessment approach at exactly this type of specificity. The knowledge about how changes in the social environment may provoke survival circuits to switch from off to on is the information that may guide providers toward effective treatment. Sometimes this information is very subtle. It may involve a certain type of glance from a parent or the tone of voice used in certain contexts by a teacher. If this is the stimuli that will repeatedly lead to the *on* switch, then providers need to know about it or they will not have enough information to know what to do.

What the DSM May Tell You about Denise and Robert

The utility of the DSM diagnosis of PTSD is only that it casts a "fishnet" that will capture many children (and adults) who have this basic developmental problem related to the dysregulation of survival states. In other words, using the symptom groupings of PTSD will identify many children who have problems regulating survival states described in this chapter. The symptom groupings of PTSD are, however, a poor way of describing and organizing the symptoms and experiences that are most relevant for psychopathology related to trauma. The most important psychopathological process that must be identified is how awareness, affect, and action fluctuate when the environment shifts and how a child adapts to these fluctuations. The symptom groups of PTSD may be a proxy for this process, but not a very good one.

Consider the DSM-5 criteria for PTSD:

1. Traumatic event
2. Intrusive symptoms
3. Avoidance
4. Negative alterations in cognition and mood
5. Alterations in arousal and reactivity

These symptom groups are, to be sure, an important part of the trauma response. They may describe certain types of emotional states and corresponding behavioral responses. The problem is that the listing of these symptom groups—which may relate to survival-in-the-moment states as we have described them in this and the previous chapter—say nothing about the critical process of how they may fit together in certain moments or the process by which they shift together in those moments. From our point of view, it is exactly this information that tells providers what they must do to help a traumatized child (or adult). We provide a lot of detail on how to gather this information in Chapter 9.

 Consider the case of Denise. We can say that she has PTSD. She has:

- Intense distress at traumatic reminders
- Flashbacks
- Restricted activities related to fear about the trauma
- Hypervigilance
- Irritability or impaired affect modulation
- Feelings of ineffectiveness, shame, despair, or hopelessness

We can also say that Denise, when confronted by reminders of sexual abuse from her mother's ex-boyfriend, transitions from a regulating state to a reexperiencing state marked by changes in awareness (has fragmented memory, becomes disoriented to place and time, becomes depersonalized), affect (panic, dread), and action (running away, curling up frozen in a ball). One of her chronic adaptations to dysregulation process is feeling continually ashamed. These states are repeatedly provoked by stressors in her social environment, including exposure to domestic violence and lack of privacy.

Similarly for Robert, we can say that he has PTSD. He has:

- Intense distress at traumatic reminders
- Flashbacks
- Restricted activities related to fear about the trauma
- Hypervigilance
- Irritability or impaired affect modulation
- Aggression
- Self-destructive and impulsive behavior

We can also say that Robert, when confronted by demeaning comments reminiscent of physical abuse, transitions from a regulating state to a reexperiencing phase marked by changes in awareness (has fragmented memory, becomes disoriented to place and time, loses awareness of surroundings and context), affect (rage), and action (aggression).

We believe that this latter way of describing Denise and Robert is truer to their experience and has much greater clinical utility.

An Alternative Classification System: The National Institute of Mental Health's Research Domain Criteria (RDoC)

There is an initiative within the mental health field that we believe has the possibility of capturing the missing information and also is truer to what we believe is the essence of traumatic stress: the National Institute of Mental Health's (NIMH) Research Domain Criteria (RDoC).

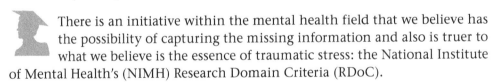

The RDoC initiative proposes that psychiatric symptoms are the overt expressions of knowable biological processes that fit together and become manifest in certain contexts.

The NIMH RDoC initiative developed because of the perceived limitation of the DSM for advancing the understanding of mental illness. This initiative's primary critique of DSM, like our critique, is that counting up symptoms and putting individuals in various categories of mental illness greatly limits our understanding of the nature of mental illness or its treatment. The RDoC initiative proposes that psychiatric symptoms are the overt expressions of knowable biological processes that fit together and become manifest in certain contexts. The thoughts, emotions, and behaviors that are the main descriptors of certain categories of mental illness are the "downstream" expressions of much larger biobehavioral processes. Central to these processes are specific brain circuits.

Upstream from these brain circuits are molecular and cellular processes that are driven by the genome and gene expression, and downstream from the brain circuits are physiological, emotional, behavioral, cognitive, and social processes. Different categories of mental illness are defined by these processes. Although the RDoC is in a very early stage of development, we believe it offers a much more accurate and useful accounting of mental illness than does the DSM perspective.

Our accounting of the core processes of traumatic stress in this chapter and Chapter 2 entirely fit within the spirit of the RDoC. As we have detailed, traumatic stress is marked by clear and dramatic shifts in state, defined by the three A's, when the present environment is perceived to be threatening based on a child's trauma history. These shifts occur in four predictable ways, defined by the four R's. We use the three A's approach to communicate a meaningful and useful way of remembering the elements that can be observed to shift in the process of state dysregulation—but, as described, "beneath the surface" there are equally dramatic shifts occurring, including neurological (e.g., amygdala firing), psychophysiological (e.g., heart rate, heart variability), chemical (e.g., cortisol, norepinephrine), and even the expression of certain genes. This information is very important for both research and clinical work. If we think of the center of dysregulation process as the survival circuit detailed in Chapter 2, then the processes of shifting states include both "upstream" and "downstream" shifts in molecular, cellular, neurological, emotional, and behavioral expressions when the survival circuit switch is turned *on*.

The RDoC of traumatic stress is captured when the brain circuitry (termed the *survival circuit*) switches on in response to specific environmental signals perceived to indicate threat, and an integrated pattern of upstream and downstream changes occur that are described by the survival-in-the-moment states.

We now turn our attention to those environmental signals: understanding the social environment.

The Social Environment and the Services System

Traumatic Stress Responses Are Embedded in a Social Context

LEARNING OBJECTIVES

- To understand how the child's natural social environment influences traumatic stress responses
- To learn about an important experiment involving rats at play
- To understand how the child services system can help when problems arise in the child's social environment

---

ICONS USED IN THIS CHAPTER

Essential Point	Academic Point	Quotation	Case Discussion

As described in the earlier chapters of this book, it's all about a "trauma system." The trauma system consists of:

1. A traumatized child who experiences *survival-in-the-moment* states in specific, definable moments.
2. A social environment and/or system of care that is not able to help the child regulate these *survival-in-the-moment* states.

In Chapter 3, we reviewed what it means to regulate survival-in-the-moment states in a lot of detail. We introduced the building blocks of this dysregulation process and described how the three A's shift across the four R's. We defined the two E's of environment—present and environment—past and their relations. This chapter provides more detail about the two E's, the second part of our trauma system. If you go back to our TST picture shown in Figure 1.1 (p. 12), you see categories of people, at various levels, that are there to support a child's regulation and growth. These individuals comprise the second part of the trauma system. It starts with those who are naturally around the child, such as parents, relatives, teachers, clergy, and coaches, and when (for whatever reason) these people are not able to support the child's regulation and growth in a good-enough way, intervention is needed through the engagement of the child services system.

This chapter is about the people around the child and the importance of their contribution to making the trauma system better or worse. Before we dive into this discussion, we make a brief digression to discuss an experiment with . . . young rats.

WE KNOW! What does an experiment with young rats have to do with the social context? Keep reading . . .

Why Do Rats Play?

Almost all young mammals play. This is interesting, in itself. As professionals concerned about the mental health of children, we know the importance of play and, in particular, when play stops or goes wrong. Some of the first treatments in the field of child mental health involved play. Why do human and nonhuman children play?

Jaak Panksepp, a neuroscientist at Washington State University, believes that play is a substrate of the emotion of joy and has important evolutionary value. Rat pups, like all other young mammals, play. Panksepp studies young rats at play and is able to quantify their play. Even in lab cages, as in their natural habitats, these rats play.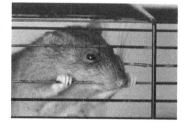

Panksepp (1998), in his great book *Affective Neuroscience*, reports on his study of young rats at play. He observes these animals playing for several days and keeps track of the number of play initiations and episodes of rough-and-tumble play they display under normal conditions.

He then introduces what he calls a *minimal fear stimulus* in this environment: a single hair from a cat. He leaves the hair in the cage for 24 hours and then removes it. What happens to play after the cat hair is introduced? What happens when it is removed?

It's important to know that these experiments are conducted with lab rats: They have never actually seen a cat. Figure 4.1 is adapted from Panksepp's experiment and shows what happens. The y-axis shows the amount of play. The x-axis shows "Day." As you can see, the young rats are happily playing for 4 days. On the day the cat hair is introduced, play stops completely. Even after the cat hair is removed, play never returns to anywhere near the level where it was before the hair was introduced.

What is at stake here? Why is this research relevant for our chapter on the social environment? What, exactly, does a lab rat experiment have to do with traumatized kids?

We, of course, understand that our human social environments are immeasurably more complex and sophisticated than that of a lab cage. It is worthwhile to consider, however, whether our need for safety and security is any different from that of young rats. What happens when threat is introduced, even briefly, into our present social environment (E-present)? It changes everything. That

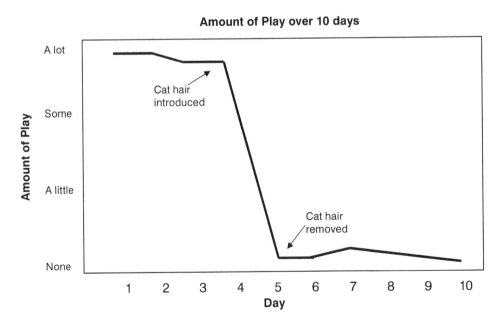

FIGURE 4.1. The introduction of cat hair stops play in lab rats. Adapted from Panksepp (1998).

safe environment of the rat cage that contained happily playing rats has become an environment of present threat. Play is gone, forever. It's worth considering how the past environment (E-past) fits into this experiment. In Chapter 3, we reviewed the integral relation between a child's reactivity to the present environment based on his or her memory of the past environment. These lab rats have never experienced a cat before. What past environment? E-past for these rats is memory sculpted over millions of years, stored in their genomes, and determining their brain's reactivity to odors that the rat itself has never experienced. Evolution is an amazing thing!

Whether a signal (even a minimal signal) of threat is based on evolutionary traumatic memory or on a memory of a child's past traumatic experience, the impact is dramatic: The survival circuit switches to *on*, as detailed in Chapters 2 and 3. Now let's consider the environments inhabited by the children with whom we work. Let's think about Denise or Robert . . .

Remember Denise?

 Denise is a 16-year-old girl with a history of sexual abuse from her mother's ex-boyfriend. While at a local mall with friends, she saw a man who frightened her. She later reported that this man reminded her of her mother's ex-boyfriend. Denise remembers becoming extremely anxious and flooded with memories of sexual abuse. She does not remember walking away. Her friends found her curled up in a bathroom stall, unresponsive.

Remember Robert?

 Robert is a 10-year-old boy with a history of severe physical abuse from his stepfather. He has a long history of extreme and impulsive aggressive behavior. While on the playground at recess, another child made a demeaning comment about Robert. Without thinking, Robert lunged at him and continued to pound him in the face with his fists until the school monitors pulled him off.

What if we told you that Denise's story continues like this?

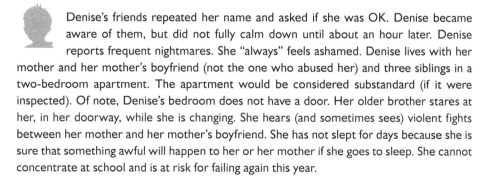 Denise's friends repeated her name and asked if she was OK. Denise became aware of them, but did not fully calm down until about an hour later. Denise reports frequent nightmares. She "always" feels ashamed. Denise lives with her mother and her mother's boyfriend (not the one who abused her) and three siblings in a two-bedroom apartment. The apartment would be considered substandard (if it were inspected). Of note, Denise's bedroom does not have a door. Her older brother stares at her, in her doorway, while she is changing. She hears (and sometimes sees) violent fights between her mother and her mother's boyfriend. She has not slept for days because she is sure that something awful will happen to her or her mother if she goes to sleep. She cannot concentrate at school and is at risk for failing again this year.

What if we told you that Robert's story continues like this?

 Robert was sent by ambulance to an emergency room in restraints. He did not finally calm down until about an hour after his arrival, when he fell asleep. He was awakened by a loud argument in his room between his father and a nurse. His father was insisting that he take Robert home because "this is a family matter—I know how to discipline my boy." Hospital security was called when Robert's father became agitated and threatening. They escorted him into another room. The psychiatrist then evaluated Robert, who reluctantly disclosed that his father beats him with a belt and sometimes his fists almost every night. His mother tries to help but she is "given a beating if she gets in his way." Robert reports that he is sure that he will either "be killed, kill someone, or kill himself" in the near future. He is in a regular, overcrowded class at school. He has been suspended 10 times over the past 6 months for fighting and is "about to be kicked out."

As Panksepp's experiment illustrates, if there is a single cat hair in the environment, nothing else matters. Similarly, if there is a real threat in a child's social environment, it makes no sense to address anything else. The child cannot possibly attend to anything else if a signal in the environment represents threat. Regarding Denise and Robert, they cannot possibly recover if the cat hair in their environment is not clearly and effectively addressed in treatment.

In Denise's case, she lives with both cat hair and cat:

1. Being watched by her brother in the doorless doorway *(cat hair, unless we believe her brother may plausibly assault her)*
2. Seeing and hearing violent fights between her mother and her mother's boyfriend *(the cat)*
3. Seeing men at the mall *(cat hair)*
4. Failing at school *(cat hair)*

Robert also lives with both cats and cat hair:

1. Receiving beatings from his father *(the cat)*
2. Seeing his father beat his mother *(another cat)*
3. Hearing demeaning comments in the schoolyard and classroom *(cat hair)*

What is simply and tragically true for Denise and Robert—and for more traumatized children than any caring adult would like to admit—is that they are living in cages full of cat hair . . . and sometimes they are living with the cat.

What is simply and tragically true for Denise and Robert—and for more traumatized children than any caring adult would like to admit—is that they are living in cages full of cat hair . . . and sometimes they are living with the cat.

Cat Hair and the Two E's

To understand a traumatized child's transition into survival-in-the-moment states, described in Chapter 3, we need to gather information about threat in the environment. The building blocks, shown in Figure 3.1 (p. 48), include a description of safety and threat in the present environment and the history of threat in a child's past environment. A child's reactivity to his or her present environment can be understood through these two E's: environment—present and past. This is all a discussion of cats and cat hair. A child who experiences a cat, even once, may be primed to react through survival-in-the-moment states when the present environment contains even a whiff of cat. Again: Exposure to a "cat" is defined as any situation where the child, or someone close to the child, may have been in serious danger. Exposure to "cat hair" is defined as any stimulus (no matter how seemingly minimal) in the present environment that may evoke memories of the child's exposure to the "cat." Accordingly, our job of assessing a child's present environment and history of past environments is primarily one of assessing the presence of cats and cat hair.

> A child who experiences a cat, even once, may be primed to react through Survival-in-the-Moment States when their present environment contains even a whiff of cat.

In Chapter 2 we quoted Joseph LeDoux (1998) saying that "the amygdala leads a hostile takeover of consciousness by emotion" (p. 226). LeDoux's statement is about switching the survival circuit to *on*. That statement is not, however, entirely true: Cat hair activates the amygdala to lead this hostile takeover of consciousness by emotion. If we want to help traumatized kids, we must know where the cat hair is and help to clean it up. To simplify the story (don't worry, we'll make it more complicated in a minute):

Cat hair → survival-in-the-moment states

What Do We Mean by the Environment?

Urie Bronfenbrenner (1979; Bronfenbrenner & Ceci, 1994) describes the social environment as an ecology with various nested and interacting levels. This is a powerful idea, and we have used it to define TST as illustrated in our TST picture shown in Figure 1.1 (p. 12). In the TST picture, you saw how the child's propensity to shift from his or her usual state to survival-in-the-moment states is influenced by various nested levels of people and organizations whose ultimate function is to support the child's regulation and growth. These nested levels include the individuals and organizations that a natural part of the ecology (e.g., families, peers, schools, teams, religious

> Each level of the social ecology plays a key role in some aspect of healthy child development, and as such, may serve an important recovery function when the child is exposed to traumatic stress.

organizations) and those that are part of the services system when intervention is needed (e.g., mental health, special education, child welfare, juvenile justice). Each level of the social ecology plays a key role in some aspect of healthy child development, and as such, may serve an important recovery function when the child is exposed to traumatic stress. In a way, these ecological levels outside the individual child represent his or her "rat cage." Signals of threat or danger at any of these levels will produce an important challenge to development, especially regarding emotional regulation. What are the purposes of these social ecological levels? They serve many purposes, but ultimately they insulate the individual from the inevitable bumps of life. Children with traumatic stress often have clear breakdowns in many of these levels. Think about Denise and Robert. Count the number of breakdowns in their environments.

Bronfenbrenner's ecological model provides a way to understand how a child is influenced by and influences his or her world throughout development. These mutual influences, or transactions, highlight ways that healthy development can be either promoted or inhibited.

Bronfenbrenner's ecological model provides a way to understand how a child is influenced by and influences his or her world throughout development. These mutual influences, or transactions, highlight ways that healthy development can be either promoted or inhibited. The insight that the children and their social ecology mutually shape each other is very important. It is not simply that, for instance, families affect how a child develops; *the arrows go the other way too*—a child affects his or her family. So our simple figure from above actually is a little more complicated:

Cat hair → survival states → more cat hair

Social environments are not static entities. They are constantly changing, responding to the child. Sometimes systems go awry and the social environment changes in ways that are not helpful and that compound the problems a child is having. Consider Denise, who has been having trouble sleeping at home and is failing at school:

 Denise continued to have trouble concentrating in school. One day during math she seemed to be daydreaming out the window, despite being called back to attention several times. Her teacher, frustrated that Denise didn't seem to be applying herself, sent a note home to Denise's mother requesting a meeting and saying that Denise was not performing up to her capacity. When her mother received the note, she became angry with Denise, telling her she would never amount to anything. When the mother's boyfriend came home that evening, her mother was still in a bad temper, and very soon the two started yelling at each other. Denise lay in bed unable to sleep; the next day she arrived at school with her homework incomplete and again unable to concentrate.

Transactions like this take place between the child and the social environment all day, every day, on every level. Consider the many ways in which transactions between a dysregulated child and the social environment can reinforce the problems:

> Parent criticizes 5-year-old Sammy harshly → Sammy enters a survival state, begins kicking and screaming → parent physically restrains Sammy

> Lauren, a teenager, becomes overwhelmed with anxiety at a crowded school basketball game and leaves abruptly → her friends think she is walking out on them and the next day exclude her from the lunch table → Lauren feels rejected, her anxiety rises, and she leaves school rather than sitting alone at lunch

> A child bumps Lucy on the playground → Lucy beats him up → teachers call in police monitors to restrain her

> Cat hair → survival state → more cat hair

The above examples illustrate how specific instances of cat hair can lead to specific episodes of dysregulation that in turn pull for harsher, more rejecting responses from the environment. Where things get really difficult is when chronic adaptations to trauma—as described in Chapter 3—begin to shape the way the child thinks and acts *even when he or she is not in a survival state*, and these, in turn, pull for negative or hostile reactions from the environment.

> Cat hair → survival state → more cat hair → persistently negative expectations of self, world, future → negative responses from people and world (more cat hair)

You see the problem.

As we described, a traumatic event does not just impact the individual. It impacts every aspect of the child's social ecology. To truly understand the impact of trauma, you must appreciate its effect on each environmental system as well as the *transactions* between systems. To effectively intervene, you must enlist those systems to collaboratively support the child.

So what do you *do* about the problem? One of the reasons that TST so powerfully affects children's lives is that it addresses not only the child at the center of the social ecology but also the surrounding layers of the social ecology. In essence, we address not only the survival response but the cat hair as well.

One of the reasons that TST so powerfully affects children's lives is that it addresses not only the child at the center of the social ecology but also the surrounding layers of the social ecology. In essence, we address not only the survival response but the cat hair as well.

In order to do this, however, we must first know where the cat hair is. As we describe in Chapters 9 and 10, it is extremely important to identify the signals of danger (i.e., the cat hair) for a traumatized child at each and every level of the social ecology and to construct intervention plans to get rid of them.

Our job is to do everything we can, to work with any member of the social ecology who can or will work with us, to remove as much cat hair (threat) as possible, and to create plans to address the cat hair that we cannot remove.

Trauma and the Social Environment

The role of the social environment following a trauma is to support the child's regulatory capacities so that the child can effectively manage the emotions following the trauma. Ultimately, we want the child to be able to adapt and function in this posttraumatic world. Members of the child's social environment will need to recreate a sense of stability, control, and order in this new world.

Trauma, however, has the potential to disrupt the very environmental systems on which the child has depended to manage and cope over the course of his or her development.

Events such as traumatic injuries or physical and sexual abuse of the child, house fires, or murders in families have the potential to impact all levels of the social ecology. The impact of the trauma might include making caregivers or loved ones physically unavailable to children through separation or loss, or by rendering them emotionally unavailable because of their own reactions to traumatic events. Robert's mother, for example, was simply unable to help him due to fear for her own life. Whether a parent's trauma(s) is ongoing, recent, or from childhood, if the parent is experiencing traumatic stress reactions, those reactions can interfere with his or her parenting in general, and with his or her ability to help the child regulate in particular. The parent may have distorted perceptions of the child's behavior, in some cases personalizing behavior that may be developmentally "normal" (e.g., a preschool-age child having trouble sitting still even when asked to do so by the parent) or a response to the child's own trauma experience (e.g., a teenager "shutting down" when asked to do something by the foster parent that inadvertently reminds the teen of his or her past abuse). A child's traumatic reactions may also bring up reminders in parents of their own trauma experiences, making it hard to respond supportively in the moment.

Larger-scale traumas, such as terrorist activities and natural disasters, more directly impact multiple levels of the child's social ecology. In these instances, the extended families, religious and neighborhood organizations, and schools that have been implicated as potential protective factors for children coping with trauma may be disrupted by the trauma and therefore be less able to serve in their important roles of supporting and facilitating the survival and healthy development of children. Similarly, cultural rituals and beliefs may be broken down by traumatic events in ways that alienate people from their histories. These disruptions then may act to exacerbate a child's experience of traumatic events and complicate his or her ability to cope in the wake of these events.

Complex Problems Need Comprehensive Solutions

What do we know so far? We know that traumatic events can be disruptive for children and families, as well as for different levels of the social ecology. The aftermath of trauma can overwhelm children's coping skills, decrease their display of adaptive behaviors, and increase their display of maladaptive behaviors. Trauma also can impair the ability of the environmental support systems to help children cope.

Clearly, interventions on the individual level are not sufficient to address all these issues. Comprehensive interventions are required to support the child and to improve the ability of the different levels of the child's social ecology to support him or her in the process of recovering from traumatic events. The TST model prescribes a way to think about which services need to be a part of the intervention, how to apply them, and how to coordinate them in order to ensure maximal success in the child's and the family's recovery from trauma. As we have noted, many different systems are involved in the growth and development of children. That means that there are many different systems that can help a child when traumatic events occur. TST recognizes the many different players (systems) in a child's life and works to weave them together so that everyone is working toward a common goal: *fixing a broken system* (more on what this means in Chapter 6 on treatment principles).

The Natural Ecology and the Services System

Broadly speaking, we can divide the social ecology into two sections: what is already there, and what sometimes needs to be there. The first section describes the naturally occurring connections that the child has with the world around him or her. Family, peers, school, and neighborhood are all part of "what is already there"—for better or for worse. We refer to this first section as the child's *natural ecology*. Because the natural ecology will always be an important part of the child's environment, it is considered an essential part of the treatment. We (and others) refer to the second section as the *services system*. The services system engages when problems develop within the child's natural ecology. Providers and agencies within the services system are there to intervene. One important note: Just because they are there to intervene doesn't necessarily mean that they are helping! As will be detailed in other chapters, a key role of a TST team is to appraise what the child needs and then to determine if the interventions the child is receiving are helpful or even necessary. As we talked about earlier, unless these agencies and the rest of the social ecology are working together toward a common goal, there could be a lot of noise but no music. Under TST we first figure out (1) who is involved, (2) who else needs to be involved, and finally (3) how can we get all those players working together toward the common goal. First, let's talk about who is involved.

> Unless these agencies and the rest of the social ecology are working together toward a common goal, there could be a lot of noise but no music.

The Natural Ecology (or What Is Already There)

Family

The family is the child's first significant environment. It is through contact with caregivers in the family environment that the child develops his or her first attachments, learns about the world around him or her, appreciates the impact of his or her behavior on the world, begins to regulate emotions, engages in social exchanges, and incorporates cultural values and beliefs. If all goes well, the family environment supports the child's development in these areas and serves as the base from which the child branches out into other levels of the social ecology, carrying these lessons with him or her. We will discuss the importance of family relationships in the next chapter, "Safety Signals."

> No matter what a family system looks like, it's an important part of a child's social environment.

Sometimes families have trouble supporting their child's development. Sometimes parents' own reactions to the child's trauma, their own problems such as substance abuse, or even their own capacity to hurt their child gets in the way of supporting the child. No matter what a family system looks like, it's an important part of a child's social environment. Under TST, the goal of working with the family is to help family members function at their best so that they can help support the child's recovery. This work can look quite different depending on the family resources. At one sad end of the continuum, the goal is to keep the family from hurting the child. At the other end of the continuum, families are active helpers, healers, and essential treatment team members. No matter where a family falls on the continuum, however, TST is about assessing the impact of the family on the child and helping to build the strengths.

But first a reality check: Although families are always an essential part of a child's social environment, providers and TST treatment teams are not. What? TST teams are not essential?

Let's phrase that a different way. Families are a basic part of a child's life, but families have a choice about whether or not to make providers, or TST teams, a part of that life. We're part of that outer layer of the social ecology—the "needs to be there?" group of agencies. Fundamentally, a family has to *want* TST to be a part of the child's social environment. So always, always, *always*, the first step in successfully working with a family is building a treatment alliance. We talk at length about this later in the book, but raise it here as a reminder: Without the treatment alliance, there is no treatment.

Peers

Next to family members, peers are the primary socializing influences in children's lives. Peers can influence all aspects of children's belief systems. Peer influences can affect children's understandings of the way the world works (information that is sometimes as likely to be inaccurate as accurate), the importance they place on education, how they negotiate and problem-solve in social situations, how they initiate sexual contacts, how they think about what are appropriate goals (from striving to attend an Ivy League school to joining a gang), and how they cope with difficult circumstances (experimenting with substance use, cutting, running away, attempting suicide).

As with family, peers can be positive supportive influences—or they can be part of the "cat hair" in the child's social environment. Think back to Denise, who was curled up in the bathroom stall. Her friends, who found her there and stayed with her until she was calm and oriented, were very positive, helpful members of her social environment. Depending on how Denise feels about it, they may be important players to bring into the TST team. Or, if not that, they may at least be important people for Denise to talk about and learn to call on when she's having trouble at school.

Now think back to Robert. Robert recently got into a fight after a peer made a demeaning comment. We don't know a lot about his other peers, or his friends, but from what we *do* know right now, some aspects of his peer environment are making it harder for him to manage at school. Depending on whether the TST team sees this as a priority problem (more on how to define priority problems later), they may decide that this level of the social ecology is an important place for intervention. Exactly how you intervene in the peer ecology will look different depending on a number of factors—for example, maybe the school needs to be more involved in monitoring the playground, maybe Robert needs to be transferred to a more structured school—but the key is to identify this part of the social environment as an area for change.

Schools

The school environment rivals the home environment as the setting in which children spend the majority of their time. Schools do a lot more than teach academic skills; they provide opportunities for children to engage in social exchanges, vocational training, athletic activities, and in some schools, religious instruction. Schools are also mandatory for children to attend! Put these factors together and it is easy to see that schools are (1) a really important part of every child's social ecology and (2) an essential element of intervention in the lives of traumatized children.

Unfortunately, the same things that make schools so ubiquitous and important in a child's life—being responsible for so many facets of so many children's development—can make it difficult for teachers or school personnel to attend to specific trauma-related needs of individual children. Not that they don't want to or can't, but many teachers or administrators simply haven't had the opportunity to learn about how trauma affects kids and how they, as school personnel, can help. As providers, we know that traumatic stress affects not only children's feelings and behavior, but also their attention, processing of information, memory, and learning. What looks like dissociation to us might look like daydreaming or being lazy to a teacher. Unless we help make these connections for teachers and school administrators, we're contributing to that age-old problem of the provider not talking to the teacher not talking to the . . . and so on.

One aspect of working with the school as a part of the child's social environment is to help teachers understand the core and associated features of traumatic reactions, such as appreciating differences between inattention and dissociation, and between hyperactivity and the increased arousal and watchfulness that might characterize reactions to trauma. Teachers could also benefit from support that recognizes the difficulties that they face in handling the challenges presented by working with traumatized children in the context of their other professional responsibilities. Think about the times that a certain child is just about all we can handle one-on-one in a therapy office setting—now imagine doing that in a classroom of 30! Depending on the situation, teachers may need some additional support to learn how to work with a traumatized child in a classroom—or the classroom itself may need to be changed. Specific ways this information might benefit children is by having their IEP note the problems of traumatic stress that need to be addressed for children, such as by providing behavioral modification plans, curriculum adaptations, coordinated counseling services, transportation, social skills training, help with activities of daily living (ADLs), summer school, in-school respite workers, supportive tutoring, and tracking and investigating the causes of school absences (e.g., trauma-related avoidance). Don't worry about how to do all of this just now—the important point to remember is that schools are a key part of a child's social environment, and if some aspect of a school is a priority problem (more on this later . . . again), then there are lots of ways to help schools provide a more supportive presence for the child.

One other important plus of working closely with the school: School personnel see the kids all day long and in lots of different contexts. Teachers can be very important partners in identifying what leads to a child's experience of dysregulation, and what helps the child to stay regulated.

> Teachers can be very important partners in identifying what leads to a child's experience of dysregulation, and what helps the child to stay regulated.

Neighborhood

As discussed previously in reference to Panksepp's work, the actual environment that a child is in can contain traumatic reminders that inhibit adaptive behavior and increase maladaptive behavior. On the neighborhood level, such traumatic reminders would include neighborhood violence and crime. Other associated features in the environment, such as vacant buildings or gang and drug activity, although not direct reminders of traumatic events, create the kind of environment in which traumatic events can continue to occur. Similarly, factors such as racism, disenfranchisement, and limited opportunities also create a sense of bleakness in the environment that can interact with traumatic reactions in a way that slows down recovery from traumatic events. Given that children spend considerable amounts of time in their neighborhoods (whether or not they have the luxury of being able to play outside or walk to school or stores without fear), their perceived level of safety in the environment is key to their ongoing adaptation to traumatic events.

It might not be realistic to include as part of a TST Treatment Plan "replace all broken windows in eight-block area" (one of our treatment principles is to "align with reality"—more on that in Chapter 6). But for starters, we can try to understand how the child feels about the neighborhood and what kinds of frank threats *do* exist there. This is all part of the assessment of the social environment, and depending on the priority problems, may be important enough to rally around. Systems advocacy, an integral part of safety-focused treatment, provides some tools for chiseling away at big systemic problems that are fundamental contributors to a child's dysregulation.

Sometimes problems with neighborhoods need to be handled by helping other layers of the social ecology—the family, the individual child—think creatively about how best to protect the child from neighborhood threats. Activities that demonstrate a sense of commitment to and pride in neighborhoods might emerge, such as establishing neighborhood watches or forging links with local police agencies to advocate for better surveillance and protection for community residents.

It's also important to keep in mind that all neighborhoods, even if they have some problems, have some very important strengths—and in TST one of the fundamental principles is to "build from strength." Just as important as your assessment of the traumatic stressors in the neighborhood is an assessment of the strengths. Are there neighborhood recreational centers, or churches, or "watch blocks," or crossing guards who everyone knows and loves? Are there neighbors whom a child knows he or she can trust? Factor these into discussions of who, in the social environment, can be a source of help.

Cultural and Religious Agencies

Many children and families have spiritual and cultural connections that are defining aspects of their social environment. Given the important role that these systems can play in a child's and family's recovery from traumatic events, it is important to attend to ways that these levels of the social ecology can be included in the child's treatment.

What comforts does a family derive from their religion or culture? How does that religion or culture suggest the child heal? In investigating the answers to these questions, you may find common points of view in the approaches to supporting people in the wake of trauma. These common views can be drawn upon to provide consistency in care provided to families.

The Internet

OK, OK, the Internet is not depicted as one of the layers of the social ecology. It doesn't fit neatly into categories such as *peer* or *neighborhood* or *universe*. But more and more we need to consider the role of *Internet ecology* (yes, we made up that term) on child development. The Internet can be a source of incredible information—or misinformation. It can expose children to violence, inappropriate sexual content, sexual predators, terrorism recruiters, or just plain-old bad stuff. Considering the extent of a child's access and exposure to the Internet is critical to understanding his or her full social environment. Happily, more and more effort is being devoted to understanding how the power of social media and the Internet can also be harnessed to promote healthy development. Ask about and follow a child's Internet use, and work with families to make sure that that layer of the social ecology is harnessed for the good.

The Service System (What Sometimes Needs to Be There)

As described, the service system is meant to step in when there are defined problems in the natural ecology. When a child's biological system breaks down, the medical system steps in. When the breakdowns become expressed in dysfunctional emotional or behavioral states in the child, the mental health system intercedes. When the child's family breaks down, such that there is need for child protection, the child welfare system intervenes. There have been many books written about each of these systems. Accordingly, we briefly summarize their roles related to TST next.

The Mental Health System

The most common setting for a TST team is within the mental health system, usually the outpatient mental health system. And yes, finally, mental health agencies can be a part of a child's social environment. If you are a mental health provider, you of course know that this system addresses the ecological breakdowns that ultimately result in a child being disabled by a wide variety of emotional and behavioral states and then classified using DSM. When these disabling emotional and behavioral states do not interfere with a child's capacity to safely get by in his or her world, the outpatient mental health system is there to help. When the child's emotional and behavioral states preclude the child's ability to safely function, the emergency and inpatient mental health system is engaged, with variants including day treatment, home-based, crisis stabilization, and longer-term residential care. This system is populated by a variety of providers, including social workers, psychologists, psychiatrists, and nurse practitioners. There are well-known cross-disciplinary "silos" within the mental health system as well as silos between the aforementioned levels of care, and well-known differences between the public and private mental health systems. Within all of these barriers to integrated care, we have not even left the mental health system! Whether a TST team is based within the mental health system or within another child-serving system, its members will necessarily include mental health providers, and it will need to interface at various times with each of these parts of this disconnected system. We discuss this process in great detail at various points in this book.

The Child Welfare System

The child welfare system is the frontline safety net for maltreated children. The various divisions of this system are in place, more or less, in every state and county of this country. Child protective services conducts the investigations to determine whether a report of maltreatment is substantiated and then to create a service plan based on the results of the investigation. This service plan may be carried out by a prevention services division that is responsible for providing support for the family to enable the child to stay in his or her home. For more serious cases of maltreatment, the child is removed from the home and placed in a foster home. The foster care division of the child welfare agency carries out this part of the services plan. The foster care division secures, trains, and oversees a cohort of foster families, and tracks all children placed in foster care. This division of the child welfare system is also closely involved in decisions related to reunification with the child's family. The foster care system usually has a specialized track to handle children with significant behavioral or medical needs, and foster families in this specialized track receive additional training and support.

TST teams have been based in both the prevention and the foster care divisions of child welfare agencies. Whether a TST team is based within the child welfare system or outside it, there are critical roles to fulfill, such as coordinating services, integrating evaluation and treatment planning information, and advocating where necessary. If a child receiving TST has a child welfare service plan, ongoing contact with caseworkers and supervisors is essential. Service plans can be developed based on a comprehensive understanding of which elements need to be included to provide adequate support for the child that facilitates recovery and to ensure appropriate delivery and coordination of these services.

Legal/Court Systems

Occasionally children's traumatic experiences will lead to involvement with legal or court systems: for instance, as a result of a child's behavioral dysregulation landing him or her in juvenile court because of a fight, an investigation of a child's abuse for the purpose of the offender's prosecution, or an immigrant family's political asylum claim. The legal process can often be drawn out and difficult for families. In TST, the role of the court and legal system may be important to consider if (1) the problem being addressed is a traumatic trigger for the child (e.g., the threat of deportation to a country where the child witnessed war); (2) the legal process itself is a traumatic reminder (e.g., the child must testify about abuse); or (3) the child is being prosecuted for something he or she did in a traumatized state (e.g., the child had dissociated at the time of a crime). Each of these scenarios presents a different reason for TST providers to be involved, and the involvement would take a different form. At the heart of any decision to become more closely involved with the legal system, however, is a fundamental question: Is the child's priority problem in some way related to the legal proceeding? If it is, then involvement as an advocate for the child or a trauma educator for the courts may be essential. As with any layer of the social ecology, this legal service system may need bolstering and insight from a trauma-trained clinician to make it the most helpful, and least hurtful, for a child. The juvenile justice consortium of the National Child Traumatic Stress Network has developed a number of resources to guide clinicians and courts toward more trauma-informed care.

Medical Care

In instances where children have experienced medical illness or injuries that require the involvement of medical professionals, connecting with health care providers and agencies will be a very important aspect of the child's care. Issues of understanding how a physical illness (e.g., an asthma attack) or a physical injury (e.g., a surgical scar or amputated limb) may serve as a traumatic reminder and the implications of such a reminder for the child's and family's adjustment to the condition and compliance with medical interventions need to be sensitively navigated in order to best help. Similarly, helping medical professionals understand the interactions between traumatic reactions and grief (as might be experienced in response to a considerable change in a child's level of function as a result of trauma) could impact the way they convey information about a child's condition to the child and family.

What Is the TST Approach to Coordinating Services?

We have identified the levels of the social ecology and outside agencies that may be involved in a child's care and talked about why each is so important in helping a child recover from traumatic experiences. Now that you know all this, how do you put it all together in a way that will really meet the child's and family's needs? As you might imagine, the process of coordinating services becomes increasingly complex as the number of services and agencies providing them increases.

First of all, more is not always better. Just because we listed a lot of different agencies and groups doesn't mean that they all need to be, or should be, intimately involved in treatment. Certainly we will want to *assess* each of those layers of the ecology and think about the strengths or, well, the cat hair, of each layer. But in terms of who is actually involved in the treatment, a careful decision needs to be made in coordination with the family. Essentially, you want to involve the players or agencies most likely to influence the priority problems that have been identified for treatment. Other people or agencies may come into play later—but let's face it, you can't do it all at once. Put scarce resources where they'll work (another treatment principle you will read about in Chapter 6) and pick the team that makes the most sense for the problem at hand.

Once you've made this selection, the TST provider plays several key roles in ensuring that all goes off without a hitch. First, the TST provider serves as the *single point of contact* for the family. That means that the TST provider is the person with the primary responsibility for working with the child and family to ensure that they are active participants in the treatment planning and development process. Second, the TST therapist sets the tone of the collaboration between the other levels of the social ecology and how they interact with the family and with each other. Thus, the tasks of the TST provider are many. Through successful balancing of these many tasks, the TST therapist helps to guarantee that the services provided to children and families are integrated, not fragmented, and that all effort is focused on a common goal.

The services administered as part of TST care build upon a foundation of strengths in the child, family, and service systems. TST provides a framework for bringing together the layers of the social ecology to provide the best help and protection possible for a traumatized child.

Safety Signals

The Importance of Safe, Caring Relationships for Traumatized Children

---

LEARNING OBJECTIVES

- To understand the importance of interpersonal relationships within TST
- To understand the importance of the therapeutic relationship within TST
- To understand how this therapeutic relationship forms the cusp between emotional regulation and the social environment

---

ICONS USED IN THIS CHAPTER

Essential Point	Academic Point	Case Discussion

Relationships are the matrix within which everything happens in TST. It is easy to get lost in our special lingo and procedures, but the bottom line is that everything stands or falls on the quality of relationships. It is usually some type of problem concerning relationships that initially brings the traumatized child to the professional for care, and it is the quality of the relationship that the professional forms with the child and family that offers the real hope for recovery. The therapeutic relationship exerts its effect in very specific ways, and psychotherapy, from any theoretical perspective, will work only if very specific qualities are present. The therapeutic relationship is the *necessary condition for all effective treatment.*

In the previous chapter we detailed the importance of the social environment for the trauma system and, therefore, for TST. When we consider the social environment, the operative word is *social*: people. The child's social environment is comprised of people and of organizations represented by people. We keep returning to the TST picture shown in Figure 1.1 (p. 12): The trauma system involves the child and those around him or her who influence the child's regulation and growth. How exactly do people around the child influence his or her regulation and growth? To answer this question, we must drill down and examine human relationships and their impact on the traumatized child and on everyone else. As we drill down, we will see that human relationships are comprised of signals between individuals. These signals may indicate threat or safety. TST is about building safety signals, which is why we have called our chapter on relationships "Safety Signals."

The Primacy of Relationships

Relationships stand at the cusp of the trauma system. They are the mediator between the child's emotional regulation capacities and the capacities of the social environment to help the child regulate emotion. How does this regulation work?

The regulation of emotional states grows out of the quality of interpersonal relationships. In very early development these tasks are not seen as capacities of the individual infant but as transactions between infant and caregiver. The caregiver's response to the infant's distress is (ideally) all about regulating that distress. Over time, as the infant increasingly develops the capacity to regulate his or her own distress, these developments are constantly refined by ongoing transactions with caregivers.

> The regulation of emotional states grows out of the quality of interpersonal relationships.

The infant's job is to attain control over the switches between emotional states so that a more desired state is maintained for longer periods of time and across different situations. The parent's role is to help the infant transition from less desired states to more desired states. When an infant cries, this means he or she is in a distressed state. Parents hear the cry and respond by distracting or soothing the infant back to a calm state. When parents intervene in this way hundreds or thousands of times, the young child learns how to self-calm and self-soothe. In situations of family trauma, abuse, and neglect, the parent on whom the infant depends for calming and soothing is either causing the distress or is ignoring it. This lack of soothing parental intercession can create lifelong difficulties with emotional regulation. The survival-in-the-moment states detailed in Chapter 3 are very much related to early interpersonal developmental processes.

If these ongoing transactions between the child and caregiving environment are distressed or neglectful, there may be critical impacts on the brain systems involved in the development of emotional and behavioral control. Because these are the systems that must develop to help the child cope with threat throughout life, damage to them creates a developmental cascade of dysregulation. Let us share a story of a girl, a ball, and a jump rope.

 Lucy is skipping rope in the backyard at home when a ball suddenly rolls by her. Running after the ball is her brother. As he runs by, he bumps into Lucy. In this moment, Lucy could have any of several thoughts run through her head:

1. "He bumped me by accident."
2. "He bumped me on purpose."
3. "He bumped me on purpose and *he could really hurt me next time*."

What Lucy does next depends, in large part, on which of those three thoughts is true for her. If she thinks "he bumped me by accident," she will likely pick up her jump rope and continue on, not giving it another thought. If, on the other hand, she thinks "he bumped me on purpose and he could really hurt me next time," she will be more likely to react with fear or anger. She may cry, run away, or hit him. In short, she may enter a survival state.

So what determines Lucy's answer to why he bumped into her? Lucy's answer to *why* grows out of a lifetime of signals of care that she has (or has not) received. What exactly are *signals of care*?

Safety Signals

These ideas, based largely on the literature on attachment theory and developmental neuroscience, show why the quality of relationships sits right on the cusp of the two components of our trauma system: emotional regulation and the social environment. This process works as follows:

Relationships and Emotional Regulation

The quality of the child's earliest relationships sets the stage for the child's ability to regulate emotion in the face of threat throughout his or her life.

The quality of the child's earliest relationships sets the stage for the child's ability to regulate emotion in the face of threat throughout his or her life. These early experiences create memories of relationships that are only available implicitly (through the rapid "low road" of emotional processing) instead of through more conscious memory processes (the slower "high road" of emotional processing). We respond to interpersonal signals in certain ways that are built on these early experiences, but often without consciously having access to these memories. This lack of access means that subtle interpersonal signals (e.g., a momentary harsh look, a detached tone of voice) can lead to a survival-in-the-moment state in a given moment without the child knowing what he or she is responding to or why. In truth, the child is responding not just to that particular harsh look in that particular context, but to an embedded pattern of memory that has been encoded through the accumulation of relational experiences with others.

Relationships and the Social Environment

Signals, both subtle and not so subtle, are ubiquitous in the social environment. When the signals are somehow uncaring or threatening, they can be the "cat hair" described in Chapter 4. Happily, signals can also be very positive influences in a child's social environment. These interpersonal signals, again both subtle and not so subtle, can remedy the emotional dysregulation precipitated by other, more negative interpersonal signals. These "safety signals" usually communicate warmth, empathy, and positive regard, and, especially, signal that the social environment is safe. Joseph LeDoux, Regina Sullivan, Christopher Cain, and others at New York University (NYU) and elsewhere are now studying the impact of safety signals on the survival circuits in animals, and that impact works very much in the way we would expect (Ostroff, Cain, Bedont, Monfils, & LeDoux, 2010; Perry & Sullivan, 2014; Schiller, Levy, Niv, LeDoux, & Phelps, 2008). Safety signals diminish the reactivity of the amygdala, promote regulation, and prevent survival-in-the-moment states.

We all live with both safety signals and signals of threat (the cat hair). The point is not to try to eliminate all harsh looks or moments of distraction when a parent fails to attend to a child (parents are, after all, human). Rather, the hope is that safety signals form a "critical mass" within a level of the child's present social environment so that he or she feels cared for. Recall from Chapter 3 that the child's survival circuit has what amounts to an on and off switch related to perceived threat in the environment. When switched *on*, a survival-in-the-moment state occurs. Safety signals act to keep the switch off, unless absolutely necessary. When a harsh look *does* come his or her way, the child will be much less likely to respond with an episode of dysregulation. In that moment it is not just the given signal that determines the child's regulation and response, but the *critical mass* of signals the child has experienced in that and other relationships. If there is no such critical mass of safety signals, the child (or anyone) will feel apprehensive, uncomfortable, and unsafe, and will be much more likely to have an episode of dysregulation when provoked.

Relationships at the Cusp of the Social Environment and Emotional Regulation

Interpersonal relationships both create the child's emotional regulation capacities and create the environments in which the child is more or less likely to respond with a survival-in-the-moment state when provoked. To repeat:

Relationships are the cusp of the trauma system. So where does the therapeutic relationship fit in all of this? The therapeutic relationship, and the whole TST team, must work to create a social environment filled with safety signals. Accomplishing this goal can be achieved on many different levels. Remember the discussion of the social ecology from Chapter 4? Every individual and institution in the

child's life contributes at least a little bit to the balance of threat signals versus safety signals. When you are working to change that balance, you are working to change the trauma system.

> The therapeutic relationship, and the whole TST team, must work to create a social environment filled with safety signals.

The therapeutic relationship can also offer a very important opportunity to understand how subtle interpersonal signals can lead to emotional dysregulation and re-regulation when it occurs in clinical session. Just as parents are human, therapists are human! That means that sometimes therapists will give off signals that the child perceives as harsh or threatening. Sometimes these signals may be fairly neutral ("Johnny, please help clean up the toys"), and sometimes these signals may be coming from real frustration or anger ("Johnny, please help me clean up the mess from my fish bowl that you just dumped on the floor!"). Either way, these are golden opportunities to closely observe how the signals the therapist sends off (the social environment) relates to the child's reaction (emotional regulation). The microcosm of what happens between the child and therapist can speak volumes about how the larger trauma system is operating.

What if a child's primary trauma is not defined as interpersonal? Are the therapeutic relationship and all of the safety signals as important? Yes! In some of our research, for example, we found that the single greatest predictor of the eventual development of traumatic stress in a child who is hospitalized for a burn is separation anxiety (Saxe et al., 2005). In other words, a burned child in the hospital is much more likely to experience traumatic stress if he or she feels anxious that there is no one there to help him or her. Any traumatized person will ask him- or herself the same question, consciously or unconsciously: "Who is here to help me through this?" In this way, all trauma is interpersonal. The critical mass of safety signals in the environment needs to adjust accordingly.

Although every relationship in a child's life is important, in this chapter we focus on two particular relationships: The parent–child relationship and the therapeutic relationship. The first of these is unquestionably more important than the second— but the second can sometimes help us to understand and transform the first.

The Parent–Child Relationship

 Trauma in children's lives comes from many different sources. Sometimes it is located outside the family and due to natural disaster, political conflict, or neighborhood violence. Sometimes it is located in the family, and the parent has been a source of violence or hurt. In the latter case, there are times when the degree of hurt is so great or the capacity of the parent to change so little that the child is removed from the parent's care. In all other cases, however, promoting safe and loving relationships between a child and his or her parent is fundamental to treatment.

One of the great challenges of helping a child who experiences extreme emotional dysregulation is dealing with the collateral damage that these episodes cause. *Collateral damage* occurs when someone other than the intended target gets hurt in the process of an attack. A child who is in a survival-in-the-moment state may intend to "attack" a threat to his or her safety. In the process the child may say hateful things about people around him or her, may physically lash out, throw and break things, or may—in countless other ways—give off messages of rejection and anger. Recall how the thought that runs through Lucy's head determines how she acts? Parents, too, have thoughts that run through their heads. For example:

1. "She hit him because she is extremely sensitive to being touched and probably felt threatened by him bumping her."
2. "She hit him because she's an aggressive, mean kid."
3. "She hit him because she's aggressive and mean, and if she keeps this up she is going to rip this family apart."

As you can imagine, the way a parent responds to Lucy will be quite different depending on the answer to the *why* that runs through a parent's mind. In the moment that Lucy (in a survival state) begins to hit her brother, what she most needs from her mother are safety signals. These signals may entail gently setting firm limits, physically removing her brother from danger, refocusing Lucy on alternative and safer behavior, or any number of other interventions that communicate "I care about you and I am going to help you stay safe." Lucy's mother is going to best be able to provide these safety signals if the thought that runs through her mind is . . . you guessed it, #1.

A very important part of TST is helping to repair the collateral damage that may have affected parent–child relationships, and that may make it difficult for a parent to respond with safety signals when they are most needed. Helping to frame how parents understand their child's behavior begins with providing information about trauma and how it affects children (a part of our ready–set–go approach, described in Chapter 11) and continues through every phase of treatment. Building positive family time—times when joy, love, and care can suffuse parent–child interactions—is critical to changing the landscape of a home so that safety signals become automatic and pervasive. Activities that promote positive family time are included in each intervention phase.

Systems are often very resistant to change. Parents may work very hard to alter the way they think about and respond to their child, but for a period of time their efforts may be met with entrenched patterns of responding from their child. One of the reasons that the therapeutic relationship can be so supportive of positive change in the parent–child relationship is that the child is sometimes more able to be flexible and try out new patterns of responding with a new person—for example, a therapist—than with the parent. This practice with the therapist then paves the way for the child to be receptive to the parent's efforts to positively transform the relationship. As you will read below, a great deal happens in the therapeutic relationship. The interactions that take place within that relationship can help to establish new patterns of relating and new expectations for relationships that can support positive transformation within the parent–child system.

The Therapeutic Relationship

For some traumatized children, the therapeutic relationship may be the first "healthy relationship" they have ever had. For this reason, in forming a relationship with you, the therapist, they may be embarking on an entirely new journey. They may expect that you will abandon them, hurt them, or abuse them in some way. And when you don't, it can be an extremely powerful and transformative experience. The safety signals you create go exactly counter to all the interpersonal signals of danger in the child's environment—present and past.

Traumatized children often have memories of relationships riddled with conflict, strife, betrayal, violence, loss, and abandonment. There are a great many consequences to these memories. Perhaps at a most basic level these memories indicate to the child that he or she is unloved and unlovable, uncared for and unworthy of care. The consequences of these memories and expectations, among other things, lead to lifelong difficulties with relationships and sense of self. These difficulties, described in Chapter 3, involve chronic adaptations to trauma that may be expressed through an avoidance of all relationships; a failure of self-protection within relationships; or patterns of strife, conflict, and violence within relationships.

There are four reasons why the therapeutic relationship is critical in TST. These are:

1. **The experience of feeling cared for is a necessary condition of the child's and family's engagement in treatment.** If the child and family do not feel sufficiently cared for in treatment, nothing you do will really matter. As we have described above, traumatized children and families tend to vigilantly appraise whether a relationship is safe enough. They will be vigilantly

scanning your words, face, and body for signals that suggest danger. They will be testing you to see if you are safe enough. When we set up the therapeutic relationship to be safe and work very hard to create an environment filled with safety signals, such efforts often work against the child's and family's entire history working with those in authority. When we say "I will help you," the child and family members will often be thinking, whether expressed verbally or not, "Sure, just like all the other therapists I have worked with who said the same thing!"

It is important to understand that this type of reluctance to form a therapeutic relationship is self-protective and should not be seen as a problem. When a traumatized person opens up to a new relationship, there is great vulnerability. It is far healthier for a child or family member to enter a relationship with wariness and self-protection than to jump right in and get overwhelmed. Providers should support the self-protection by saying, for example, "I don't blame you for not wanting to do this given what I understand you have been through"; or perhaps "I don't expect you to trust me right away—you don't even know me yet. Hopefully, over time I will earn your trust." In the next chapter on treatment principles we recommend that the provider "insist on accountability, particularly your own." We will only be able to earn a family's trust and therefore to enable a therapeutic relationship if we are vigilant about our *own* accountability to each family. If we are able to do this, *we* will have earned the possibility of forming a therapeutic relationship. Chapter 11 explores engaging with the family in treatment and forming the treatment alliance. We call this process *ready–set–go* because we cannot really start treatment until there is a treatment alliance, and we cannot form a treatment alliance unless the family feels sufficiently cared for.

The invitation to a safe and healthy relationship will be tested in many different ways. Clinicians should expect this testing and manage it by, again, understanding and respecting that this is a form of self-protection.

2. **Information exchanged within the therapeutic relationship may offer a critical window into the child's emotional regulation problems within interpersonal relationships.** Interpersonal signals, no matter how subtle, can frequently be a stimulus that leads to emotional dysregulation in a child who has experienced interpersonal trauma (abuse, assault, etc.). It is sometimes hard to know exactly what leads to dysregulation in the life of an abused child. Directly observing how these signals can work within the therapeutic relationship opens the possibility of knowing how they work in all relationships and then doing something about them.

> Interpersonal signals, no matter how subtle, can frequently be a stimulus that leads to emotional dysregulation in a child who has experienced interpersonal trauma.

This point is illustrated in the following case:

Serena is a 7-year-old girl who was referred to treatment due to oppositional behavior both at home and at school. She was recently brought to the emergency room because she threatened to stab one of her teachers with a knife. Serena is currently in her fifth foster care placement. During the initial intake evaluation with Serena's foster mother, the therapist discovers that Serena had been severely beaten by her biological mother until the age of 4, at which point she was removed from the home. She had been transferred from foster home to foster home due to the fact that she was "difficult to handle" and would often initiate physical fights with other children in the home. During the first therapy session, the clinician introduces Serena to the toys in her office and tells her that the toys need to be cleaned up before the end of the session. Serena throws several toys onto the floor and yells at the therapist, "You clean up this mess!" When the therapist offers to help Serena clean up the mess that she made, Serena says, "If you don't clean this up right now, I'm going to smack you." The therapist calmly explains that the therapy room is a safe place where no one gets hurt and no one is allowed to hit anyone. She then says to Serena, "Even if you make a mess, I'm not going to hit you. Lots of kids worry that if they do something bad, they might get hurt, but that doesn't happen here." Serena paused to look at the therapist and slowly started to clean up the toys.

The therapist needs to be a keen observer of the subtle interpersonal transaction between self and child. Such careful observation nets critically important information about how subtle interpersonal signals can lead to dysregulation outside the session. Serena threw the toys and yelled at the therapist after being given a subtle warning about cleaning up the toys. We do not know much about Serena's history, but it is not a great leap to imagining that she was regularly threatened to get her to clean up or do other chores. Serena may be thinking, consciously or unconsciously "or else . . . what?" "What will the therapist do if I don't clean up?" This question may then lead, with lightning speed, to linkages between other episodes in which she was found to be "difficult to handle." When we see dysregulation occurring right in front of us, caused by an interpersonal signal we have given, it gives us a golden opportunity to understand the child.

Serena also illustrates other points about the therapeutic relationship described above. This is the first session of treatment, and Serena is busily appraising whether the therapist is safe or trustworthy enough. Serena needs to know that she will be cared for even if she is "difficult." The therapist's response to this difficulty can be judged according to whether she "passed the test" in the moment.

Many of these ideas have been described within the psychodynamic literature as *transference*: the transference of attributes, thoughts, and feelings toward the therapist related to experiences prior to the therapy. These are powerful ideas and should always be considered in our efforts to understand and help the children and families with which we work.

3. **The experience of feeling cared for can be transformative.** As described, a strong therapeutic relationship can often counter the negative impact that previous neglectful or abusive relationships may have had on the child. Safety signals diminish a life history of signals of danger. The experience of feeling cared for is often so novel that it directly addresses such critical human needs as gaining a sense of self-worth and value.

One of the most important lessons that a traumatized child can learn in therapy is that he or she is worthy of attention—the good kind of attention. In fact, many of the children we see have never had an adult pay more than a few minutes of attention to them, unless it was due to their misbehavior. Consequently, with the establishment of a strong therapeutic relationship, children eventually learn that they can get their needs met without having to "act out." We also see many children who have internalized their neglect and abuse experiences so that they come to believe that they deserve to be treated this way. The therapeutic relationship can be reparative in that children can now experience a relationship filled with positive interactions and mutual trust, the impact of which they can take with them beyond the therapeutic experience. The therapeutic relationship can help them to form an internal model of what a "healthy" relationship looks like and feels like so that they can replicate it in the future. In short, the simple experience of being cared for can be transformative for a traumatized child.

Importantly, safety signals do not always look like "being nice" in the eyes of a child or family. Let's return to the scene where Serena and the therapist are talking about cleaning up the toys, and imagine a different—but still caring—scenario.

> The therapist calmly explains that the therapy room is a safe place where no one gets hurt and no one is allowed to hit anyone. She then says to Serena, "Even if you make a mess, I'm not going to hit you. Lots of kids worry that if they do something bad, they might get hurt, but that doesn't happen here." Serena, however, seems unable to take in what her therapist is saying. She proceeds to pick up toy after toy and hurtle each at the wall, yelling "I'm gonna kill you!" Serena does not respond to the therapist's calming statements or requests to put the toys down, but instead begins to hit her head repeatedly with a hard plastic toy. The therapist then observes, "It seems like you're having a hard time keeping yourself safe right now. I'm going to call security and ask them to help walk us down to the emergency room where I know we can keep you safe." Serena continues to yell, now screaming, "I hate you! I don't want to go to the hospital again!" When security arrives a few minutes later, Serena angrily throws the toy on the floor but then walks calmly with the two men out of the office and to the emergency room, where she is evaluated and later hospitalized.

In this scenario, the therapist doesn't give Serena what she wants. In fact, the therapist takes a hard stance on behalf of maintaining Serena's safety, and if Serena can't keep herself safe, then the therapist will do whatever it takes to make sure the *system of care* keeps Serena safe. In that moment when

the therapist refused to stand by and watch Serena hurt herself, she communicated a powerful signal of safety. Another example of a safety signal
that might be hard to provide in the moment, or feel "mean," is reporting
suspected child abuse to authorities. Even when the child pleads with you
not to make a report and says "I was just kidding!", standing for safety and
being willing to temporarily be the "bad cop" show the child that you and
the surrounding system of care are very serious about keeping her safe. These
decisions accumulate to create that critical mass of interpersonal signals and
system-of-care signals that ultimately shows the child that he or she is held
within a truly caring environment.

4. **The emotions experienced by the clinician can have powerful benefits
    and costs.** The experience, on the therapist's part, of contributing to the
    transformation of a traumatized child can be particularly sustaining despite
    the difficulties of the work. On the other hand, working with children who
    have experienced trauma, sexual and physical assault, and abuse can elicit
    very uncomfortable feelings in the therapist. Feelings of hopelessness, with-
    drawal, anger, aggression, or sexual arousal are part of the human mix of
    working with traumatized children. It is very important to be aware of these
    feelings, to think about them and to consider how they might impact the
    treatment. In the psychodynamic literature the therapist's responses to the
    patient are referred to as *countertransference*. Whichever term is used, it is
    extremely important to be aware of these feelings so that they do not get
    enacted with the child. Such enactment often occurs when our feelings lead
    us to withdraw or retaliate in even subtle ways. These behaviors then become
    perceived as signals of danger and a very difficult trauma-related transac-
    tion ensues. In Chapter 7 we discuss the importance of the treatment team
    for addressing this common countertransferential problem. In Chapter 6 we
    discuss one of our principles—"Take care of yourself and your team"—as a
    means of minimizing the likelihood of enactment.

It is always a good idea to think about how you are reacting to a particular
child. Most likely, others are reacting to that child in a similar way. For example, is this a child who makes you feel irritable as soon as he or she enters the
office? Is there a specific behavior that seems to trigger your reaction? This
may be something that you can address with the child directly in therapy. Or
is this a child who makes you feel extremely sad because he or she appears to
be so lonely and withdrawn? The child may not be able to tell you verbally
how he or she is feeling, but your own reactions can often tell you even more
about the child's internal experience.

Traumatic Reenactments

 Among the most painful transactions that can occur in the therapeutic
relationship concern what are called *traumatic reenactments*. In essence,
the child and/or parent—and the therapist—engage in a process of

interaction that resembles the traumatic experience that is the focus of treatment. Traumatic reenactments can happen to the best clinicians and within the best of therapies. Although enactments may seem like obvious things to avoid, they can start very subtly, but move very quickly in intensity. Although they are clearly an expression of the therapeutic work related to the child's and/or family member's psychology, they cannot develop without engaging the clinician's psychology as well, usually at an unconscious level. Traumatic reenactments are usually marked by the clinician and child and/or parent assuming increasingly rigid and affect-laden roles related to well-known trauma-related interpersonal transactions. Karpman (1968) offered the most influential description of this process, initially described as the *drama triangle*, to capture the intensity that can develop within therapeutic relationships and their rupture. Many trauma specialists have adapted this triangle for understanding traumatic reenactments. It is for this reason that we refer to it here as the *trauma enactment triangle* (FIgure 5.1). It is a useful tool to prevent traumatic reenactments and to understand them once they occur.

Karpman described the interpersonal transactions that can occur within the therapeutic relationships in which the participants assume increasingly rigid roles. Enacting these roles within the therapeutic relationship sets the stage for traumatic reenactment, as the therapeutic transactions become increasingly intense and emotion-laden. There is one main rule for the transactions that occur in this triangle: Once a "player" enacts one of the three roles, he or she will eventually enact all of the roles (e.g., a rescuer feels victimized; a victim acts aggressively). How might this happen? Imagine this scenario in a session with an adolescent:

ADOLESCENT: I can't believe I'm telling you this. I've never told anyone before. You're such a good listener. I know that you can help me. I was never able to talk to Dr. Smith. He was such a jerk.

YOU: (*thinking*) You know . . . she's right. I am a good listener . . . and I am really good at working with kids like this . . . and Bob [Smith] really is a jerk. She's a pretty good judge of character (*laughs to self*).

YOU: (*saying*) Tell me more.

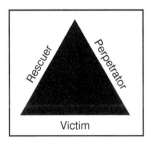

FIGURE 5.1. The trauma enactment triangle.

ADOLESCENT: Well, you know how difficult it is for me to trust people. But you're different. You have integrity. I know you'll be there for me no matter what.

YOU: I am here for you.

Congratulations. You've just entered the trauma enactment triangle. It's so easy to go there. The first step can be so subtle, especially if you feel, like most providers, underappreciated. Do you know what your statement "I am here for you" meant for this adolescent? Or do you know what she meant when she said, "I know you'll be there for me no matter what"? Do you know what actually happened that made her think Bob Smith is a jerk? Do you think it's possible that you might do something that will make her believe you broke your promise to "be there for her no matter what"? How will she react to that? Might she feel victimized by you? Might she put you in the Dr. Smith category of jerkness (at best)? How will you feel then? You know where we are going with this.

We're not saying that any of this will necessarily happen with this type of transaction. But it might. Again: The process can start subtly but can get intense very quickly. There's also nothing bad about entering the trauma enactment triangle. We've all been there. The experience also gives you a painful, but invaluable, opportunity to understand the people you work with (and yourself) a little better. Your efforts to restore the therapeutic relationship once reenactments happen can also be invaluable. If you think you may be moving into the triangle with a child and family, your TST team and your supervisor can be very helpful. Here's an example of the type of help we mean.

One month later:

YOU: (*agitated*) I . . . she . . . he . . . just can't . . . I just can't believe that she . . . he . . . did that.

SUPERVISOR: (*concerned by your tone*) What's going on? What happened?

YOU: (*still agitated*) I just got a call from Bob. She's seeing him again!

SUPERVISOR: (*confused*) Who's seeing him again? Bob? You mean Bob Smith from outpatient?

YOU: (*still agitated*) Yes, Bob Smith from outpatient. Mia. You remember my patient Mia . . . 16-year-old with abuse history . . . we talked about her a month ago . . . *Mia* . . . ring any bells??

SUPERVISOR: (*a bit annoyed*) Yes. I remember. It sounded like treatment was going really well. I remember you told me how much she opened up to you and how much you were glad the trusting relationship was developing. We're talking about the same Mia, right?

YOU: (*still agitated*) Right. Well, Bob called and he said Mia called him up and said she wanted to go back to treatment with him. Believe it or not, he even met with her for a session and didn't even call me! He worked with her for about a year, but from her point of view he didn't help her at all. Then I get this call, completely out of the blue.

SUPERVISOR: OK. Now I'm beginning to get it. So, what happened in your sessions that may have led to this turn of events? I can imagine this would be upsetting given how things were going in the very recent past.

YOU: (*a bit calmer*) I don't know. I've actually only seen her once since I told you about that really good session. It was the afternoon of our staff meeting. I remember because . . . remember . . . that meeting went late, about 10 minutes over. We were hearing about the new electronic record initiative and Nancy [clinic director] wouldn't let us leave.

SUPERVISOR: Oh, yes. I remember.

YOU: (*still a bit calmer*) So I was about 10, maybe 12, minutes late to the session with Mia. Her appointment was right after the staff meeting. I remember she seemed a bit upset at the beginning. I tried to talk to her about it. I told her our staff meeting went over and sometimes this happens. She just kept silent. She said hardly anything, maybe one sentence all session and she wouldn't look at me. I did my best and tried hard to engage her, but she wouldn't budge.

SUPERVISOR: Then what happened?

YOU: Toward the end of the session she said, "Can I go now?" I said, "Mia, I think we should talk about this." She just got up and quickly walked out.

SUPERVISOR: What do you think was going on for her?

YOU: I don't know. I guess putting on my therapist hat (*laughing to self, a bit*), I can imagine that she was pissed that I came late. But it was only 10 minutes. And do you know how many times I stayed after the session, 10, 15, even 20 minutes because she needed it? And in this last session, she was soooo aggressively withholding (*stopping self*) . . . I know . . . I know . . . maybe those overtime sessions were boundary issues . . . but she can be soooo engaging. And maybe what I see as aggressively withholding is an expression of something in our relationship and . . . (*long, thoughtful pause*) . . . and then—I guess—I did make that promise.

SUPERVISOR: Promise? What do you mean?

YOU: Well . . . I just thought of this a minute ago . . . no . . . I actually thought of it right after that very good session Mia and I had. . . . Whatever . . . the point is . . . in that really good session she was saying really positive things about me. You know. Things like "You're a really good therapist," "I've never told anyone this before," "You have such integrity," and . . . I guess . . . and this is embarrassing. . . ."Bob's a jerk" . . . am I so shallow that I'd get sucked in by all this?

SUPERVISOR: (*Smiles and nods empathically.*)

You: And then . . . I guess . . . that promise. Towards the end of that session she said something like "I know you'll always be here for me." I remember feeling a bit uncomfortable when she said it, but I can't quite put my finger on that feeling of discomfort. But then I said . . . and looking back I know I shouldn't have . . . but then I said, "I'm here for you." And then . . . I guess . . . I wasn't there for her during those first 10 minutes. Boy. I wonder what that meant to her?

Supervisor: (*Smiles and nods empathically.*) Yes.

You: Thank you! You're a really good listener. This really helped me. You really helped me get to the heart of the problem. My other supervisors are such jerks . . .

Supervisor: (*Laughs.*)

You: (*Laughs hard.*)

And that's what it looks like to enter and exit the trauma enactment triangle. It's easy to enter the triangle and it's much harder to leave. As you saw, the emotion can get pretty intense, and the roles—rescuer, victim, perpetrator—can get very rigid and shift quickly in the transactions. A seemingly innocent comment that is made with the intention of emitting a safety signal ("I'm here for you") can quickly become a signal of threat ("I abandon you after promising to be here for you"). It's important to be mindful of the process, in all its subtlety, and have people around you—like teams and supervisors—who can help.

Closing Thoughts on Safety Signals

Many of the stimuli that lead to emotional dysregulation in the traumatized child concern subtle interpersonal cues that signal danger as only the child would know, given his or her trauma history.

The term *safety signals* is the TST way of emphasizing the key ingredient in interpersonal relationships with the traumatized child. Many of the stimuli that lead to emotional dysregulation in the traumatized child concern subtle interpersonal cues that signal danger as only the child would know, given his or her trauma history. It is therefore extremely important for the TST clinician to be keenly aware of how these signals may lead to dysregulation in the child's social environment, including within the therapeutic relationship. As described, if the trauma system is riddled with signals of danger, the child's only hope is to experience, finally, a critical mass of safety signals to feel safe in an ongoing way. If this transformation can occur, it offers the child a dramatically increased chance at a future of health and happiness.

We now turn our attention to Part II of this book, Getting Started, to begin to understand how this trauma system can be transformed.

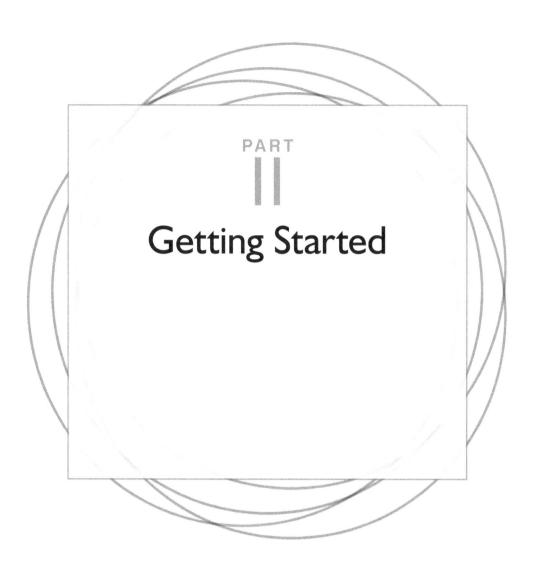

PART

II

Getting Started

Ten Treatment Principles

The Principles That Guide TST

TST is guided by 10 treatment principles. These principles are based on some of the foundations described in the previous chapters, and their implementation is described in the chapters that follow. Table 6.1 shows the 10 principles. The rest of this chapter discusses them.

TABLE 6.1. Ten Treatment Principles

1. Fix a broken system.
2. Put safety first.
3. Create clear, focused plans that are based on facts.
4. Don't "go" before you are "ready."
5. Put scarce resources where they'll work.
6. Insist on accountability, particularly your own.
7. Align with reality.
8. Take care of yourself and your team.
9. Build from strength.
10. Leave a better system.

Principle I: Fix a Broken System

As we noted in Chapter 1, the trauma system is defined by:

1. A traumatized child who experiences *survival-in-the-moment* states in specific, definable moments.
2. A social environment and/or system of care that is not able to help the child regulate these *survival-in-the-moment* states.

The trauma system is a broken system. TST is devoted to fixing this broken system. Many people have asked us how TST is different from other models of treatment. We always say: TST uses a lot of elements from other types of treatment. What is different about TST is its relentless focus on fixing the trauma system. TST assembles interventions in a clear, integrated, and organized way in relation to this focus. A corollary to Principle 1 is:

> If it is not about the trauma system, it is not TST.

Treatment within TST always boils down to fixing a broken system. If a provider or team cannot clearly see how an intervention addresses helping a child regulate survival-in-the-moment states, helping the social environment and/or system of care to help the child regulate these states, and, ultimately, improves the interaction between these two, then the intervention is not part of TST.

The nine other principles are all about what it takes to fix a broken system.

Principle 2: Put Safety First

All kinds of risks are involved when providers enter the trauma system. The child can be at risk to hurt him- or herself or other people. The child can be at risk to be hurt by family members or others in the social environment. Sometimes, even the provider can be at risk for harm, particularly during the safety-focused phase of treatment, but risk can occur during any of the phases. The important emphasis in Principle 2 is for providers and teams to stay vigilant about assessing risk and proactive about reorganizing treatment based on the results of this assessment. A provider, prepared to focus a session on emotional regulation skills, for example, elicits information from the child about suicidal ideation or about child abuse. Accordingly, all plans stop in order to address safety. This principle is, of course, simply good clinical care, but in the messiness of treatment, it can sometimes be missed.

In other words, when a safety concern is raised, all treatment resources are devoted to addressing the safety concern. The treatment plan is not resumed until the safety concern is over.

Principle 3: Create Clear, Focused Plans That Are Based on Facts

TST is about focus. It requires the gathering of specific clinical evidence to decide about the child's
level of emotional dysregulation and the level of
instability in the child's environment and system
of care. Chapters 9 and 10 describe the framework

> A disorganized assessment will lead to an unfocused treatment plan, which will lead to ineffective treatment.

that must be used to assess and develop a treatment plan for a child and family
within TST. This framework can be used only if facts are gathered methodically
and clearly. A disorganized assessment will lead to an unfocused treatment plan,
which will lead to ineffective treatment.

Once the team develops a clear notion about the treatment plan, it must
be communicated to the family as part of ready–set–go (described in
Chapter 11). This plan forms the foundation for building a treatment
alliance and troubleshooting practical barriers to care. It also contributes to
transparency—an openness and honesty with ourselves and the families about
the treatment. The construct of transparency is very important within TST.
Unless everything is clear to all stakeholders (not the least of whom is the provider and the TST team members), treatment will not work.

Once the plan is set up, it is very important for the team to marshal a high degree
of focus on the specific treatment goals. A TST provider needs to be tenacious—
sticking to the plan like a dog to a bone! But whereas the provider's focus on
the plan must not waver, the plan itself needs to be flexible in response to new
information or new circumstances. Clinical evidence is continually gathered in
TST and the plan revised based on new evidence. This point is part of Principle 2
regarding changing the plan when there is new evidence of safety concerns, but
it is also relevant to any type of new evidence. The TST provider and team are
always proactive about gathering clinical evidence and redoing the plan based
on new evidence. What remains constant is a dedication to focusing the plan on
the most critical elements for fixing the trauma system.

The need to proactively revise the plan is especially important when treatment
is not working. When things are not going as planned, the team members must
always ask themselves: "What am I missing? What are we missing?"

If team members are not asking "What are we missing?" at least twice per meeting, then they are surely
missing something!

> If the team is not asking "What are we missing?" at least twice per meeting, then the team is surely missing something!

Principle 4: Don't "Go" before You Are "Ready"!

As we explore in Chapter 11, before treatment can really begin, three components must be in place:

1. There must be the beginnings of an alliance with the family about a specific treatment plan.
2. There must be a troubleshooting of practical barriers to treatment (e.g., transportation, child care, appointment times).
3. There must be some psychoeducation regarding traumatic stress responses and what involvement with TST will entail.

 It is a common mistake in almost every type of psychotherapy to dive into treatment without a clear treatment alliance with the family. In our consultations with many clinicians who are doing TST, the most common reason for treatment failure is that the ready–set–go process is not properly completed. Often when providers think they have a good alliance with a family, it is based on their idea that the family likes them and they like the family. Under TST, liking each other is not enough!

The treatment alliance in TST is very specific. *It specifies that the family and the provider agree to work on a problem that addresses something that the family is motivated to change, and that the family and the provider agree that the TST Treatment Plan can help to change that problem.* In Chapter 11 we outline the ways in which the ready–set–go process can be completed and the parameters by which the team can know that the child and family are, indeed, ready. Of course, building a solid alliance takes time (particularly with families that do not easily trust strangers [you!]). Accordingly, we do not believe that a treatment alliance must be absolutely and completely in place before anything else is done. It is a question of how much alliance is enough to *go*.

We ask a lot of families in TST. For family members to be motivated to do what we ask them to do in TST, they must have clarity on two points:

1. That the treatment plan addresses an important source of their pain.
2. That the treatment plan can, to some degree, alleviate their pain.

If family members do not have clarity on these two points, why in the world would they want to work with us?

Principle 5: Put Scarce Resources Where They'll Work

TST addresses difficult and complex problems within the child, the social environment, and the system of care. Frequently, these problems have existed for years before the TST team is put in place. Accord-

> Treatment will only work if the team is strategic about its resources.

ingly, it is presumptuous to even suggest that a treatment can change everything. Even if a treatment team were given endless resources, they still wouldn't be able to change *everything*. And nobody has endless resources. In reality, mental health resources are very limited. So how can we begin to help?

We have suggested a series of intervention modalities that we believe can help (e.g., home-based care, emotional regulation skills training, psychopharmacology, advocacy) and put them into a framework in which they fit together and strengthen each other. We believe that this framework is a significant advance over previous interventions for child traumatic stress—*but this framework is still not sufficient*. We can't, and shouldn't, give every service to every person. We need to be strategic about the way we use our resources.

Mental health interventions are expensive. Mental health clinics and agencies struggle to make ends meet. Giving the limited (scarce) resources contained within a clinic or agency and placed on a TST team, these resources must be allocated with a high degree of strategy. Milton Erickson, the founder of strategic therapy, said that psychotherapy is like helping with a logjam. The question is finding the right log to kick. The TST provider, like the good strategic therapist, is always searching for the right log to kick that will get the rest of the logs flowing down river. The TST provider is also a good economist and knows that there are not unlimited resources that can be used to find and kick the right log. Therefore the TST clinician and team are always asking "How can we get the best solution at the least cost (or the best flow for our kick)?"

As we describe in Chapter 7, the treatment team is the holder of these scarce resources and is entrusted to use them strategically and effectively. This principle is true in the context of a given child and family, for whom the team must make decisions about the use of its home-based psychotherapy, psychopharmacology, and advocacy resources. It is also true at a macro level, where a team must decide, given its limited resources, how many children will be able to get the various service elements at a given time. These types of decisions are not easy, but they do set the stage for effective (and efficient) interventions.

Principle 6: Insist on Accountability, Particularly Your Own

Why should family members trust you?

Why should family members trust you? Family members may have been violated by those in authority and may have long histories of adversarial relationships with, for example, teachers, social service workers, court officers, police, or previous mental health clinicians. Why should they trust you? You are usually of a different class, race, or ethnic group. If they do trust you on your first meeting, sometimes that may even signal a "red flag."

We discussed the issue of trust in detail in Chapter 5. What is most important in building trust is accountability: doing what you say you will do. This point is very important. We all know that *actions speak louder than words*. When a provider enters the therapeutic relationship with an individual who has been traumatized, frequently there is the unspoken scanning of the clinician for evidence that he or she will be "just like everyone else." A provider's failure to keep his or her word, no matter how unavoidable the circumstances, is a sure sign, from the family members' perspective, that their fears are real.

As providers, we must understand that accountability is extremely important and that our communication, via our behavior more than our words, is critical. When we fail, addressing our failure up front and with authenticity will help a great deal. We are building trust in people who have no implicit reason to trust us, and we are modeling something very important for the building of other positive relationships and for good parenting. Some of the ideas mentioned earlier about transparency and alliance building are very important for communicating to families the value of accountability. The root of the word *accountability* is *count*. Accountability is about the indispensable question that providers and families ask (to themselves) of each other, "Can I count on you?"

The root of the word *accountability* is *count*. Accountability is about the indispensable question that providers and families ask (to themselves) of each other, "Can I count on you?"

The other part of insisting on accountability is insisting on the child's and family members' accountability, as well as others in the child's social environment and system of care (including professionals). An important reason for our development of the TST Treatment Plan (introduced in Chapter 10, included in Appendix 4) is to elicit accountability from everyone who is involved in implementing the treatment plan, including family members. The TST Treatment Plan outlines the treatment plan and specifies who is responsible for what, and it includes a space for signatures. The only way that TST providers can be in a position to insist on the families' accountability is by being meticulous about our own.

This principle is extremely important because family members may never have had an experience in which expectations were communicated in such a clear way. What are these expectations? Family members are expected to fulfill their specified part in the treatment plan. This part may include activities that are very difficult to complete. However, if the ready–set–go part of treatment is properly instituted, family members will know what they have to do, why they have to do it, and how it can benefit them and their child. Additionally, they will have agreed to do the specified activity beforehand. These agreements can include such challenges as the following:

- Stopping the use of drugs and starting drug abuse treatment.
- Asking a partner to leave and completing a restraining order.
- Calling the police to help with a violent child or partner.
- Taking psychiatric medications regularly.
- Participating in a Child Welfare investigation.
- Allowing a home-based team into the home.

Every session of TST includes a check-in period to ascertain if the tasks agreed to previously were completed. When agreements are kept, family members are given a lot of credit. When agreements are not kept, the inaction is discussed explicitly, including going back to the original treatment agreement and evaluating whether family members will be able to keep that agreement. This discussion may include renegotiating the treatment alliance, troubleshooting practical barriers again, reexamining the treatment plan in light of new information, or providing further psychoeducation. The important point is that agreements are attended to and accountability is expected. TST providers must be vigilant about this principle if their hard work creating a treatment plan and building an alliance is to pay off.

Principle 7: Align with Reality

 Align with reality? What does this mean? Whose reality? Providers and families must work within the bounds of reality no matter how strong the pull is to enter a fiction of a simpler, happier world.

In Chapter 1, we used the analogy of walking past a child drowning in a river to describe the trauma system. Principle 7—align with reality—is exactly about this analogy. There is a clear reality to a child drowning in a river. The child's life will end soon if

> In the trauma system, actions that do not align with reality become steps along the riverbank, past the drowning child. Never go there.

definitive intervention is not provided within the needed time. There are facts that must be considered and acted upon. The distortion of facts, in the context of wishful thinking, will result in great harm. In the trauma system, actions that do not align with reality become steps along the riverbank, past the drowning child. Never go there. We discuss Principle 7 in more detail than the others because we believe it is extremely important and often missed.

- Decisions that conform to the practical realities of the given situation (i.e., that align with reality) are more likely to succeed. A decision to place a child in a supportive classroom with 2:1 supervision ratio and an emphasis on teaching Latin may be just what the child needs, but if that classroom doesn't exist—if it isn't *real*—the plan will fail. Similarly, although it might be easier to believe the parent when she says "Oh, Jinny is lying about my hitting her!" we can't believe her just because it's easier. If we don't base our decisions on what is real, we won't succeed.

- The high level of emotion contained within a trauma system can interfere with making decisions that conform to the practical realities. Everyone inside this system (including the TST provider) can make this kind of mistake.

- The TST provider has an important role to play in helping children and families take into account the practical realities of their situation and to build skills toward making reality-based decisions.

- The TST Treatment Plan is built within the bounds of practical realities and is a map of the best decisions possible—given reality.

Consider the following case illustration:

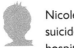 Nicole, a 14-year-old girl, recently was discharged from a hospital after a serious suicide attempt. You see her for a first visit after the discharge. Just prior to the hospitalization she had disclosed to her mother that her mother's boyfriend had sexually abused her. The Child Welfare investigation is ongoing, but her mother has said that this abuse is "impossible." The night before this visit Nicole and her mother had a big fight about the allegation. Nicole's mother called her a "liar"; Nicole called her mother a "bitch." Nicole then went to her bedroom and cut her arms. At this visit, Nicole and her mother are both agitated and angry. You raise the possibility of Nicole's going back to the hospital. Nicole becomes more upset, saying that she hated the hospital and could never stand to be "locked up again." She says that she learned her lesson and will never hurt herself again. She begs you not to send her to the hospital and says she will call you if she has new thoughts of hurting herself. Nicole's mother, in frustration and anger, states, "I don't care what you do with her." There are no other friends or relatives that can be identified to help.

Commentary

This case brings up a number of reality-based concerns. What decisions best reflect the practical realities of this clinical situation? Nicole's understanding of reality is that she has "learned her lesson" and does not need to go to the hospital. Furthermore, she "contracts for safety" by promising to call you. What is the practical reality?

This is an adolescent who was recently hospitalized following a serious suicide attempt in the wake of disclosure of sexual abuse. She impulsively cut her arms after a fight with her mother, who disputed the reality of the abuse. Nicole is currently quite agitated, and her mother is not displaying evidence of being able to help minimize risk. There are no other members of the social environment who can be engaged to help. The clinician's appraisal of the reality of risk is that it is very high. Thus, aligning with reality, the clinician initiates another hospitalization—it is a prudent decision. If the clinician were to convince herself that Nicole is able to keep herself safe and to let Nicole go home, it would be like walking by Nicole drowning in a river. We know what will happen.

Sometimes clinicians are concerned about the impact of aligning with reality on the treatment alliance. There are, of course, risks here, but risks that are mitigated by how the alliance was initially constructed. Presumably, with Nicole, this alliance would include working together to minimize the risk that she would hurt herself. According to Nicole's understanding of her current reality, she is not at risk. On the contrary, your understanding of the practical realities suggests very high risk. An important corollary of Principle 7 is:

> The alliance with the patient is always constrained by the alliance
> with reality.

The TST provider must always ask him- or herself about the practical realities of the clinical situation, despite huge pressures to ignore them (as illustrated in this case). The TST provider must never deviate from this understanding. In this way, TST is a treatment model that is strongly grounded in reality.

 After Nicole is hospitalized, you have a session with her mother in which you review Nicole's suicide attempts and her allegation of abuse by the mother's boyfriend. Nicole's mother becomes angry at you for bringing up this issue. She says, "You're not going to believe her, are you?" You ask why she believes the abuse is "impossible." She says that she knows how to "read people" and can tell that her boyfriend is not an abuser. She also says that Nicole "lies about everything." She has complied with the Child Welfare request that her boyfriend not come to her apartment, but she admits that she has met him elsewhere two or three times since this request was made. When asked about their relationship, she says he is the "perfect gentleman." When asked, she admits that he hit her "once or twice when he was using—but he's clean now." You raise the concern about what it means for Nicole that her mother believes the abuse is "impossible" even before the Child Welfare investigation is completed. Her immediate response is, "I can't believe a word that kid says."

Commentary

One of the main factors that interfere with good decision making when working with the trauma system (and elsewhere) is the difficulty in distinguishing a wish from reality. From the details presented, Nicole's mother so strongly wishes that her boyfriend had not abused her child that she is not even willing to consider the possibility that it might be true. This wish can be motivated by, among other factors, guilt for letting a dangerous man into her home or for her own urgent need for companionship. Her decision to reject the possibility that her daughter might be telling the truth is not prudent because it raises the real risk that she will not protect her child from a man who might be dangerous, and it does not include the reality of her future relationship with her daughter. The TST provider aligns with reality by keeping these facts on the table. The function of aligning with reality is not unlike the psychoanalytic notions of the ego's main function of helping individuals understand reality in the face of their wishes, emotions, and impulses.

After meeting with Nicole's mother, you call the Child Welfare case worker to get information on the investigation. The case worker appears stressed and rushed, and says that the case is being "screened out." She says that she tried to interview Nicole during her first hospitalization, but Nicole would not speak to her. Furthermore, staff at the unit confirmed that she "does lie," and that they had difficulty trusting her. The case worker also interviewed the mother, who, consistent with what she had told you, reported that her boyfriend could not possibly have abused Nicole and that Nicole was never alone with her boyfriend. The case worker also reported that the mother's boyfriend completely denied the abuse. When you bring up issues such as the boyfriend's past domestic violence and drug abuse, the mother's possible motivations for believing the abuse is "impossible," Nicole's possible reasons for not wanting to be interviewed on one occasion, and the need to integrate a full psychological evaluation in this decision, the case worker replies, "It's too late, the decision has already been made."

Commentary

None of us is immune to factors that can interfere with our ability to align with reality. The case worker may not have had the time needed to conduct a reasonable evaluation. Nevertheless, the decision making of this worker does not reflect the practical realities of the current situation. Accordingly, you protest this decision and, using advocacy skills, write a letter to the director of the Child Welfare area office, outlining the realities.

Obviously, TST providers are only human and do not have the market cornered on access to reality. Furthermore, when the TST provider enters the trauma system and is confronted with the many reality-bending emotions contained within it, it can be difficult to "see" the practical reality of a given situation and to make good decisions. Accordingly, we have built certain safeguards into TST. These include team discussions and decision making (reviewed in Chapter 7), supervision, and the clarity of a structured treatment model. Furthermore, the next principle addresses ways to manage emotion so that prudent decision making is enhanced.

> When the TST clinician enters the trauma system and is confronted with the many reality-bending emotions contained within it, it can be difficult to "see" the practical reality of a given situation and to make prudent decisions.

Team decision-making processes that adhere to Principle 7 are peppered with such questions as "Is it practical?", "What is the reality?", and "Can it work?"

 Given the difficulty of discerning practical realities across language or culture, it is, of course, important to obtain consultation when indicated or, even better, to have diverse cultural groups represented on the team.

Principle 8: Take Care of Yourself and Your Team

When oxygen levels drop on an aircraft, there is always an announcement to parents to put on their *own* oxygen mask before their child's. Why? Isn't a parent's main concern during an emergency the safety of his or her child? The airlines have wisely discerned the basic reality that for parents to most effectively attend to their child's safety, they must be strong enough to do it by ensuring that *they* have enough oxygen.

The trauma system is like an oxygen-poor environment in which it is easy to get weakened, sick, disoriented, and hurt. In order for providers to manage what they must do to *fix a broken system* (Principle 1), they must take care of themselves and be sufficiently cared for by their team, agency, and organization (we review some of these ideas in Chapter 7).

> The trauma system is like an oxygen-poor environment in which it is easy to get weakened, sick, disoriented, and hurt.

Trauma service providers face some of the following challenges on a daily basis:

- Facing the cruelty of life by hearing stories of children assaulted, tortured, and murdered.
- Facing the randomness of life by hearing stories of children unexpectedly injured or ill.
- Trying to help children and families in great need, without a lot of resources to help.
- Experiencing the extreme emotions that trauma elicits and which are sometimes directed at the provider.

- Making decisions that contribute to a parent losing custody of his or her child.
- Making decisions that contribute to the child staying in the home, when the provider is unsure whether the home is really safe.
- Making decisions related to whether a child will hurt him- or herself or someone else.

Such ubiquitous challenges can corrode the humanity in us if we are not careful. In particular, repeatedly bearing witness to the harm that one person can cause to another, particularly to a child, can lead to withdrawal, burnout, and personal life stress. Clinicians with their own histories of trauma can be especially vulnerable.

The emotional toll that this work takes can affect clinical decisions. It is hard to make good decisions when one is burned out or fed up. Similarly, emotions related to this work can lead to the provider's withdrawal from the child or family or to an overly punitive stance by the provider. Chapter 5 described ways in which this relationship can adversely affect therapists and influence clinical decision making. Chapter 7 describes ways in which the team can be organized to take care of its members. All teams must be on top of how its members are responding emotionally and contribute to the effort of making this important work rewarding and fulfilling.

Principle 9: Build from Strength

People are resilient. Our families are resilient. People have, over time, developed ways of coping with their situations that are adaptive, notwithstanding other ways of coping that may be highly maladaptive.

> Cultures have developed rituals over the centuries to help their members manage adversity; these resources should never be ignored.

Given the degree of emotion and need expressed by some children and families, it is easy to see them as driven by pathology. However, the strengths and ways of coping that children and families have developed over time comprise powerful means of managing emotion and should be explicitly integrated into care. This notion of strength-based care is often given lip service in mental health systems but is, truly, an effective approach to treatment. Traumatized children often have many social, intellectual, artistic, or athletic skills that can help them a great deal to manage their emotion. It is not only individual strengths but also community and cultural strengths that can be used. Cultures have developed rituals over the centuries to help their members manage adversity; these resources should never be ignored. This point is consistent with Principle 3 to *put scarce resources where they will work.* Given that mental health treatment resources are scarce and expensive, it is highly strategic to integrate individual, family, and cultural coping mechanisms into the treatment plan. However, before these can be integrated, the provider must, of course, know what they are. In Chapters 9 and 10 we discuss ways of assessing strengths and integrating them into the treatment plan. *Building from strength* is also a principle that is important for alliance building. Why would anyone want to ally with us about anything if they believe we only see their weaknesses? When children and families see that *we* see their strengths as well as their vulnerabilities, they are more apt to feel that we view them as people worthy of care and want to work with us toward maximizing this care.

Principle 10: Leave a Better System

The operative word here is *leave.* Notwithstanding the considerably complex problems that TST is meant to address, it is not intended to be a long-term support for a child and family. There are significant downsides to long-term treatment, not the least of which is the development of dependence on the treatment team. We are always mindful of the great wisdom contained in the imperative:

The operative word here is *leave.*

> *If you give a man a fish, you feed him for a day,*
> *If you teach a man to fish, you feed him for a lifetime.*

TST is about teaching people to fish. *Never do for a family what you believe family members can do for themselves.* This does not mean that the TST provider and team do not do things for children and families. Families are in great need, particularly early in treatment, and TST providers are accordingly very active. The guiding principle is that, over time, children and families should be doing more and more for themselves. Our job is to (1) enter the trauma system, (2) assess the problem with focus, (3) construct a treatment plan that strategically allocates intervention resources, (4) conduct the plan mindful of the changes that need to be made for treatment to end, and (5) leave children and families with the skills necessary to do enough of this work on their own, and with services in place that maximize the chance of their sustaining lasting change.

Principle 1, *fix a broken system,* is about intervening in the trauma system when:

- A traumatized child is not able to regulate survival states.
- The social environment/system of care is not sufficiently able to help the child regulate these survival states.

Principle 10, *leave a better system*, involves imagining, from the start, what needs to be in place in the child's emotional regulation capacities and the capacities of the social environment/system of care in order for treatment to end.

Will we leave a perfect system? None exists on earth. Our goal is to leave a system that is *good enough* to help the child manage emotion when he or she is faced with a reasonable range of stressors and reminders.

- *Leaving a better system* means giving the child the right emotional regulation skills (Chapter 13), cognitive processing skills (Chapter 14), and some semblance of meaning and perspective toward the traumatic event or events (Chapter 14).
- *Leaving a better system* means giving parents the right skills to help their children manage emotion, to protect them from threat, and to advocate for themselves and their children within the system of care (Chapter 12).
- *Leaving a better system* means instituting processes within the system of care to help and protect the child after treatment ends (Chapters 8 and 12). Such processes might include a more appropriate IEP or social service plan.

Leaving a better system can have important public policy implications. Although TST is not explicitly about changing public policy, the TST team comes face-to-face with public policy issues every day. The specific focus on advocacy, systems of care, and the mental health needs of traumatized children gives the TST team unprecedented information that can be useful for improving public policy. Similarly, it is our hope that using an intervention model that is comprehensive, focused, integrated, and testable can influence other treatment providers and public policymakers in efforts to build a better system for addressing the needs of traumatized children.

The Treatment Team

*How to Build a Multidisciplinary Treatment Team
(and Keep It Going!)*

LEARNING OBJECTIVES

- To learn why a treatment team is a necessary part of TST
- To learn how the treatment team contributes to treatment fidelity
- To learn how to use the treatment team to support its members

---

ICONS USED IN THIS CHAPTER

Essential Point	Quotation	Case Illustration	Useful tool

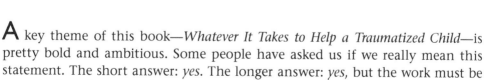

A key theme of this book—*Whatever It Takes to Help a Traumatized Child*—is pretty bold and ambitious. Some people have asked us if we really mean this statement. The short answer: *yes*. The longer answer: *yes*, but the work must be organized so that providers will be able to do *whatever it takes*. What does this mean? The short answer: the TST treatment team. The longer answer: the rest of this chapter.

We thank Erika Tullberg for her contribution to this chapter.

If it takes a village to raise a child, it at least takes a team to provide intervention after a trauma. TST, by design, is not a treatment that can be accomplished by one lone therapist in an office. We think treatment is best done by a web of providers that together form a net to support kids and families during the toughest times. Not only that, but our net of providers helps *each other* during tough times. There's a Somali proverb that says if you have five sticks and hand them to five people, each person can break the stick. If you have five sticks in a bundle and hand them to one person, the sticks will not be broken. So it is with the TST team. Providers are stronger and better able to hold onto hope and patience during the difficult periods of treatment if they aren't standing alone. And by standing together, we will be able to do whatever it takes to help a traumatized child.

A well-functioning TST team is critical for the success of a TST program. In Chapter 8 we provide ideas for how this team should be built within a formalized organizational plan. In this chapter, we detail the importance of the team and offer guidelines for its operation. As we illustrated with the TST picture shown in Figure 1.1 (p. 12), the TST team supports the child and those around the child to foster his or her regulation and growth. How, exactly, does the team do this?

But first . . .

Why Bother with a Team?

Just ask Marlene:

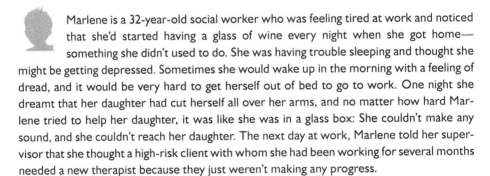

Marlene is a 32-year-old social worker who was feeling tired at work and noticed that she'd started having a glass of wine every night when she got home—something she didn't used to do. She was having trouble sleeping and thought she might be getting depressed. Sometimes she would wake up in the morning with a feeling of dread, and it would be very hard to get herself out of bed to go to work. One night she dreamt that her daughter had cut herself all over her arms, and no matter how hard Marlene tried to help her daughter, it was like she was in a glass box: She couldn't make any sound, and she couldn't reach her daughter. The next day at work, Marlene told her supervisor that she thought a high-risk client with whom she had been working for several months needed a new therapist because they just weren't making any progress.

What is going on here? Is it possible for a provider to dread going to work? Marlene should be looking for a new profession, right? Perhaps Marlene's story hits close to home. Perhaps you have sometimes felt like staying away from your work with traumatized children. Why? BECAUSE YOU ARE HUMAN! Maybe you've never experienced what happened to Marlene, but chances are that if you work with traumatized kids long enough, *some* of those things will ring true: feeling depressed, losing hope for a client, feeling like a failure, having nightmares, using unhealthy coping strategies, or having trouble separating work from home.

We can make a pretty good guess that Marlene's dif-   BECAUSE WE ARE HUMAN!
ficulties are making it hard (if not impossible) for her
to give the best care to her clients. We can also make a pretty good guess that her clients' difficulties are at least part of what is affecting Marlene. This all-too-common scenario is a perfect recipe for burnout.

These problems have been called countertransference, vicarious traumatization, secondary traumatic stress, or just plain hopelessness and are very common in working with traumatized children. Why? BECAUSE WE ARE HUMAN! Add in a few dealings with ineffective service systems or a resource-poor agency, and it is downright amazing that we don't *all* burn out!

The Balance between Product and Process

 There are two overarching goals on the TST team:

1. To provide effective care for traumatized children and families (TST Principle 1: *Fix a broken system*).
2. To take care of the people who are providing this care (TST Principle 8: *Take care of yourself and your team*).

Within the treatment team both of these goals must be attended to. If the team does not attend to the structure of effective care (are the TST assessment and intervention done adequately?), then the team might as well be meeting to talk about last night's hockey game. If the team does not attend to the emotional needs of its members, the team conference room will be empty before too long. Effective care is the TST product. Providing this care in a sensible way is the process. There are no hard and fast rules about this balance. The team leader and the team members must always be mindful of this balance. It often helps during a team meeting if some of the following questions are asked:

- "Are we doing TST correctly?"
- "Are we sticking to the TST principles?"
- "Are we holding ourselves accountable for what we said we'd do?"
- "Are we following the treatment plan?"
  - "If not, is there new information that needs to be incorporated into the treatment plan?"

- "Is our treatment working?"
  - "If not, what are we missing?"
- "What can we do to make our treatment better?"
- "How is everyone doing?"
- "Are we taking care of ourselves and our team?"
- "What can we be doing to support our therapists better?"
- "Are people remaining hopeful?"
- "Is the meeting too heavy?"
- "Is there anything else we can do to make the meeting more bearable?"
- "What's going well?"
- "Who brought these delicious cookies?"

Bearing Witness

Clinicians are witnesses. Clinicians may work with patients who are repeatedly flooded with memories and emotions of prior abuse and trauma. The repeated reliving of traumatic experiences is a tragic remnant of the traumatic event. Clinicians may be the first person to hear of these events. Implicit to the notion of bearing witness is the burden of tolerating what one hears and sees. Bearing witness means making empathic contact with another human being who has experienced horror. It means lessening the burden, a little, by being there and listening. Bearing witness means hearing and seeing the depths of what one human being can do to another. It brings us a little closer to horror. The humanity in each of us cannot help but be touched and affected. The way that bearing witness affects the clinician is different for different people. Although we all have expert clinical training we are mostly just human beings who will respond to the horror in another in human ways. The deleterious consequences of working with those who have experienced violence are simply a natural outgrowth of our own humanity. If this clinical work does not have a profound personal effect on a clinician, that is something that clinician should pay attention to. (Saxe, Liebshutz, Edwardson, & Frankel, 2003, p. 157)

> "Bearing witness means making empathic contact with another human being who has experienced horror" (Saxe, Liebshutz, et al., 2003, p. 157).

TST is designed to provide treatment to individuals in some of the toughest conditions out there. TST is for kids who have experienced horrific traumas, and often lots of them. It's for families that have trouble engaging in treatment. It's for service systems that aren't able to help and might, in fact, be hurting. TST is conducted by providers who must bear witness to all of these things. TST demands a lot of its providers—that you think (and work) beyond the office and beyond the 50-minute-hour. So TST needs to also be concerned with how to keep its providers going.

The good news is that TST has built into it some routines and procedures that make doing therapy in a tough world a little bit easier. It's got systems for facilitating communication between agencies. It's got guidelines for advocating within systems. But most importantly, it's got a TST *team*.

How Does the TST Team Work?

Within TST, the team meets on a weekly basis. The TST team meeting is for all the TST providers who see any TST family. This is a chance for all TST providers who see different cases to come together and talk about their various experiences. Team meetings last between 1 and 1.5 hours, depending on how many cases need to be discussed. The team should have a leader or team of leaders identified, who have the responsibility of both ensuring that the team is *doing* TST, and also that the team members are taken care of and able to keep up the hard work. The leader of the TST team meeting should be a senior clinician who has strong clinical skills, is well versed in TST, and is attuned to team members. In sum, the team leader needs to be both a teacher and a cheerleader. The team itself can consist of social workers, psychologists, psychiatrists, nurse specialists, home-based clinicians, advocacy attorneys, and trainees.

This format probably sounds very familiar. We, of course, did not invent the multidisciplinary treatment team meeting, but we do think it is a necessary condition for effective treatment and have thought a lot about how this type of team can be best structured to fit within TST.

Team meetings follow this basic structure:

1. Set the agenda.
2. Discuss new intakes.
3. Discuss ongoing cases—crises and updates.
4. Talk about something good that happened.

We'll talk a little bit here about what happens, practically, during each section of the meeting—the content. Then we'll talk more generally about how to make the meeting supportive—the process.

I. Setting the Agenda

Setting the agenda is a pretty straightforward part of the meeting: Who has new intakes? Who has an ongoing case? Who has something good to share? The practical side of agenda setting is to make sure that the meeting is paced to allow for everything to get addressed. But this is also an important time to take the pulse of the group. Some days people have lots to say—and this is usually a good sign. People are actively working on their cases, ready for and open to input, and willing to share with the group. Usually this means that they have some energy to hear new ideas and feel supported by the group. *Bingo*, that's what we want our providers to feel.

Some days, however, it's ominously quiet when it's time to set the agenda. It could be, of course, that there were no new intakes and everyone's cases are just cruising along with no problems, nothing to talk about. Unfortunately, however, this is rarely the case. Instead, people may be thinking "I have tried everything with Kenny—I just can't listen to another suggestion. They don't get it, it just won't work!" Or "If I talk about Lori and this school issue, they're just going to tell me to get in contact with the teacher—and I don't have time for that this week!" Or maybe even "I've done such a bad job on this case, I'm too embarrassed to tell people. I mean, I just don't even know what the problem is!"

So pay attention during agenda setting. If the room starts to have that weirdly quiet sound, and people are carefully looking away from the eyes of the agenda setter, it may be time to take stock of the team culture. It could be time for the team leader to engage in some cheerleading, or bring in some pizza, or check over the level of support that people have been getting in response to their case presentations (more on these points later). Just as therapists need to take some responsibility for getting their clients to engage in treatment, a team leader needs to take some responsibility for getting team members engaged in the TST team meeting.

2. Discussing New Intakes

A new family comes in for an intake. You sit with them for an hour or 2 or 3, depending on your intake model, and are supposed to come out at the end with a clear sense of the problem and treatment plan. Chapter 10 (treatment planning) contains all the details of how we handle this stage in TST.

Yet, although our providers know the material in Chapter 10 really well, they talk about every single new case that comes to our clinic in the TST team meeting. We do this for several reasons.

First, the provider is only one person with one perspective. A good provider presenting a case will most likely have an excellent sense of a child's development, mental health symptoms, and what treatment approach seems appropriate. A legal advocate listening to the case presentation may pick up on the fact that the housing is substandard and that there are resources for improving this—as the advocate points this out, the clinician begins to think about how the quality of the home may be contributing to the child's posttraumatic symptoms. A home-based provider notes that he or she is familiar with the neighborhood and that there is a lot of gang activity near the family's current home. The team concurs that the stability of the environment is "distressed," and advocacy for better housing in a safer neighborhood becomes a priority. A psychiatrist wonders whether a medication evaluation could potentially provide some immediate change in behavior to help stabilize the child while the longer-acting advocacy is taking place. And so it goes, with the different perspectives gradually building a well-rounded treatment plan.

Another reason all new cases are discussed during TST team meetings is that it is a way of introducing them—a sort of "We have a new member of the family" approach. Down the road, a new complication may come up with treatment, or some great progress will be made, and when the clinician says "Hey, remember that boy I talked about who came in with the BB lodged in his head?", the team can nod and be curious, and ask "What *did* happen with that boy?" Once a client is talked about on the TST team, he or she is part of the family, and we can all be there to struggle through the challenges and celebrate the successes.

> Once a client is talked about on the TST team, he or she is part of the family, and we can all be there to struggle through the challenges and celebrate the successes.

Finally, and perhaps most importantly, we have an idiom on our team that we stand firmly behind. It's something that a supervisor once told to a trainee, who became a supervisor and then told it to a trainee, who then became a supervisor and. . . . It's this:

Never worry alone.

> Never worry alone.

Pretty simple, but very important. With a treatment like TST, you are bound to be working with some very high-risk cases. TST does a lot to keep kids out of the hospital and provide intervention in the least restrictive environment. We think this is great for kids, but it also means that providers need to be very watchful, curious, and concerned about how clients are doing. The better you know a family, the better able you are to sense when things are heating up or seeming unusual and worrisome. But new intakes have lots of unknowns, and can be difficult to judge for safety. The last place we want a TST clinician to be is staring at the ceiling in the middle of the night worrying about a decision that he or she made. The entire team reviews all intakes to make sure that all team members have evaluated the risk level carefully, and that the clinician is not worrying alone.

3. Discussing Ongoing Cases

Once a case is "part of the family," it's important for the team to stay up-to-date on major changes, complications, or progress. Sometimes a TST team becomes its own miniseries, with weekly updates full of drama and intrigue—except that with a miniseries you can just watch, and when you're on the team, you are an active participant in solving the problems and supporting the other providers.

High-risk cases should be discussed on a regular basis. As with new intakes, this practice helps bring many perspectives to bear on a critical case. It also helps to have more than one set of eyes on the risk level. Remember . . .

Never worry alone.

> Communication between providers and agreement on goals and the treatment plan are essential to making TST work.

Finally, another key reason for discussing high-risk cases on a regular basis is that frequently these cases have the most providers involved. Communication between providers and agreement on goals and the treatment plan are essential to making TST work. Being able to use 5 minutes of the team meeting to say "Hey, I got a call this morning from Mom who thought that I was dealing with the housing issue . . ." can make all the difference in providing integrated, focused care.

4. Talking about Something Good That Happened

Picture this. Three new intakes: a 16-year-old girl who was raped, a 14-year-old Somali boy who saw his father murdered in the war, and an 8-year-old boy who just reported that his mother was beat up by her boyfriend last night. Two ongoing cases—that one with the gang-involved adolescent, and that other one with the girl who witnessed her mother's rape. Feeling good yet? Ready to head out of the meeting and greet the world?

Probably not. Leaving a TST team meeting week after week with your tail dragging and head down is not going to help anyone feel inspired to keep fighting the good fight. And we know that people who are repeatedly exposed to hearing about trauma can begin to get pretty jaded as a self-protective mechanism. They can start withdrawing psychologically from the people they need to help, or they can develop harsh and overly judgmental attitudes about them. Don't create a process on the team that allows this to happen. Take care of team members. Reserve a little bit of time at the end of the meeting for something good. If someone has a good story about a case, great! Put it on the agenda as a way to end the meeting. If nobody has a case that is uplifting, just have somebody share something from outside of the work arena. Or encourage people to identify things that *other* team members have done well (as we often find it easier to see the positive in each other than in ourselves). Just make it good. Bring in readings, make a note of good movies or books that the team might be interested in, or just get the team thinking about some little tidbit of good news. We don't mean to invite Pollyanna onto the team, but neither do we want to have the Grim Reaper holding court.

What Separates the TST Team from the Spanish Inquisition?

In addition to providing support and ideas for providers, the TST team has a very important function of making sure that the interventions offered are faithful to the TST model. Adopting TST on a treatment team means changing a culture. There's a language that goes with it, a way of doing things, and a list of things that are and are *not* TST.

 For the team that is trying to adopt the TST treatment, it can be helpful to rate cases that are presented based on how closely they adhere to the treatment model. When a provider presents his or her case, someone is ticking through the list of actions to make sure that what is supposed to be done is being done.

We started doing this on our team, but pretty quickly ran into a problem: Who wants to present a case when you're about to be judged? The very environment that was supposed to feel supportive to a therapist suddenly was charged with criticism and corrections. Uh-oh. The therapist burnout index just went up.

When we thought about it a little bit more, it seemed that if the intervention wasn't consistent with TST, or if the therapist wasn't feeling supported, then that was a problem with the *team*. So we came up with a list of TST activities for the *team*: a set of do's and don'ts for when we are listening to someone's case. Are team members listening actively? Are they noting the progress of the case or positive actions of the therapist? Are they coming up with concrete suggestions that are consistent with TST? Are they acknowledging the very real challenges the therapist is facing?

> The culture of the TST team is what makes or breaks the TST treatment. If the team is supportive, understanding, and well versed in how to make TST work, then the therapist on that team is going to be able to provide good treatment.

The culture of the TST team is what makes or breaks the TST treatment. If the team is supportive, understanding, and well versed in how to make TST work, then the therapist on that team is going to be able to provide good treatment.

 A team leader can do a lot to encourage a culture of support on the team. Here are a few ideas:

- Mark successes or accomplishments with a sense of celebration (food never hurts).
- Be quick to point out the successes and achievements.
- Be ready to remind people of the larger context in which the work takes place: the possibility of making a real difference in a kid's life.
- Don't be afraid to acknowledge how hard it is, and how much we are asking of people. Admitting that at times you get discouraged or feel burned out too can encourage more open discussion.
- Lighten things up a little and use humor if you can.
- Strike the right balance between focusing on "product" and "process."

But What Could Possibly Go Wrong?!

Well, OK, it turns out nothing is ever quite so simple. There are, in fact, a few challenges that present themselves in establishing and running a TST team. In fact, we feel compelled to admit here that one of the most difficult, challenging, strenuous, arduous, nearly insurmountable problems of implementing TST presents itself in relation to the TST team. We hope you have a tremendous amount of training, inner fortitude, and perseverance because we are about to share with you this challenge:

Scheduling

One of the greatest assets of TST is the way it brings together people from different disciplines, from different agencies, those who do community-based care with those who do office-based care, administrators and providers and . . . boy, is it a headache to find a time when everyone is free and sitting around the same table. The challenge is real! But instead of telling you how to solve it, we are simply going to tell you that you do need to solve it because TST is about doing whatever it takes to help traumatized kids. The team is essential.

Here are some common challenges to scheduling:

- "But that is unreimbursable time. You can't really mean that I [the administrator] free up all those people to sit around and do nothing!"
  - "They are not doing nothing! They are engaging in learning the model, enhancing care for the children they serve, providing more efficient and effective care, eliminating the need for the three phone calls to other providers they had to fit into their day somewhere, and they are less likely to burn out and vanish on you next week, leaving you to hire and train someone anew. This is not nothing!"

- "But we have other meetings we are required to hold by the state [or funder, or agency, or . . .]"
  - "We recognize that the TST treatment team meeting can rarely replace other required meetings. But neither can those meetings replace the TST team meeting! Can you (1) lengthen the meeting time and accomplish all the goals, or (2) schedule another meeting time?"
- "We're really never in the same place at the same time. Can't we just call in?"
  - "Well, yes, you can listen to the Red Sox game on the radio too, but does anything really replace popcorn and beer in the stadium? Sometimes teams have reverted to this option but there is a cost to it. Nuanced communication, team building, the ability of the team leader to spot flagging spirits . . . sometimes a Herculean effort up front to get people in the same room at the same time on a weekly basis can prevent far greater problems down the road."
- "I'm only paid for the cases I work on. How about I just show up on the weeks I have a case I need to discuss?"
  - "The TST team is not just about getting feedback on your own cases. It is about learning the model, sharing your perspective with other providers, and *being part of a team*. If this barrier is preventing people from showing up regularly, administrators need to carefully consider what they can do to make it possible for providers to come, every week, no matter what, to the team meeting."

It's really important to hold the TST team meeting . . . did we mention that?

Even once the TST team meeting has been scheduled and team members' attendance time protected, a few challenges still remain. Next we provide a summary of some of the most common challenges and some thoughts about how to handle them.

I. "We can never get through all of the cases!"

True, you never can. That's OK. Try to divide the meeting into three sections: (1) new cases, (2) urgent updates, (3) nonurgent, scheduled check-ins. Don't let any one section, or any one case, take over the meeting.

Over time, providers will get more efficient at presenting new cases in a format that quickly communicates the information most necessary to TST. There are a few known hazards to keeping on schedule. First, cases in crisis can often pull the entire team off track and hold them hostage for the duration of the meeting. For sure, these cases need to be discussed thoughtfully. But here team leaders need to be very active in helping to reign in comments. The team leader should jump in and point the team toward the *most urgent issues*. Often the most urgent facet of a case involves a safety issue. Any other issues should be secondary to the discussion of safety. The team leader may also need to summarize action item steps and move the team from conjecture to action. For example, "So, it sounds like what we need to know is whether the boyfriend is, in fact, coming over despite the restraining order, and the answer to that question will determine our course of action. Let's park the what-if discussion until we have the facts. What is the plan for getting the answer to that question?" Finally, the team leader needs to honor the clock. As hard as it may be to cut off a discussion, sometimes it must be done because there are other kids who need to be discussed too, and they also deserve the team's attention. Here is where good backup supervision is critical, because the team leader can then say: "I recognize there are a lot of really complicated, important issues that we need to sort out here, and we haven't had time to get to them all. Let's make sure that some of the remaining issues can be discussed in supervision with Cheryl later today."

2. "We've been up and running for a couple of months now, but Jerry just doesn't seem to get it!"

Sometimes a team member may have trouble shifting his or her perspective and practice. This difficulty can have a variety of reasons: Perhaps the person hasn't fully grasped the model, or is entrenched in other ways of working, or perhaps thinks that this new-fangled trauma-informed treatment stuff is just unnecessary. Whatever the reason, having a team member who isn't on board can be a drag on the whole team.

A well-run team should help to shape and reinforce TST principles that encourage, over time, even the toughest Jerrys to become facile in implementing the model. Sometimes, however, really understanding why Jerry is not on board is best done outside of the team meetings. A supervisor can, in a nonjudgmental way, engage the reluctant provider in a conversation about his or her practice. For example: "I notice that in the team meeting, you prefer to talk about your cases in diagnostic terms rather than by using the TST Treatment Planning Grid (described in Chapter 10). Tell me your thinking about that. . . ."

Remember that when we engage in ready–set–go with parents, we focus on the fact that TST must be seen as something that could plausibly help with what the family most cares about; that it might actually "work" for the problems they want solved. The very same point is true about providers. TST takes work—it requires change effort, and the willingness to be a novice again on the part of the provider. What do providers gain from it? We frequently hear from providers that TST has solved some of the problems that they *do* care most about in their work:

"I feel a sense of order and clarity with my hardest cases now, I know where to start."

"For so long it felt like the tool I was using didn't fit the problems of my clients. Now I can do what it takes to really help."

"I feel hope again that I can make a difference!"

"I don't feel alone with the problems now."

If a provider isn't adopting TST, try to understand what he or she cares about and consider whether TST could help.

If a provider isn't adopting TST, try to understand what he or she cares about and consider whether TST could help.

3. "We had such a great discussion, but now how do I communicate that to the powers that be?"

A TST team must be supported by the organization within which it works. We've seen many situations where the work was not sufficiently supported, and it became a near-impossible task to get the work done. One of the reasons that we built a formalized process of organizational planning is to try to make sure that this tremendously difficult work is properly supported. As detailed in Chapter 8, the leaders of the organization are required to participate in building this plan, and a leadership team is assembled that meets regularly to manage this plan. Accordingly, there should be "built in" processes for communicating what is needed to the "powers that be." If we go back to the TST picture in Figure 1.1 (p. 12), we can see that (1) the TST team supports the child and those around the child for his or her regulation and growth, and (2) the organization supports the team in supporting the child and those around the child for his or her regulation and growth.

Regardless, clear channels of communication and a comprehensive understanding of TST are necessary for good leadership.

4. "We ended with something good, but . . . it's just not enough. How, really, do I take care of the team?"

The most important process for taking care of the team is a formalized and well-implemented organizational plan, endorsed by agency leaders for supporting the team for the difficult work ahead. As described above, this organizational process is a required component of TST treatment. Organizations may not see this attention to the emotional needs of employees as a part of their responsibility. From our point of view, this is a big mistake and can significantly erode the effectiveness of the TST team. Problems such as absenteeism, staff turnover, staff conflict, substance abuse, and depression can be consequences of what has, broadly, been called *secondary traumatization*. In Chapter 8, we describe how to work with organizations to minimize the secondary traumatization of their members. In this chapter we describe the team processes that should be instituted to accomplish this work. Again: Each of these processes *must* be supported by the organization:

  a. *Encourage and support self-care.* It is easy to forget that we are human. It is easy to lose sight of our own human needs as we work to address the daunting human needs of the children and families who come to us for care. Team members should be encouraged to be attuned to their own needs and to attend to them. Tried-and-true self-care practices such as eating right, exercise, getting adequate sleep, spending time with friends and loved ones are very important. Team members should be encouraged to pursue these and other activities that they have found to be helpful and meaningful, such as meditation, dance, yoga, sports, artistic pursuits, or connections with religious and cultural communities and practices.

  b. *Be attuned to the emotional state of team members.* The impact of trauma does not exclude the personal lives of team members. Of course, team members have partners, parents, children, friends, and other loved ones, and ongoing and past personal difficulties may be evoked in uncomfortable (and sometimes unconscious) ways by the experience of working with traumatized children. Relational conflict, separation, divorce, illness, death, or injury of a loved one can impact the way a child's trauma resonates with specific team members. Bearing witness to trauma may have resonance to deeply felt human beliefs and activities, and impact a person's spirituality, sexuality, and sense-of-self. Team members with their own history of trauma can be particularly vulnerable to having conscious (and unconscious) emotional reactions to the work, including traumatic stress responses. Team leaders, members, and supervisors should be mindful of all of these possibilities and note when specific team members may be having difficulty. A team member's absenteeism, withdrawal, or uncharacteristic behavior may be a warning sign. Attitudes and decisions toward the child, family, or others that seem overly intrusive, harsh, withdrawn, distant, or neglectful may also represent warning signs. As we introduced in Chapter 5, the team should build a culture so that team leaders, supervisors, and other members can check in with, and offer support for, team members who may be having difficulty. Such support may include referral to personal psychotherapy. To build such a culture, team leaders and supervisors should aspire to set a tone that normalizes uncomfortable emotional reactions as an expectable part of the work, including thoughtfully revealing their own uncomfortable emotional reactions. Building such a culture powerfully creates a more trusting, vibrant, and effective team.

> The impact of trauma does not exclude the personal lives of team members.

c. *Watch for traumatic reenactments.* If insufficient attention is dedicated to the emotional reactions (conscious or unconscious) of team members, the stage is set for traumatic reenactments within the team and even the broader organization. In Chapter 5, we described the *trauma enactment triangle* as a transactional process that can unfold within the therapeutic relationship when the provider, child, and/or family members assume increasingly narrow roles as rescuer, perpetrator, or victim, which then shift over time. Enacting these roles within the therapeutic relationship sets the stage for traumatic reenactment, as the therapeutic transactions become increasingly intense and emotion-laden. Recall the main rule governing the functioning of the trauma enactment triangle: Once an individual enacts one of the three roles, he or she will eventually enact all three roles (e.g., a rescuer feels victimized; a victim acts aggressively). Here's something to consider: The trauma enactment triangle can also be enacted within teams of providers. How might this work? Perhaps a team member is having particular difficulty concerning a child, based on the team member's own personal experiences. Perhaps that team member decides to take an overly punitive and intrusive clinical stance to the child's mother, based on this experience. Perhaps that stance is not well aligned with reality, and other team members do not believe that such a stance is clinically appropriate. Perhaps another team member voices concern in a team meeting, and the affected team member reacts defensively and with great anger. Perhaps that other team member begins to feel victimized by the angry response and the accusation that was made to him or her. Perhaps . . .

You see how this kind of situation can unfold, and there are so many combinations and permutations of the trauma enactment triangle. Indeed, the trauma enactment triangle can even creep outside of the team to the broader organization. Perhaps the team members feel victimized by a decision from their CEO. Perhaps . . .

How can you avoid the painful process of traumatic reenactment on the team? Do your best to create a trusting culture that addresses the emotional needs of members. Understand that even in the best of teams, traumatic reenactments can occur. Note when team process seems uncharacteristically intense, conflict ridden, blaming, or disengaged. Be curious about what is occurring. Build processes to facilitate the team's capacity to stop the discussion, step back, and ask what is going on—and then to openly investigate whether the team process is a reflection of a traumatic reenactment. Use the information to improve the functioning of the team and the understanding of the child and family being discussed.

Final Thoughts on the TST Team

In a way, the same type of care that is necessary for working with traumatized families is also necessary for the clinical teams that work with these families. In essence, teams need safety, containment, and structure.

The TST team functions as a container. If the team is organized right, team members will feel contained; they will feel that they have a safe place to go to discuss their work. Make sure there is plenty of safety signals communicated throughout the team meetings. Never presume there are enough. When there are enough safety signals, you will see the evidence in the spirit of teamwork that grows on the team. We must never forget that team members are being asked to manage powerful posttraumatic emotions. This type of emotion can be destabilizing not only for the children but also for providers, supervisors, teams, and agencies. In a way, the same type of care that is necessary for working with traumatized families is also necessary for the teams that work with these families. In essence, teams need safety, containment, and structure. If these elements are in place, the work becomes much more effective.

CHAPTER

8

Organizing Your Program

What It Takes to Support a TST Program

LEARNING OBJECTIVES

- To understand how TST addresses agencies' main priorities
- To learn how to use the TST Organizational Planning Form
- To learn how to create a TST leadership team
- To outline the implementation of TST

ICONS USED IN THIS CHAPTER

Essential Point	Useful Tool	Case Discussion	Danger

 Susan is a 45-year-old clinical director of a busy mental health clinic. For a long time she has been concerned about the quality of the services her clinic offers. She believes the most important problem concerns her clinic's ability to help families with significant ongoing environmental stressors. She worries about what happens to the kids after they leave the clinic following their appointments. She worries about the kids who don't return and what happens to them. She tries not to think about her clinic's 45% "no-show" rate. She attended a TST training and believes that the TST model may really help her clinic.

That's what we like to hear! A person, like Susan, hears about TST and decides it's exactly what the clinic that she runs needs. Susan has amazingly excellent taste and has made exactly the right choice! Here we are. Let's walk into the sunset together . . . we know, we know . . . TST Principle 7: *Align with reality.* There goes that pesky principle again!

What does TST Principle 7 have to do with Susan (and with us)? Keep reading. . . .

 Susan knows that for a TST program to be implemented, she will need the support of her boss, Linda, the Vice-President of Clinical Services. She gets a headache thinking about how she will be able to get Linda's attention. Each of their weekly meetings over the past 6 months was devoted to Linda's concern about the "red ink" in their organization, which Linda explains is related to Susan's 45% no-show rate. Linda is also very concerned about the new state initiative that requires all staff to be trained (without reimbursement) in a new assessment instrument called the Pan-modality Assessment for Children and Adolescents (the PANACEA). The state funding of her agency is contingent on all staff implementing the PANACEA with all families.

Susan had intended to bring the TST idea up at her next meeting with Linda, but Linda spent the whole hour talking about how Susan needs to increase her "show" rate and to get her staff fully trained to use the PANACEA. At the end of the meeting, when Linda asked Susan if she had anything for the agenda, Susan said, "No nothing . . . just what we've already been talking about." As she said these words, she noticed her head beginning to throb.

Susan walked back to her office feeling hopeless about ever getting Linda's attention for her idea about a TST program. She then thought of telling her staff about her TST idea and imagined what their reaction was likely to be. How could she even think to ask them to do one more thing? Her staff was working extremely hard and morale was pretty low. Two of her best people had left over the last few months for reasons related to "stress." Susan worries that even a mention of this new TST idea would lead to more staff deciding to leave.

Her mind wandered . . . why did she develop this stupid TST idea in the first place? Why did she ever take this stupid job in the first place? Why did she ever join this stupid profession in the first place? Why didn't she just follow her childhood passion and join the Roller Derby?!

Don't Join the Roller Derby!

We need you. The field needs you. Kids and families need you. If you are reading this book, we presume you want to do things a little better. We also presume that Susan's story is, at least, not unfamiliar to you. In our experience, Susan's story is very common. Early on we learned the hard way. We received enthusiastic calls from people like Susan who told us we were exactly what they needed. We liked hearing that! And sad to say, we believed them, as we believed Susan. So how'd it go? Here's what happened: We trained her staff, set up her program, worked with her team over months, and then we discovered that our . . . brilliant . . . ideas . . . were . . . not . . . working! So we asked about Linda . . . and . . . boy . . . did . . . we . . . learn . . . a lot.

There's nothing wrong with Linda, Susan's boss. She's not evil or incompetent. She doesn't hate kids. She cares. She wants to do the best for her staff and the families that her program serves. There's only one thing that Linda is missing: An understanding of how the program that Susan is so excited about will help her with the areas that she (Linda) sees as most important. That's it. If only this one little area could be addressed, then everyone would be happy. How do we make everyone happy?

Well . . . we know that Linda is very worried about a couple of areas. The clinic's no-show rate is killing her. Her feet are held to the fire by the state mental health office to implement the dreaded PANACEA. If Linda is like most senior administrators, she may be at least as stressed out as Susan and may even believe her job is on the line if she doesn't deliver in these two areas. Here's something most people who work for Linda don't know: She's also thinking about joining the Roller Derby! Linda: Don't do it! We need you.

There are many similarities between Susan and Linda. There is also one critical difference. *Linda has decision-making authority on the mobilization of her organization's resources, and Susan does not.* If Linda says something needs to happen, it needs to happen. Although Susan has some clout in her organization, she has to do a lot of begging and pleading to get things done. Linda does not. Sooo . . . how to get Linda's attention? There's only one way.

Susan must help Linda to see that the TST program she is pleading with Linda to support will help in those areas that Linda sees as most important. That's it. No pathways to success through any other route are available.

Pulling the Thorn Out of Linda's Paw

How to reach Linda? That may seem like quite a tall task. Linda is usually near the top of her organization and the notion of reaching her often seems intimidating. There is one secret to reaching Linda. If you effectively address her main source of pain, you have the best chance of getting her attention. You remember what happened when Androcles pulled the thorn out of the lion's paw. It's a little like that . . .

What are the thorns in Linda's paw? It's her no-show rate and her PANACEA.

How to remove her thorns? TST!

If you can imagine how TST can help Linda with her no show rate and with PANACEA, and she becomes convinced that TST can help with these "thorns" in a better way than the way Linda is currently trying to remove them, then Linda—like Androcles' lion—will become your friend for life.

Ninety percent of children in TST treatment were still in treatment after 3 months, compared to only 10% who were in treatment as usual.

As a matter of fact, TST has been used many times to pull out just these types of thorns.

A clinic's no-show rate, for example, is usually pretty terrible when children are in need of what we have termed *safety-focused treatment*. What if TST included an engagement strategy to keep families coming back (it does) and utilized home-based treatment in situations when families are unlikely to follow through with clinic-based treatment (it does, as well). TST can remove this thorn! In fact, one of our outcome studies found that 90% of children in TST treatment were still in treatment after 3 months, compared to only 10% who were in treatment as usual (Saxe, Ellis, Fogler, & Navalta, 2011). TST has also been used to integrate state/countywide assessment initiatives like we imagine PANACEA would offer.

Here's a number of "thorns" that TST has been used to remove from the "paws" of people like Linda:

- Improve no-show rates.
- Improve staff retention and satisfaction.
- Improve compliance with state/county data initiatives.
- Improve compliance with state/county evidence-based and trauma-informed treatment initiatives.
- Improve clinical outcomes.
- Improve family satisfaction.
- Reduce secondary traumatic stress among staff.
- Reduce critical incidents.
- Respond to state audit related to below-standard practice.
- Provide enhanced collaborative care.
- Improve cross-system collaboration.
- Improve out-of-home placement rates.
- Reduce foster care placement disruptions.
- Improve academic performance and school attendance.
- Reduce use of restraint and seclusion as forms of intervention.
- Reduce use of atypical antipsychotic medication.
- Reduce number of psychiatric hospitalizations.

Do you know what particular type of thorn is in the paw of your Linda, and can you imagine how TST can help remove it? Successfully implementing your TST program must start with the answer to these two questions.

As we discuss in Chapter 11 on family engagement, there is an integral connection between the process of pulling the thorn out of Linda's paw and pulling the thorn out of a child's and family member's paws to engage them in treatment. People are people. People will engage in the things that give them value based on how *they* define their needs. The process of engaging the individuals you need at the organizational level and those you need at the clinical level is very much the same. Whatever we do—clinically or organizationally—it must address the issues that are most important to the people whose engagement is needed. We call this, whether in the clinical or organizational context, addressing people's major source of pain. There's only one way that *anyone* dedicates significant energy to addressing *any* issue in a sustained way with a new approach: The person can see that if he or she directs energy toward the new approach, there is a good-enough chance that something he or she sees as a very important problem can be improved—and improved more effectively than the approach he or she is currently using to address that problem. In this regard, Linda is no different than Susan, who is no different than any parent or child with whom you may work, who is no different than you, who is no different than us. That's it.

> People will engage in the things that give them value based on how *they* define their needs. The process of engaging the individuals you need at the organizational level and those you need at the clinical level is very much the same.

Establishing the TST Organizational Plan That Will Pull the Thorn Out of Linda's Paw

Let's assume you've gotten your Linda's attention in the way we just described. You have to be ready to answer her first question. If she asks this question, it is a clear indicator that you've done your job well. Here's the risk: If she asks this question and you stare blankly back at her, she will pull her paw (with its thorn in place) so far away from you that you will know that you will never get a crack at this thorn or any other thorn for a very long time. You *must* be ready for her question. Here's the question that Linda will ask you:

"So, what do you need me to do?"

What will you answer? You'd better have something good because the quality of your answer will determine the confidence Linda will have that you will be a good-enough thorn remover for her paw that is aching.

You must do your homework. To prepare to answer Linda's one question, you must first ask yourself eight questions. The answers to these questions will form the basis for your answer to Linda and for the TST organizational plan that you will eventually develop with your Linda and all other key players for your desired TST program. The questions you should ask and the TST organizational plan you will create are not meant *only* for your Linda. Your Linda is, of course, critically important, but the TST organizational plan is meant for any and all people whom you will need to implement your TST program. We ask these questions in response to someone like Linda, but they could be asked of anyone you need in your organization.

We provide the eight questions you must ask yourself next. Each question provides key information for the development of the TST organizational plan that is described at the end of this chapter. Table 8.1 lists each question and where its answer fits within the TST Organizational Planning Form included in Appendix 1.

TABLE 8.1. The Questions That Define the Components of the TST Organizational Plan

Your question	Where your answer belongs in your TST organizational plan
1. "Am I sure I have a good-enough understanding of how Linda would define the thorn that I think is in her paw?"	TST Organizational Priority Problems
2. "How do I imagine that the TST program will be able to effectively remove the thorn in Linda's paw?"	TST Organizational Solutions
3. "Who is needed to help make my imagined TST program work?"	Partners
4. "How will my TST program operate?"	Operations
5. "For whom is my TST program intended, and how will we scale it up for this intended group?"	Population
6. "How will my people get trained to do TST and to monitor its quality over time?"	Training
7. "How will we pay for our TST program?"	Finances
8. "What does success look like and how will we know it if we see it?"	Evaluation

I. "Am I sure I have a good-enough understanding of how Linda would define the thorn that I think is in her paw?"

Remember, this is how *she* would define the thorn, not how *you* would define it. Think it through. Make some hypotheses. Check them out with colleagues or other supervisors. Ask Linda. Remember: It's only when you have a clear-enough understanding of how the thorn is defined by Linda that you will be able to answer the second question.

2. "How do I imagine that the TST program will be able to effectively remove the thorn in Linda's paw?"

TST has been used to remove a lot of thorns. All the thorns listed on page 132 were addressed with a TST program. Think it through. Talk to colleagues. Call people who are participating in TST programs. Seek consultation. Call us. We love thinking through these questions. The more precisely you can see how TST will help, the more clearly you can communicate this benefit to Linda and the more effective you will be designing your TST program. As you think through the answers to the first two questions, you might want to begin to develop a TST leadership team of people in your organization and in partnering organizations that you need to make your imagined TST program work. This point leads to the third question.

3. "Who is needed to help make my imagined TST program work?"

You need Linda. That's obvious. Who else? It all depends on where the program is located within your organization as to whether you need partners from other organizations to make it work. If you imagine the base of the program to be an outpatient clinic, who needs to be at the table to allow this to happen? Who has the expertise about the way things really work? Do you need the clinic director (if that's not you)? Do you need the medical director? The director of social work? The training director? Similarly, if you are planning to base your program in a residential, inpatient, substance abuse, or child welfare facility (or anywhere else), you need to have the key players (or at least their representative) responsible for the relevant programs at the table. What about individuals who represent partnering organizations? If you intend to partner with an agency that provides home-based services, for example, you need to have someone from that organization on your team. Will another agency be providing psychopharmacological services? Same thing. What about state or county public agencies that are central to the success of your program? You may want to include representation from those agencies. The next question, of course, is about the programs you need represented.

4. "How will my TST program operate?"

Answering this question is critical. You need to establish a team of professionals to work together to deliver TST. If you recall from Chapter 1, TST requires four essential services: (1) skill-based therapy, (2) home-based care, (3) psychopharmacology, and (4) legal advocacy. Where will you find these services? The professionals who provide these services need to be represented on your team. Most agencies do not have all services provided in house. Therefore, many agencies form collaborations with others to provide these four service elements on their TST team. A given agency may provide both psychotherapy and psychopharmacology but not home-based care, for example. Another agency may provide home-based care and office-based therapy but not pharmacology. The missing service is often provided by an agency "down the street," and the pharmacology or home-based needs of a given agency are managed by referring children to the other agency. What happens, of course, is that care becomes disconnected. What were to happen if the missing service provided by the agency down the street was not handled as a simple referral. Instead, what if the agency *joined* the TST project, handled (and billed for) the service as it usually handled it, *but* with an integrated treatment plan created by all providers, irrespective of the agency, participating in the TST treatment team. That is how, from our perspective, integrated care can be achieved.

What will your TST program ultimately look like? Although there is a great deal of variation among TST programs, there are some common features.

- Your TST program will be centered on a team of providers that either works for a single agency or works for more than one agency that have agreed to collaborate with each other.
- This TST team will meet approximately every week to review new cases and monitor the care of ongoing cases. This team will have at least one leader who is responsible for directing the team members to deliver TST with sufficient fidelity to the TST treatment model (as described in this book). This team will integrate assessment information to develop a TST Treatment Plan, develop the engagement strategy for this plan, and monitor the quality of implementation of this plan.
- A defined intake process will determine that the right people are referred to the program and that the process of assessing their needs is implemented according to TST assessment requirements. This intake process should have a defined inclusion and exclusion criterion for the TST program. As described in Chapter 1, TST uses very general inclusion criteria:
  - (1) a child with a plausible trauma history who has (2) difficulty regulating survival-in-the-moment states that might plausibly be related to the trauma history.

- A leadership team is formed that is responsible for developing the overall TST organizational plan (as defined in this chapter) and for monitoring the quality of the implementation of this plan over time. A specific evaluation process (explained later in this chapter) is part of this plan, so that the leadership team can make decisions about the quality of the implementation.

5. "For whom is my TST program intended, and how will we scale it up for this intended group?"

As described above, TST has fairly general inclusion criteria. We designed TST to be used for a great many kids. Over the years we have developed confidence that it can help for most any kid who has a plausible trauma history, has problems regulating survival-in-the-moment states, and/or has developed maladaptive views of self, world, and future that can plausibly be related to the trauma history. These straightforward criteria mean that you don't need all the details about the trauma history. You don't need to be 100% confident about all aspects of the trauma; you just need to have enough information from the child's records or from what the child says and what others say about the child to believe that a trauma history is *plausible*. Not every child with a trauma history develops survival-in-the-moment states or maladaptive worldviews. Kids are resilient. TST is intended for children who *do* develop survival-in-the-moment states and/or maladaptive views based on their plausible trauma history. Does this mean you have to be 100% certain that their problems are related to specific experiences in their past? Of course not. You simply need to have enough information to indicate that their problems in the present are plausibly related to their history of past trauma.

> TST is intended for children who *do* develop survival-in-the-moment states and/or maladaptive views based on their plausible trauma history.

This definition probably applies to a lot of kids treated by your agency. Most places that implement a TST program develop their own, more restrictive criteria to manage the number of children that TST might help. It's very hard, right from the beginning, to take on a new program for most of the kids your agency treats. Programs sometimes start small and then decide to expand over time. What are some of the ways in which programs have developed more restrictive criteria to both manage the numbers of children and to use TST for children of the highest priority? Here is a sampling of various restrictive criteria:

- Children at risk for psychiatric hospitalization
- Children "stepping down" from hospitalization
- Children at risk for out-of-home placement
- Children with a PTSD diagnosis

- Children with comorbid substance abuse
- Children who are high users of services
- Children with high no-show rates
- Children with multiple foster care placement disruptions or who are at risk for a disruption in placement

6. "How will my people get trained to do TST and to monitor its quality over time?"

Since we have declared TST to be public property, anyone can implement TST without license. Most programs that want to implement TST, however, seek out consultation and training.

Real, sustained change in how work is done usually takes more than reading a book and even participating in a daylong training. Over the years we have found that sustained and faithful implementation of TST is best achieved through a collaborative process between TST experts and agencies that want to implement TST that includes the following components:

1. *Organizational planning* to help the organization best configure answers to the eight organizational planning questions outlined in this chapter.
2. *On-site TST training* to help all providers and key administrators learn and practice the TST model and also to consider how to implement the model in a way that best fits the strengths and needs of the agency.
3. *Weekly TST consultation*, to help shape understanding of, and fidelity to, the model through real-world cases.
4. Establishment of a *leadership team* to monitor and refine the implementation of the TST program based on the organizational plan.

7. "How will we pay for our TST program?"

Remember our warning from Chapter 1: *Beware the trap of grant funding.* There is no surer way to torpedo your program than establishing it purely through grant funding, only to see the program end when the grant funding disappears (and it almost certainly will). In our experience, programs that are based on grant funds almost never go through the very tough process of figuring out how to finance them after the grant expires—and it is that very tough process that makes or breaks the sustainability of a program. Linda knows this very well. She may even expect you to propose grant funding as the financial source for the TST program. Here's where you really have a chance to impress her. Do your homework. Present a sustainable financial plan that is largely based on reallocating existing resources. Fortunately, we have designed TST to help you create this sustainable financial plan. We have thought of the services that are contained within TST based on what may be conventionally financed in most places. We hope that you will first look to existing services your agency provides and, if needed, partner with another agency with which you already work if it provides a necessary service that your agency cannot easily provide. You will likely need a small amount of funds to start, but if you think it through, obtaining this small amount of funds is doable and sustainable. For what services are these extra funds used?

> Present a sustainable financial plan that is largely based on reallocating existing resources.

Expenses that are occasionally paid out of grant funds include:

- The initial TST training and consultation
- The evaluation of the TST program
- The time for the TST attorney to work with team members on advocacy
- The time for selected members of the team (particularly the attorney and psychiatrist/psychopharmacologist) to attend team meetings

Where do these funds come from?

- Small grants (OK for these purposes)
- Agency training funds
- Philanthropic donations
- Linda's discretionary funds

 Imagine how much your credibility and influence will grow if you are able to have something like the following conversation with your Linda:

LINDA: So what's this about a TST program? We really don't have time for such a program. How are things going with your no-show rate and the PANACEA training?

YOU: That's exactly why I'm thinking about TST. I think it can really help with both our no-show rate and PANACEA.

LINDA: What do you mean?

YOU: Well, TST has a terrific treatment engagement approach that I've heard people have used to reduce no-show rates. In fact, they've published a study that found that way more families that received TST stayed in treatment than those who did not receive TST. We can also make the PANACEA a requirement for our program and even use it to evaluate TST.

LINDA: OK. Well. You'll have to convince me exactly how TST can be used for these purposes, but I think that conversation is a nonstarter.

YOU: Nonstarter? Why?

LINDA: Do I need to remind you about that large Institute for Mental Health Services grant and what happened when it ended? Remember all the people we laid off? We're not going to make that mistake again. Focus on your no-show rate. I have another meeting.

YOU: I remember well. No grant funding here. Just 5 more minutes. I'll never mention TST again after those 5 minutes if you're not interested.

LINDA: (*Looks at watch.*) Five minutes, then I gotta make a call.

YOU: OK. Look. We have a lot of families with very complex problems. We spend a lot of our time spinning our wheels. A lot of that time is uncompensated because we are on the phone doing collateral work, chasing people down. Most of these kids have significant trauma histories. We need to do better with them. I also think it will help our bottom line.

LINDA: How?

YOU: We already provide psychotherapy services. We already provide pharmacology. It's a big drag that our therapists and psychiatrists hardly talk to each other. I think TST will help with that. We bill for these services. No additional expenses here. We send the families we worry most about for home-based care to Maple Street Family Services because they have the home-based contracts, but who knows what they do in those homes. When the insurance runs out, they finish their work, send the families back to us, and way more often than not, I can't see the benefit. Then we have to start over. What a waste. I talked to Judy, my counterpart at Maple. She's sick of the situation too, so we made a plan.

LINDA: A plan?

YOU: Yes. One of Judy's teams has been focusing on trauma and is also interested in TST. We already refer about two families a week to that team, and most of their caseload comes from us. We've agreed to have our outpatient team and her home-based team work together under a TST umbrella. They'll come to us and attend a weekly TST meeting. We'll all train together to make sure that care is integrated. That's what TST is all about. One integrated treatment plan per family. Everyone bills the way they always bill. The only additional expense is the training and the weekly team meeting. Last month I remember you mentioned the need for a team meeting for the cases we are most worried about—the TST would be for those cases.

LINDA: OK. So let's say—just for the moment—that I believe everything you've just said. Let's say I buy it. TST helps for no-show and for PANACEA and doesn't cost too much or require a grant. I'm not saying I buy this, but let's just say I do. So if I buy this—I'm not saying I am buying this, mind you— but let's just say, just for the moment, that I buy it. Well. So. Well. If I buy it, *what would you need me to do*?

BINGO: That thorn is halfway out of her paw. Congratulations!

8. "What does success look like and how will we know it if we see it?"

Here is your chance to pop that thorn completely out of Linda's paw. It's how we think of evaluating any TST program. What does success mean? How can we operationally define success and then create the process to measure how well we are doing over time and adjust the program to make sure we are successful? We know from Susan and Linda's exchanges that success will have to involve implementation of the PANACEA and reduce the no-show rate. There may be additional indicators of success, but let's stick with those two for now. How would Linda define success using both of these indicators? Regarding the PANACEA: Is it 100% compliance after 1 year? 80%? 60%? What is the base compliance rate now? What does Linda hope to achieve? What about the no-show rate? What is the no-show rate now? What type of improvement would Linda find acceptable? What would blow her away if you were to achieve it? Whatever the answers to these questions, make sure that you anchor the evaluation process for your program in the indicators of these answers. What if you were to achieve these goals? This is the best way we know of to make sure a program is sustained over time. The best evaluation process does not only examine the thorns in Linda's paw. Your other stakeholders have paws too, with a host of possible thorns. What thorns are currently in your paws (besides Linda's relentless focus on no-show and PANACEA)? The leadership team that is assembled to formulate the TST organizational plan should form some type of consensus on the list of thorns to remove and to develop a feasible evaluation plan to track. These should all be included in the TST Organizational Planning Form.

> How can we operationally define success from the beginning and then create the process to measure how well we are doing over time and adjust the program to make sure we are successful?

 Imagine the following conversation with Linda (following the previous conversation). Imagine the possibilities if you could pull this one off (we believe you can).

YOU: I've been thinking a lot about the PANACEA and the no-show rate. As I've said, I believe TST can help us with both, but I really want to know more about how success for TST or for any other program would look to you.

LINDA: What do you mean?

YOU: Well, I know we need to improve our no-show rate, but I want to understand what you would regard as the right improvement target. I'm committed to using TST to help us achieve improvement, but I want to be sure I understand what *you* would regard as a success. Our no-show rate, for example, is now 45%. I know this is terrible, but, from your point of view, what's a realistic target that we could celebrate?

LINDA: I know we're not going to go to zero any time in this century. Boy, if we could get our no-show rate below 30%, it would be so great. Last year I asked Alex [the financial director] what no-show rate would allow us to balance the budget. The red ink is killing us, and I can't stand Edna [the board of trustee chairwoman] droning on and on about our deficit. If we could just get that number below 30%, it would really shut Edna and the rest of the board up. Boy. That would be great.

YOU: So, organizing our TST program to reduce no-shows from 45 to 30% in 1 year. OK. Let's do it. I'll make sure it's included in our TST organizational plan, and I'll work with Dr. Brown [the TST trainer] to organize our program to have the best chance of achieving this goal.

LINDA: What are you doing for dinner tonight?

Establishing an Organizational Plan That Will Work

In the previous sections, using the example of Susan and Linda, we detailed the principles necessary to establish an effective organizational plan and the basics of completing one. A copy of the TST Organizational Planning Form is included in Appendix 1. Table 8.1 lists the components of this plan in relation to the types of questions that need to be asked and answered. In this section we provide some practical advice on getting your plan established and implemented, including managing some key trouble spots we have encountered over the years.

Leadership Team

It's very important that a leadership team is established that collaboratively develops the plan and takes ownership of implementing the plan toward success. The membership of the team should be comprised of, at the very least, managers who represent elements of programs critical to the TST program's success. If a program is based in a mental health clinic and requires the involvement of psychotherapists and psychopharmacologists, the clinical and the medical director should be part of the leadership team. If the clinic operates a home-based team, the manager of that team should be included. If there is collaboration with another agency for a key element of the program (e.g., home-based care), the manager of the home-based unit from the partnering agency should be part of the leadership team. Certainly managers representing any partnering agency should be included. Depending on the nature of the program, include the key managers whose decisions are necessary for the program's success. Leadership teams in residential programs, for example, should include managers of milieu staff as well as clinical staff. Programs constructed in partnership with state/county agencies have found it very helpful to have managers from those agencies included on the team. Wherever the program is based, managers of key program components should be included.

Refining the Plan and Establishing Buy-In

Once the leadership team, in conjunction with a TST expert, has established its organizational plan, it is important to develop a process of sharing the plan with those who will be responsible for implementing it. Providers who implement programs usually have knowledge about how to get things done, which managers typically don't have. This process of sharing the plan, getting feedback, and integrating it into a refined plan is very important for getting it right and achieving the necessary buy-in from everyone involved.

Owning the Plan

The work of the leadership team only gets started with the completion of the organizational plan. There should be processes in place to delineate (1) regular meetings of the leadership team, (2) monitoring of whether the plan is being implemented properly, and (3) decision-making steps for adjusting the plan or managing the program based on this information. The leadership team may see, for example, that although the plan is being faithfully implemented, the program is not operating as expected. Was something important missed in the construction of the plan? The leadership team should be very proactive and self-critical about asking and answering such a question. It's important to make decisions about the progress of the TST program using objective information rather than subjective impressions. The best way of doing this is to establish a formalized evaluation plan based on (1) objective indicators of success that are well aligned with the goals of the program and (2) information about the degree to which fidelity is being achieved within the TST program.

Common Organizational Planning Trouble Spots

Organizations are complex and unique. Accordingly, it's hard to fully predict trouble spots at the beginning of the planning process. Nevertheless, the following sections describe some of the common ones we have encountered.

"You don't really mean that we need to find a psychiatrist for the TST team? Do you??"

Actually—yes, we do. We also understand the challenge. Stick with us for a bit. There's a way to manage a psychiatrist/psychopharmacologist's time that can create greater efficiencies in practice and improvements in the quality of care. We'll discuss pharmacology practice within TST in a lot more detail in Chapter 15. First, let's see if we have a shared understanding of an important problem. In many settings psychopharmacology practice is disconnected from other practices the child receives. Psychiatrists have little time to gather the background information about a child's history and the social context in which emotions and behaviors identified as problematic are expressed. Without this type of knowledge—and especially without access to real-time information about changes in the social context that may influence the "symptoms"—children are prescribed more medications than they need. What if this type of information were readily available to the psychopharmacologist through his or her participation on the TST team? Communication between providers about exactly this information is a key part of TST team process. Moreover, providers have more opportunity to informally communicate information just before and after the team meeting. We know the challenge. There's clearly an expense to a psychiatrist participating in a team meeting that may not be reimbursed through conventional means. There's also an unreimbursed cost to organizations for the time providers (including psychopharmacologists) spend chasing each other down. And there's clearly a cost to children for being treated with more medications than needed. We'll talk more about this point in Chapter 15. We understand that some agencies are simply not able to make this work. This may be an argument for the application of limited amounts of grant funds to enable a psychopharmacologist to participate in the TST team meetings. It's really important.

"You don't really mean that we need to find a lawyer for the TST team? Do you??"

Actually—yes, we do. We've seen, on many occasions, the power of an advocacy attorney to enable a vital decision to activate the services a child needs. We've seen judges' decisions, child welfare service plans, and IEPs account for what is needed by virtue of having an advocacy attorney participate in the TST team and advise the team on the right strategy. We'll review the attorney's role and practice within the TST team in much more detail in Chapter 12. For now it's important to know that:

- The attorney performs a consultative function to the team and never represents the child.
- The attorney is expected to commit 1–2 hours per week to the TST program.
- The right attorney may be found in many venues, such as pro bono work assignments from law firms, legal aid clinics, lists of retired attorneys, and law school collaborations.

Mental health organizations typically do not think of an advocacy attorney as a member of a multidisciplinary treatment team, and sometimes these organizations prefer not to move out of their comfort zone to find one. The right attorney, however, will allow the work of the team to have much greater impact. Please do your best to integrate an advocacy attorney. It's really important.

"You don't really mean that we have to invest in taking care of our people? Do you??"

 Actually—yes, we do. Doing the work required of TST brings providers closer to the reality of the horror of what people can do to each other, particularly the horror of harm to a child at the hands of a caregiver. This work will impact any caring human. Providers on TST teams will work with many traumatized children and hear a great many additional accounts of trauma related to other children discussed on the team. Your people will be impacted and therefore need the right support. As described in Chapter 7, this type of impact has been called *secondary traumatic stress* (STS), and your people need the right support to mitigate its impact. To this end, a TST organizational plan should include processes for addressing secondary traumatic stress; we include some suggested approaches here:

> A TST organizational plan should include processes for addressing secondary traumatic stress.

- Provide staff members with training on STS, how to identify it in themselves and their colleagues, and strategies for mitigating its impact.
- Provide supervisors with training on identifying and addressing STS.
- Build into supervisory practice a routine discussion about the impact of the work and checking in with employees on a regular basis as to how they are functioning, and providing support when needed.
- Create an organizational culture in which discussions about the impact of the work, and strategies for addressing its impact on both the individual and organizational levels, are encouraged.
- Offer employee the time to engage in wellness activities such as meditation, yoga, massage, walking, etc., during the workday.

We understand there is an expense to organizations for providing this type of support and that many organizations are having great trouble keeping their financial books balanced. On the other hand, there is also a clear cost to organizations related to staff absenteeism, turnover, depression, drug abuse, and boundary violations. These issues are in the mix related to secondary traumatic stress. Please do your best to integrate processes to care for your staff within your organizational plan. It's really important.

Owning Your TST Program

Every TST program is unique. It is designed for your needs to fit your specific organization and the problems you aim to address. Of course, there are commonalities between TST programs as defined by our 10 principles and implemented with adherence to the TST fidelity standards, but TST is a pretty unique intervention model that encourages you to adapt and innovate such that the program will meet your needs. In Chapter 16 we detail how adaptation and innovation works within TST, including examples of how agencies have embraced and benefited from this powerful process. For now it's important to know that your program will be designed by you and will be unique to your organization. To really own and sustain your program, it's important that you design it mainly based on existing resources and conventional ways in which services are delivered and financed in your region, as reflected in your organizational plan. It's important that you select a group of supervisors and team leaders that will be equipped to carry your program and train your own people after you are fully set up. TST consultants can help you with all of these areas, but ultimately TST becomes a program *for you* and *by you*.

Closing Thoughts on TST Organizational Planning

So now you know how to construct a TST organizational plan. We began by describing your role as a "Susan" and how you might be successful with a person like Linda. In the process we described how, in order to prepare to address Linda's needs, you must think through many details about how to operate your TST program. This undertaking obviously requires a lot of time and effort—but what, really, are the alternatives? Imagine all the time and effort wasted on planning, developing, and implementing a program that never gets off the ground or never sticks. That's a lot of heartache and missed opportunities. It's important to note that even though we are focusing on you (Susan) and your Linda, TST organizational planning must integrate the needs of all of the key players to make it work. Take a careful look at the TST Organizational Planning Form in Appendix 1 and get planning—and maybe—just maybe—you won't have to join the Roller Derby!

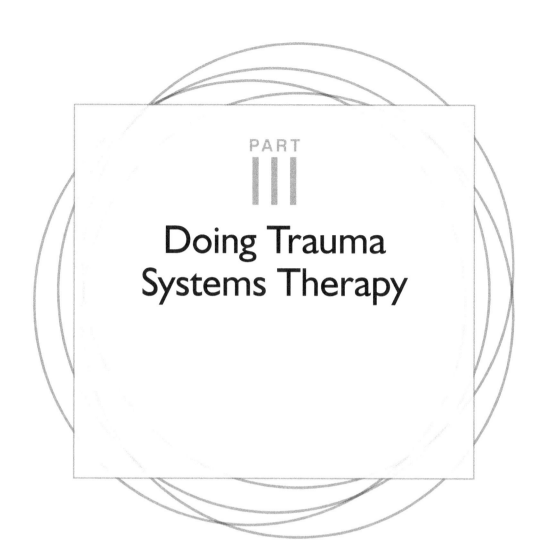

PART

III

Doing Trauma Systems Therapy

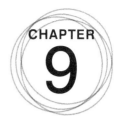

CHAPTER

9

Assessment

How to Gather the Information You Need to Know What to Do

LEARNING OBJECTIVES

- To learn how to gather the information you need to answer the five TST treatment planning questions
- To learn how to complete a TST Assessment Form
- To understand how all this information is necessary for developing an effective treatment plan

---

ICONS USED IN THIS CHAPTER

Essential Point	Useful Tool	Case Discussion	Danger

---

*A*ssessment is about how to know; it is about gathering the type of information that will give us the knowledge required to decide what to do. *Treatment planning* is about making decisions regarding what to do based on this knowledge. *Treatment engagement* is about how we partner with the people who come to us for help, based on this knowledge. Accordingly, assessment, treatment planning, and treatment engagement are tightly integrated and critically important within TST. This chapter is about assessment, and Chapters 10 and 11 are about the other two, respectively.

> *Assessment* is about how to know; it is about gathering the type of information that will give us the knowledge required to decide what to do.

What, then, is the information we will need to make decisions about the treatment plan that we will use to engage children and families? It is the information we need to answer these five questions.

Section 1: What problem(s) will be the focus of the child's treatment?
The information we need:
a. Moment-by-Moment Assessments of episodes involving problematic emotion and/or behavior
b. Exposure to traumatic events
c. Other problems that may need to be addressed in treatment, including:
   i. Comorbid psychiatric or developmental disorders
   ii. Enduring trauma-related cognitions
   iii. Current social problems that impact the child's health and development

Section 2: Why are these problems important and to whom are they important?
The information we need:
a. The functional impact of the identified problems
b. The level of concern about these problems from the child, the family, and others
c. The identification of what is most important/concerning to the child, the family, and others

Section 3: What interventions will be used to address the child's problems?
The information we need:
a. The child's vulnerability to shifting into survival-in-the-moment states
b. The ability of the social environment to help and protect the child

Section 4: What strengths will be used to address the child's problems?
The information we need:
a. The child's strengths
b. The family's strengths
c. The strengths in the social environment

Section 5: What will interfere with addressing the child's problems?
The information we need:
a. The child and family's understanding of trauma, its impact, and mental health intervention
b. The practical barriers to treatment engagement

This chapter is about gathering the information we need to answer these five questions. You'll have to wait until the next chapter to learn how to use this information to answer these questions. We devote a whole chapter to gathering the information because, if it's gathered well, the answers to the five questions are very straightforward. If it's not gathered well, the answers may never come—or worse, they may be wrong. Let's get the information right and then everything will follow. In this chapter, we take each of these questions in turn and review details about the information you will need to answer them. We recommend that you use the TST Assessment Form, included in Appendix 2, as you read through this chapter. This form includes several tools, organized according to the information needed to answer each respective question. In Chapter 10, we detail how to use this information to answer each question (please be patient, it will be worth the wait!).

 TOOL: TST Assessment Form

What it is: A tool that guides the process of gathering the information you need to know how to engage the child and caregivers in treatment and to build an effective treatment plan.

When to use it: Upon first meeting the child and family and throughout the assessment process. This is the tool to help gather and organize information that will eventually be used to make the treatment plan; to be revisited as new information emerges, if treatment is not progressing, or if a child is transitioning to a new phase of treatment.

Target goals: To ensure that the necessary information is gathered so that a sound treatment plan can be built and families successfully engage.

Section I: What Problem(s) Should Be the Focus of This Child's Treatment?

In order to determine the problem or problems that should be the focus of TST treatment, we need to gather three sorts of information. First, we need to understand, at a sufficient level of detail, the episodes of problematic emotion and/ or behavior that usually are the reason a traumatized child is referred for treatment. Second, we need to have sufficient knowledge about the child's trauma history to help us understand why he or she may express problematic emotions or behaviors in specific contexts. Third, we need to determine if anything else should be addressed in treatment.

The Episodes of Problematic Emotion and/or Behavior

 Traumatized children are usually referred to treatment because someone is concerned about an episode (or several episodes) involving the problematic expression of emotions and/or behaviors. Usually, there is concern about repeated episodes expressed by these children. We have to develop an understanding of these episodes that is sufficiently detailed to point to what might be done to help. Once we arrive at this level of understanding about these

> We have to develop an understanding of these episodes that are at a sufficient level of detail that will point to what might be done to help.

episodes, our knowledge can guide our selection of a problem, or problems, that will become our focus for treatment. As we describe throughout this chapter, our understanding must be *specific enough* and *actionable enough*. How do we get to this level of understanding?

 Consider four traumatized children who were referred to treatment:

- A teacher is concerned about Jason, a 5-year-old boy who repeatedly yells at and pushes other children.
- A foster parent is concerned about Emily, a 10-year-old girl who repeatedly expresses wanting to die and bangs her head against the wall in this context.
- A guidance counselor is concerned about Briana, a 15-year-old girl who repeatedly cuts her arms and legs.
- A mother is concerned about John, an 18-year-old teen who uses alcohol and assaults adult men when intoxicated.

> If survival-in-the-moment does underlie the problematic expression of emotion and/ or behavior for a child, we will have the specific and actionable information that we need.

What is our understanding of why each child needs treatment and is it at a level of detail sufficient to help? As we described in Chapters 2 and 3, we are focused on specific moments: those survival-in-the-moment times. Does survival-in-the-moment* underlie the problematic emotions and behaviors expressed by each of these four children? Maybe, maybe not. This is what needs to be assessed. As we discuss, if survival-in-the-moment does underlie the problematic expression of emotion and/or behavior for a child, we will have the specific and actionable information that we need. We must understand the moments. How do we do this?

Becoming a TST Detective

A TST provider must become a detective, of sorts. Consider the expression of emotion and behavior in the four children who were referred for treatment.

---

*A word about language: The term *survival-in-the-moment* accurately describes what we mean by a child's switch to a survival-laden emotional state the moment a threat is perceived in the present environment. The term can also sound awkward in some contexts. Accordingly, we sometimes refer to this same process as *survival states*. The terms are interchangeable.

Does survival-in-the-moment underlie any of these episodes? We have to gather the facts about what happened in each moment or we are just guessing. And gathering these facts is frequently not as easy as it might seem. As described in Chapter 3, the traumatized child shifts to survival-in-the-moment on occasions when there is a traumatic reminder in the present environment: what we described as "cat hair" in Chapter 4.

Children who shift into survival-in-the-moment frequently do not understand how and why these shifts occur. They may not even be aware that they have perceived cat hair in their environment. All they may know is that they became very upset, and/or those around them became very upset about what they did. Frequently those around the child have no idea why the child's emotions or behaviors changed so dramatically. Why should they have this knowledge? They do not have the child's trauma history and, even if they did, frequently the traumatic reminders are pretty subtle. As we have described, sometimes such minimal stimulus as a glance, a tone of voice, or even an odor will do. How do we help these children, and those around them, to discover why and how they feel or behave as they do? As detectives, we need to look for clues. Our tool for finding these clues is called the Moment-by-Moment Assessment. Remember from Chapter 3 that it's all about a switch? The *switch* refers to what turns the usual regulating state "off" and the survival-in-the-moment state "on." Cat hair flips the switch—if only we can find the cat hair within the haystack of information from the child's present environment (to mix metaphors a bit). We need clues. Where will we find them? They are hiding within the moments.

> How do we help the child, and those around them, to discover why and how they feel or behave as they do? As detectives we need to look for clues... Where will we find them? They are hiding within the moments.

The Moment-by-Moment Assessment

We introduced the idea of Moment-by-Moment Assessment in Chapter 3 and provided two examples of such an assessment in that chapter. We provide more detail on how to conduct this critical assessment next. Please read this section with a copy of the TST Moment-by-Moment Assessment Sheet (found in Appendix 2) readily available. The Moment-by-Moment Assessment is the primary tool used in TST to discover the problems that will become our focus in treatment. These problems are organized around our derived understanding of *what flips the switch* that leads to a child's transition from a regulating state to survival-in-the-moment states. We know that the signal of cat hair is central to this transition. We know that very often this signal is not readily apparent to the child or to those around him or her. We also know that cat hair is hiding in the moments. We have to look at the moments. How do we find the cat hair in the moments? We conduct Moment-by-Moment Assessments!

> The Moment-by-Moment Assessment is the primary tool used in TST to discover the problems that will become our focus in treatment.

Using the TST Moment-by-Moment Assessment Sheet

The TST Moment-by-Moment Assessment Sheet (found in Appendix 2) is the primary tool we use to conduct Moment-by-Moment Assessments. During the assessment process, you should focus on at least three episodes of problematic emotion and/or behavior that have occurred in the recent past. Use an assessment sheet for each of these episodes and for any episode the child experiences throughout the course of treatment. The TST Moment-by-Moment Assessment Sheet is divided into two sections. The first section, called *Step 1: Finding What Flipped the Switch*, is meant to help you get a quick read on the episode and what may have caused it. The second section, called *Step 2: Understanding What Happened When the Switch Was Flipped*, is meant to help you gather the details you need to fully understand the episode.

TOOL: TST Moment-by-Moment Assessment Sheet

What it is: A tool that helps you gather and record information about a child's episodes of problematic emotion and/or behavior.

When to use it: During the assessment process, to identify and assess at least three episodes that have occurred in the recent past. And throughout the course of TST treatment, whenever an episode occurs.

Target goals: To fully understand the episodes that define why the child needs treatment so that accurate TST Priority Problems can be identified.

To successfully conduct a Moment-by-Moment Assessment, you should:

1. *Focus only on those episodes when the child expressed problematic emotions and/or behaviors.* The episodes define the moments you need to understand. Think about the four children referred to treatment for problems with controlling emotion or behavior, described earlier. What—exactly—happened? You might have an explanation about what happened. Others might as well. Throw all your explanations out the window (for now). There will be plenty of opportunity to find an explanation later. Now is the time to gather *facts* about what happened: who–what–when–where (and not why). The explanation about what happened will turn into what we will call the child's TST Priority Problem (described in Chapter 10). These TST Priority Problems are constructed in such a way as to provide the specific and actionable information that you need. For now: Don't short-circuit the process. Gather the facts that will become the basis of your explanation and priority problem.

> Priority Problems are constructed in such a way as to provide the specific and actionable information that you need.

2. *Know that your understanding of the episode will come from the patterns that can be seen from the facts, in the moments.* This is how the TST Priority Problems are constructed. They are based on patterns you see between the moments. Episodes that may first appear completely disconnected may actually have a deep connection that can only be seen in the patterns that emerge through the facts. Consider two episodes involving Briana, the 15-year-old girl who cut her arms, described earlier. These episodes may seem completely unrelated. In the first, she cut her arms after going on a school field trip to the art museum. In the second, 2 months later, she cut her arms after going with friends to a movie. Parents, teachers, friends, and Briana herself had plenty of explanations about why she cut her arms, but none included what emerged from openly exploring the facts from these respective episodes in a Moment-by-Moment Assessment. In the first, the girl noticed a painting of a male torso. In the second, a scene in the film included a man removing his shirt. Briana remembered feeling nauseous for brief periods of time in the art museum and in the movie theater. She remembered feeling nauseous again later in the day of each episode, just before she cut herself. It was only during Moment-by-Moment Assessments of each episode that she remembered that her nausea began when she saw the painting and the movie scene, previously described. When she was asked why the image of the male torso and the scene of the man removing his shirt were so difficult for her, she immediately described memories of her uncle removing his shirt before he sexually abused her. As she relayed this memory, she began to feel nauseous. Then she remembered feeling nauseous when her uncle removed his shirt. Cat hair—to be sure—hiding in the moments.

3. *Don't make this more complicated than it needs to be.* As a first pass, we just want basic information of how a child's emotional state shifts in specific moments, and what may have led to this shift. This is the information we are looking for in Step 1 of the Moment-by-Moment Assessment Sheet: *Finding What Flipped the Switch.* To complete this step, here's all you need to do: Consider any episode of problematic emotion and/or behavior. First, consider the period of time just before the episode. What was the child doing (**Action**)? What was he or she feeling (**Affect**)? Where/what was the child's focus of attention/thought (**Awareness**)? Here we see the three A's discussed in Chapter 3.

> As a first pass, we just want basic information of how a child's emotional state shifts in specific moments, and what may have lead to this shift.

4. Second: Consider what was going on in the environment just before the episode that may have provoked a change from the child's usual state to survival-in-the-moment. Consider the period of time during the episode: What of the three A's changed during the episode? Record this information where it belongs on your Moment-by-Moment Assessment Sheet. Third: What (or who) pulled the switch? Here's your chance to go detective. You have to look

for clues. You know cat hair can be any stimuli, even hardly *detectable* stimuli. But you are now a *detective*. Take out your magnifying glass to find the cat hair that pulled the switch. What was going on in the present environment just before the problematic emotion and/or behavior began? What was going on in the present environment just before Emily, the 10-year-old girl described earlier, started banging her head against the wall and saying she needs to die? What was going on just before John, the 18-year-old boy described earlier, started to punch his baseball coach? What sights, sounds, tastes, touches, or smells did the child perceive just before he or she expressed the problematic emotion and/or behavior? Don't dismiss any of these stimuli too quickly. Any one may be relevant. None may be relevant. Record these facts in the appropriate box in Step 1 of the TST Moment-by-Moment Assessment Sheet. They are your clues. They may well point to what pulled the switch.

5. *Repeated assessment deepens the understandings of the problem(s).* The first section of the TST Moment-by-Moment Assessment Sheet (Step 1) gives you a quick, first-pass read on what may have flipped the switch. You may begin to see the patterns from this first-pass read that will form your TST Priority Problems. The more episodes you can read, the more likely you are to see the patterns. Similarly, the more detail you can discern about an episode, the more you are likely to see the patterns. More detail about the episode will also, eventually, lead to a more precise and effective treatment plan. What type of detail are we talking about?: the detail we derive from *Step 2* of the Moment-by-Moment Assessment Sheet, *Understanding what happened when the switch was flipped.* Recall from Chapter 3 that survival-in-the-moment involves the child's switch from his or her usual/Regulating state to the three survival-in-the-moment states of Revving, Reexperiencing, and Reconstituting (the four R's). Each of these states has characteristic patterns of the three A's. The optimal level of detail about a given episode is to capture how the three A's transition across the four R's. The second section of the Moment-by-Moment Assessment Sheet provides an opportunity to record this information. Interview the child and any observers about the episode in question, and see if you can capture information of how the three A's shifted across the four R's and record the Revving, Reexperiencing, and Reconstituting information on Step 2 of your Moment-by-Moment Assessment (you've already recorded the information for Regulating in Step 1). Recall that Revving happens immediately after the switch is flipped: Emotion is escalating, but the child has not yet lost full control. What are the child's three A's here? Record your answer in the appropriate box on the assessment sheet. Recall that Reexperiencing means that the child has lost control. He or she may experience the environment and him- or herself back in the time and place of the trauma. What are the child's three A's here? Record your answer in the appropriate box on the assessment sheet.

> The more *episodes* you can read, the more likely you are to see the patterns.

Recall that Reconstituting means the child is regaining control but is not yet back to Regulating. What are the child's three A's here? Record your answer in the appropriate box on the assessment sheet. The features of the present environment may be different in each of these R's. Record any distinguishing feature of the present environment during each "R" in the appropriate box on the assessment sheet. The more Moment-by-Moment Assessments you conduct with a child over time, the easier it is to see the details required for Step 2 of the assessment sheet. In your first few Moment-by-Moment Assessments with a child, you may only be able to gather the information for Step 1. That's fine. Do your best. The details will eventually come as you get to know the child and his or her episodes using the Moment-by-Moment Assessment Sheets. And it will be really important for you to be able to see these details. We hope you will carry stacks of these sheets with you at all times (you never know when one may come in handy!).

6. *Approach all of this assessment with an attitude of humility and curiosity.* The attitude you bring to the Moment-by-Moment Assessment is really important. If you begin with the assumption that you know what it will reveal, you are likely to miss something big. You may be an expert in many things. But you are not an expert about what happened during the moments of an episode before you have diligently gathered the facts. In most cases, you were not there. Moreover, you were not there when the trauma happened. You do not have access to the sights, sounds, touches, smells, and tastes that were associated with the traumatic event or events— any of which, or none of which, may be relevant to understand the child's transition to survival-in-the-moment during the episode in question. Do not assume anything. You do not know. Gather the facts. They are that important!

> You may be an expert in many things. But you are not an expert about what happened during the moments of an *episode* before you have diligently gathered the facts.

Additional Guidelines for Conducting Moment-by-Moment Assessments

1. It is unusual to be able to gather all the information necessary to be confident about the priority problem based on one episode of problematic emotion and/or behavior. Fortunately (or unfortunately) children give us many opportunities to assess these episodes and their patterns. Make sure you identify at least three episodes to assess during the assessment period and do your best to complete a Moment-by-Moment Assessment Sheet about each episode. For example: "You've told me your concern about Briana's cutting of her arms and legs. Let's focus on three times this has occurred. It's important to know as much as possible about each episode so that I can

> Make sure you identify at least three *episodes* to assess during the assessment period and do your best to complete a Moment-by-Moment Assessment Sheet about each *episode*.

best know how to help you. Let's start with the last time Briana cut her arms or legs." Then, any time Briana has a new episode of cutting her arms or legs, fill out a new Moment-by-Moment Assessment Sheet.

2. It is always best to gather information from multiple reporters about a given episode. This can involve interviewing the child, parent, teacher, or anyone who may be able to provide relevant information.

3. The assessment of younger children may rely more on the reports of observers. A skilled clinical interview with a younger child (or a less verbal older child) may involve playing or drawing about the episode.

4. A child's entry into a survival-in-the-moment state during a clinical session is a particularly valuable opportunity for assessment, because the provider can see what has precipitated the episode and how the child appears during it.

5. Carefully track the child's emotional state during the Moment-by-Moment Assessment. This is useful both to protect the child from getting overwhelmed, and to gather information about how certain themes may lead to the dysregulation that is right in front of you. You may see this shift if the child becomes:

   a. less engaged or less verbal,
   b. more agitated or aggressive,
   c. if he or she suddenly needs to stop the interview, or
   d. if his or her train of thought becomes less organized.

Sometimes these shifts are very subtle, but the information is extremely important.

6. Get help if you are struggling. If you are not able to gather accurate information about the child's episodes in a timely way, your treatment will never address the most important drivers of the child's problems. Here's a good warning sign that you may be struggling: *You are not able to get sufficient information for Step 2 of the Moment-by-Moment Assessment Sheet after assessing two or three episodes.* If you find yourself in this situation, get consultation, talk to your supervisor, review with your team. Here are some common reasons you may find yourself "stuck on Step 1."

Here's a good warning sign that you may be struggling: *You are not able to get sufficient information for Step 2 of the Moment-by-Moment Assessment Sheet after assessing two or three episodes.*

   a. You are not being systematic enough about gathering information concerning what happens after the child switches to survival-in-the-moment. In particular, you are not clearly distinguishing the revving, reexperiencing, and reconstituting states and gathering the information that distinguishes between the present environment and the three A's that characterize these three states of survival-in-the-moment.

   b. You are relying too much on one information source about the episode. The Moment-by-Moment Assessment Sheet is where you record information about the episode from *whatever sources are most relevant and informative.* Providers sometimes believe the Moment-by-Moment Assessment is only about data gathered from the child and then express frustration that they are not able to gather the required information because the child is resistant or not sufficiently verbal. Of course, do your best to gather information from the child (including the use of play and drawing), but prioritize the gathering of information from other sources, if you are stuck.

c. You are using the Moment-by-Moment Sheet as a rigid clinical interview. Gathering this information requires skill in clinical interviewing. It requires adjusting your approach based on the needs of the person in front of you, so that we are both

> The Moment-by-Moment Assessment Sheet is a place to record relevant information in defined categories; it is not a clinical interview.

gathering the needed information and maintaining empathic contact at all times. This adjustment requires flexibility and discretion. The Moment-by-Moment Assessment Sheet is a place to record relevant information in defined categories; it is not a clinical interview. Some programs have nonclinicians participate in the process of gathering moment-by-moment information. That is fine, as long as clinicians on the team carefully oversee this work. All this information about the episode in question becomes integrated for the completion of a Moment-by-Moment Assessment Sheet.

In Chapter 3, we discussed survival states related to Robert and Denise. We provide a Moment-by-Moment Assessment Sheet for a different episode for Denise next.

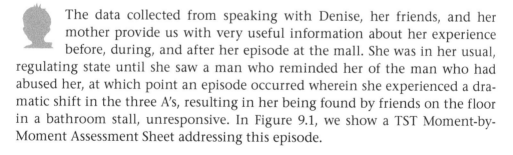 The data collected from speaking with Denise, her friends, and her mother provide us with very useful information about her experience before, during, and after her episode at the mall. She was in her usual, regulating state until she saw a man who reminded her of the man who had abused her, at which point an episode occurred wherein she experienced a dramatic shift in the three A's, resulting in her being found by friends on the floor in a bathroom stall, unresponsive. In Figure 9.1, we show a TST Moment-by-Moment Assessment Sheet addressing this episode.

Moment-by-Moment Assessments are one of the most critical tools of TST. They are the primary means for determining how stimuli in the present environment lead to survival-in-the-moment responses. Effective Moment-by-Moment Assessments yield a good understanding of the fundamental patterns of links between the environment and a

> Moment-by-Moment Assessments are one of the most critical tools of TST. They are the primary means for determining how stimuli in the present environment lead to survival-in-the-moment responses.

TST Moment-by-Moment Assessment Sheet

Child's name: *Denise*   **Record number:** *41399*   **Date:** *3/24/2015*

Step 1: Finding what flipped the switch

<u>Instructions</u>: What flipped the switch, such that the *episode of problematic emotion and/or behavior,* happened? <u>First</u>: Consider the period of time just before the *episode*. What was the child doing (**A**ction)? What was he or she feeling (**A**ffect)? Where/what was the child's focus of attention/thought (**A**wareness)? <u>Second</u>: Consider the period of time during the *episode*: What of the **three A's** changed during the *episode*? <u>Third</u>: Consider the present environment throughout this process. Record any feature of the *present environment* that you think may have been related to the *episode* (whatever it is). Any of these features may turn out to be responsible for flipping the switch. If assessment revealed sufficient detail about the **four R's**, you can skip the "During the Episode" box and complete Step 2.

Before the Episode *(possible "usual state"/regulating)*	**During the Episode** *(possible "survival-in-the-moment")*
Action: *In the mall with her friends, shopping, laughing.*	Action: *Ran away from friends, then found lying on floor of bathroom in shopping mall.*
Affect: *Enjoying being with her friends. Calm and relaxed.*	Affect: *Not sure. Probably terrified.*
Awareness: *Looking for "sales." Wanting to find the "best" pair of jeans.*	Awareness: *Seemed worried about man finding her.*

Features of the Present Environment *(possible "switch"/"cat hair")*
Saw a tall man with a red beard at the mall.

Step 2: Understanding what happened when the switch was flipped*

<u>Instructions</u>: Once you have understood what flipped the switch, you may be able to see important details about the *episode* in question. If the *episode* represents *survival-in-the-moment,* the child will have switched from a *usual state* (**R**egulating) to the three *Survival-in-the-Moment* states of **R**evving, **R**eexperiencing, and **R**econstituting. Each of these states will be characterized by changes in the **three A's**. Consider the *episode* assessed in Step 1: Record information in your *present environment* during these respective states. See Chapter 9, Section 1, of the TST book for details about conducting this assessment.

FIGURE 9.1 A TST Moment-by-Moment Assessment Sheet for Denise.

Revving	Reexperiencing	Reconstituting
Action: *ran suddenly*	Action: *Lying on floor in mall bathroom, rocking back and forth.*	Action: *Beginning to sit up. "I could move my arms."*
Affect: *Panicked*	Affect: *Dread*	Affect: *Still frightened, a bit calmer. No dread.*
Awareness: *I can't breathe. I'm going to die.*	Awareness: *Thinking "he" is going to find me and rape me. Flashbacks*	Awareness: *Confused, a bit worried about safety. Checking for Bob.*
Present Environment: *In clothing store. Sees man who looks like "Bob."*	Present Environment: *On floor of stall in bathroom.*	Present Environment: *In bathroom with friends. Out of stall.*

Was the episode you have assessed an expression of survival-in-the-moment?	How confident are you in your answer to this question?
☒ Yes	☒ Very confident
☐ No	☐ Confident enough
	☐ Not so confident
	☐ Not at all confident

*In the first few Moment-by-Moment Assessments of a child's episodes, you may not be able to see these details. The more you get to know a child—through these Moment-by-Moment Assessments—the more you will be able to see how a child's **three A's** change across the **four R's**. Seeing these details is very important for planning an effective treatment.

FIGURE 9.1. *(continued)*

child's dysregulation; a good understanding of these patterns of links, in turn, allows for the development of focused, effective, and powerful interventions. They are the primary means we have to understand why a child needs treatment, at a level of detail to know how to help them.

Exposure to Traumatic Events

In the previous section, we provided a lot of detail about how to understand the episodes that lead to the child's need for treatment. We provided all this detail because you need to arrive at an understanding based on sufficient information about each episode, as it occurred. However, the information you need to fully understand these episodes is not based solely on what happened in those moments. There is information from the child's trauma history that will also influence his or her response, in the moment. This information from the child's past should be understood and, when relevant, used in the approach to the child's treatment. We introduced these ideas in Chapters 3 and 4 in discussing the two environments, or the two E's: the *present environment* and the *past traumatic environment*. Our Moment-by-Moment Assessments collect a lot of information about the present environment. Here we are looking for signals of threat when and where the episode occurred. These are the signals—the cat hair—that flip the switch. As we described, a TST detective solves the mystery of what flips the switch by discovering the cat hair in the moment. But this leads to another mystery: the mystery of *why*? Why does this particular stimuli lead to such a large emotional and/or behavioral response for this particular child? Why does this child behave as if his or her survival is at stake in response to a stimulus that does not appear to bother other children? To answer these questions—and to solve this mystery—we need to understand the child's past traumatic environment.

> A TST detective solves the mystery of what flips the switch by discovering the cat hair in the moment. But this leads to another mystery: the mystery of *why*? Why does this particular stimuli lead to such a large emotional and/or behavioral response for this particular child? Why does this child behave as if his or her survival is at stake in response to a stimulus that does not appear to bother other children?

Why Does the Switch Flip for a Particular Child?

The present becomes our anchor for understanding the past. And our anchor is already fully in place because we have fully assessed the present environment through Moment-by-Moment Assessments. We are developing a very good understanding of what in the present environment flips the switch. This understanding becomes our anchor for understanding our second mystery, the mystery of *why*? Traumatic experiences are complex. Just because we know that a particular child was sexually abused, physically abused, or was struck by a car, doesn't mean we know what it was about the experience, or experiences, that will set up the child for survival-in-the-moment reactions in the future.

Consider the full experience of a sexually abused child: What was most threatening to him or her?

- Betrayal by father
- Disbelieved by mother
- Worries about dying during the event
- Worries about pet being killed by father, as threatened
- Pain during event
- Disgust over type of acts performed during event
- Being called ugly during the event

> We first presume nothing and then we gather the facts.

For a given child who was sexually abused, all of these experiences—or none of these experiences—may be important. We do not know. As always, we first presume nothing and then we gather the facts. And the facts we have already gathered will help a lot.

What if our Moment-by-Moment Assessments for this sexually abused child revealed that almost every episode of survival-in-the-moment followed an experience with a male who said or did something that was untrustworthy? We might then *infer* that

> in·fer·ence: The act or process of reaching a conclusion about something from known facts or evidence.
>
> *Merriam-Webster Dictionary*

the element of the sexual abuse experience of being betrayed by father was the most threatening. Alternatively, what if our assessments revealed that survival-in-the-moment reactions repeatedly followed an experience in which the child felt others regarded him or her as ugly? We might then *infer* that this element of the sexual abuse experience was the most threatening. This is called trauma *inference*. It is how we come to understand the component of a child's traumatic experience that is most threatening *to him or her*. It is how we solve the mystery of *why*. This knowledge will certainly be invaluable in helping us to help our children. In the next chapter we discuss in greater detail how we make a trauma inference. Our job for this chapter is to make sure that we collect the information about a child's trauma history to allow us to make such an inference. Record this information in Section 1.b of the TST Assessment Form.

Other Problems That May Need to Be Addressed in Treatment

By far, the most important problems to address in TST relate to how we understand the shifts to survival states. As we discuss in the next chapter, these are defined in a very specific way related to the patterns we discover about these episodes (TST priority problems). Other problems may need to be addressed during our treatment. Here's a warning, however: The more "other" problems that you identify, the less effective you will be at addressing *any single* problem in treatment. Remember Principle 5: *Put scarce resources where they will work*. You do not have unlimited resources to address problems in treatment. In all likelihood, your resources are pretty limited. Make these resources count. Only choose problems to address in treatment that you think are *really* important. That said, there may be problems other than TST priority problems to address. We put these other problems in three categories, described next.

Comorbid Psychiatric or Developmental Disorders

As you well know by now, our main way of defining problems is through understanding survival-in-the-moment reactions. As we have described, our first pass at understanding any episode of problematic emotion/behavior is to determine if it was based on survival-in-the-moment. As we noted in Chapter 3,

> Our first pass at understanding any episode of problematic emotion/behavior is to determine if it is based on survival-in-the-moment.

many symptoms may be better understood through survival states than through a diagnosis of a psychiatric or developmental disorder that was made with neither the integration of information about a child's trauma history nor with the integration of information about the context in which the "symptoms" were expressed.

This problem can take many forms. Consider the following children with trauma histories:

- *A child diagnosed with attention-deficit/hyperactivity disorder:* Careful Moment-by-Moment Assessments revealed that all occasions of hyperactivity, inattention, and impulsivity occurred within survival states.
- *A child diagnosed with bipolar disorder:* Careful Moment-by-Moment Assessments revealed that all occasions of "rapid cycling" among irritability, aggression, and grandiosity occurred within survival states.
- *A child diagnosed with "preschizophrenia":* Careful Moment-by-Moment Assessments revealed that all occasions of paranoia, hallucinations, and disorganized thought occurred within survival states.

Sometimes, children with traumatic stress also have these, and other, comorbid disorders. You certainly don't want to miss them. You also certainly don't want to treat a child for one of these comorbid disorders when the symptoms are entirely expressed within survival-in-the-moment behaviors. It is beyond the scope of this book to detail the assessment of psychiatric and developmental disorders. Please make sure you are sufficiently familiar with the assessment of these disorders when you assess a traumatized child. If you are not sure whether a child has a comorbid disorder, it is a good idea to consult with the psychiatrist associated with your team. (Chapter 15 describes recommendation for the psychiatric assessment.) Record the results of your assessment in Section 1.c.i of the TST Assessment Form.

Enduring Trauma-Related Cognitions

Sometimes children with traumatic stress have enduring negative cognitions about themselves, the world, and the future that may make them more vulnerable to become dysregulated in certain situations (e.g., a youth with an enduring belief that he or she is unlovable becomes dysregulated when he or she perceives rejection from others). It is important to try to assess for these patterns of potentially problematic cognitions and beliefs. This can be done by asking children about their beliefs related to their behaviors and then looking for patterns or themes. Some examples are self-blame, blaming others, negative expectancies related to one's future, believing oneself to be bad or unworthy of love, having a pessimistic outlook, thinking the world is unsafe, and feeling hopeless or fatalistic. Record the results of your assessment of such cognitions in Section 1.c.ii of the TST Assessment Form.

Social Problems

 The families with which we work often have a plethora of social problems: Poverty, divorce and separation, homelessness, unemployment, neighborhood gang violence, family violence, parental mental illness and substance abuse, and immigration and displacement are just some of the challenges faced by these families. Some social problems are straightforwardly remediable; others are not. Some social problems strongly impact the child's shift to survival-in-the-moment; others do not. If we are going to be effective, we must be highly strategic about the social problems that we choose to address. Again, we do not have unlimited resources. Therefore, if we choose to spend time and resources addressing one problem, we should be aware that it will take away from the time and resources we have to address another problem. Be careful here. List social problems in Section 1.c.iii of the TST Assessment Form that you think you might choose to address in treatment. In Chapter 10, we describe how to make your decisions over what to choose to address. For now, just list the social problems. We'll get to the tough choices in the next chapter.

> Some social problems are straightforwardly remediable; others are not. Some social problems strongly impact the child's shift to survival-in-the-moment; others do not. If we are going to be effective, we must be highly strategic about the social problems that we choose to address.

Section 2: Why Are These Problems Important and to Whom Are They Important?

We've gathered the information to answer the first question about identifying the most important problems to be addressed in treatment. Now we need to gather the information that will tell us why any of the problems we might address in treatment is so important. In the next chapter, we use this information to decide on the problems we will address, and their order of priority. What should be assessed here? We need to gather the information about what may be at stake if the child does not receive an effective treatment: What will be the impact on the child and the family if this were the case? This type of knowledge is important if we need to advocate for services, and it is also important in engaging children and families in treatment. With this knowledge, we can be clear in our communication to the child and family about why it is so important for them to engage in treatment. Although *we* may believe the problems are important, we should not presume that other people share this belief. Someone referred the child to treatment, presumably because he or she shared this concern. Who and why? Finally, we hope the child (of sufficient age) and family members share our concern, but we need to understand their level of concern. Irrespective of the level of concern they have about the problem we have identified, what are they most concerned about (whatever it is)? What is causing them pain? What are their goals and desires? The problems we have identified may have great impact on these concerns, pain points, goals, and desires. We can make this connection, if we know what they are.

The Functional Impact of the Episodes of Problematic Emotional/Behavioral Expression

What is at stake here? How much of a problem is the child's problems? And who has a problem with the child's problems? We need to have answers to these questions to justify the interventions we might recommend, advocate for needed interventions, and to engage the child and family in whatever we might recommend. There are several areas in which this impact may occur, so it's important to get a read on each of them. We also need to get a read on the urgency of the possible impact. Is the problem a matter of life and death? Will it affect the child's physical health? Will it affect his or her school or home placement? Will it affect the child's future? Here are some important areas to consider. Record your read on the impact of the problem(s) in Section 2.a of the TST Assessment Form.

- Impact on learning and school
- Impact on family relations
- Impact on peer relations
- Impact on health
- Impact on the child's future

The Level of Concern about These Episodes from the Child, the Family, and Others

In TST, we never presume anything. We gather the facts to know. We may wish the child and his or her caregivers are as concerned about the problem, as we are: but that is not always the case. If the family joins our concerns, that will become the foundation of our treatment alliance. If they don't share our concern: why not? Are we missing something? We must enter this discussion with curiosity. Let's leave our value judgments at the door. A disconnect over the level of concern is something to understand and may deepen our knowledge about the problem. It may also give us a clue on how to establish a treatment alliance over a concern we do share. Who else is concerned? Perhaps a teacher, coach, neighbor, grandparent, pediatrician, or member of the clergy shares our concern. These are our partners. We may need all the help we can get.

> We must enter this discussion with curiosity. Let's leave our value judgments at the door. A disconnect over the level of concern is something to understand and may deepen our knowledge about the problem.

Maybe the child and family are as concerned as we are. Maybe they are not concerned at all. At this point, this is only information that we will consider how to use. Whether the child and family are concerned, or not, we need to understand what does concern them the most. What is the most important to them? What gives them the most pain? What makes them the happiest? What are their goals, priorities, and desires? It is with this knowledge that we will build a treatment alliance and find a point of concern that joins us.

Why What Is Most Important to the Child and the Family Is So Important

Why is what's important to them so important? It is critical for our approach to engage children and families. If a person is in pain about anything, he or she can only think about the vehicle that will plausibly relieve that pain. Accordingly, we must understand the child and the family's respective sources of pain (whatever they are) and figure out how our TST intervention strategy (whatever it is) will become the plausible vehicle to relieve the pain. This information will anchor our treatment engagement approach, described in Chapter 11, called *ready–set–go*. For now, record what is most important and why it is important to the child and the family in Section 2.c of the TST Assessment Form.

 Some tips on recording what is most important to the child and the family and why:

1. Make sure to gather the information separately for the child and any relevant family member. Never presume that they are aligned about what is most important or why it is important.

2. Make sure that whatever you hear is authentic. The people we assess may be highly motivated to please us, or be embarrassed by their desires and goals, or may not think they are relevant, or (tragically) may have never been asked about this before. We may be hearing what they believe we want to hear. Make sure they feel safe enough to tell you. Make sure you get it right. You want to know what is most important to them and why. Your whole engagement strategy is dependent on this. Make sure you get it right.

> Make sure to gather the information separately for the child and any relevant family member. Never presume that they are aligned about what is most important or why it is important.

3. Make sure the goals, pain sources, and concerns are sufficiently specific. Ultimately, you will be tracking the degree to which your work will help the child and family achieve what is most important to them. Beware of vagueness (e.g., "I want to be happy," "I want to be at peace," "I want to be a success"). Push back, a little, so you are sure to understand with

enough specificity. Consider the following dialogue with the mother of
Edward, a 16-year-old boy referred for aggression, marijuana abuse, and
school truancy:

THERAPIST: You've said that what is most important to you is to
be happy. Of course, I want that for you too, but what does
"happy" mean for you? What would indicate happiness for you?

EDWARD'S MOTHER: I'm not sure. I feel so lonely since my divorce. I've
gone on a few dates, but nothing seems to stick, especially after they
meet Edward. When they see his disrespect, they run for the hills.

THERAPIST: So having a stable partner would help you to feel less lonely
and happier. I understand now. Thanks for letting me know something so important. I also hear your concern about Edward's behavior and its effect on your ability to find and keep a stable partner. I'll
definitely want to try to help you with this.

4. Make sure the goals, pain sources, and concerns are achievable. If you
select something that cannot be achieved within the bounds of reality,
you are setting people up for failure (and they've had enough experience
of failure). Consider the following dialogue with Edward:

THERAPIST: So I understand the thing most important to you is to
become a policeman.

EDWARD: Yeah. All my life. So cool. I want the badge.

THERAPIST: I can tell how important this is to you, wanting to get that
badge, all your life.

EDWARD: Yeah.

THERAPIST: So I'm not sure if you know this. Maybe you do. But Edward,
to get into the police academy, you need to graduate from high
school, and you've missed half this school year. The way this year
is going, you won't be promoted to the next grade. And you've also
been arrested twice for marijuana possession and once for assault. I
expect that record can really get in the way of getting into the police
academy.

EDWARD: I dunno.

THERAPIST: So, Edward, I want you to achieve your goal to get a badge. Of
course, I do. But maybe we can set some goals for the shorter term, to
get you on your way, so you have the best chance of being accepted
into the police academy.

EDWARD: What do you mean?

THERAPIST: Well, maybe we can set goals like going to school every day,
staying away from marijuana, and no fighting so you won't be
arrested again. Of course, you know that getting arrested will keep
that badge away from you.

Section 3: What Interventions Will Be Used to Address the Child's Problems?

We've now gathered the information that helps us understand the problems for which a child needs treatment, the functional impact of these problems, and how these problems may address what is most important to the child and family. We now need to gather the information that will help us decide which interventions the child and family need. Again, decision-making is left for the treatment planning chapter. In this chapter we gather the information that will help us make these decisions. Here's where we are going with all of this: The interventions the child needs will be based on the level of risk in his or her trauma system. Some children will need very intense treatment, given the level of risk within their system. Other children will need less intense treatment. It all centers around the information we gather about their trauma system.

> The interventions the child needs will be based on the level of risk in his or her trauma system. Some children will need very intense treatment, given the level of risk within their system. Other children will need less intense treatment. It all centers around the information we gather about their trauma system.

Remember the two dimensions of the trauma system?

1. A traumatized child who is vulnerable to shifting into survival states when threat is perceived in the present environment.

2. A social environment (including caregivers as well as providers within the services system) that is not able to *help* and *protect* the child, given this vulnerability.

These two dimensions of the trauma system—the child's vulnerability to shifting into survival states and the capacity of those in the social environment to help and protect the child—are assessed in all children. Then, based on the results of this two-dimensional assessment, we decide on whether the child needs one of three phases of TST treatment. How do we define and assess the two dimensions of the trauma system?

> These two dimensions of the trauma system—the child's vulnerability to shifting into survival states and the capacity of those in the social environment to help and protect the child—are assessed in all children.

Dimension I: The Child's Vulnerability to Switching into Survival States

You've learned a lot about assessing survival-in-the-moment states through Moment-by-Moment Assessments. These episodes of problematic emotion/behavior that you have learned to assess are not necessarily survival-in-the-moment reactions. That is what you needed to assess. In this section we define

> These episodes of problematic emotion/behavior that you have learned to assess are not necessarily survival-in-the-moment reactions.

three categories of a child's vulnerability to switching into survival states that have significant implications for how we organize treatment. The categories are:

1. No survival states
2. Survival states
3. Dangerous survival states

No Survival States

When a child fits in this category, it means that we have examined the episodes of problematic emotion and/or behavior with Moment-by-Moment Assessments and do not find that survival-in-the-moment underlies them. This means that the three A's do not all shift when the child perceives threat in his or her present environment. A child in this category has pretty good control over his or her emotional states, even when exposed to a stimulus that is a reminder of a past trauma. He or she may become upset and express negative emotions such as anger, sadness, fear, shame, or guilt, but also has a good ability to maintain regulation and go back to a state of calmness and engagement with the environment. A child may fit into this category even if he or she does have shifts in all three A's, but the shifts are so minor or fleeting that we can find no impact on the child's functioning.

> A child in this category has pretty good control over his or her emotional states, even when exposed to a stimulus that is a reminder of a past trauma.

A child with no survival states:

- Does not display episodes of survival-in-the-moment (shifts in awareness, affect, and action) when a threat is perceived in the present environment.
- If the child does display shifts in awareness, affect, and action when a threat is perceived, neither the episode itself, nor the anticipation of such episodes, results in any problem with the child's functioning.

Survival States

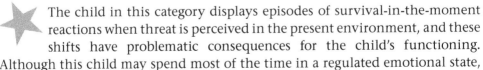

The child in this category displays episodes of survival-in-the-moment reactions when threat is perceived in the present environment, and these shifts have problematic consequences for the child's functioning. Although this child may spend most of the time in a regulated emotional state, shifts to survival-in-the-moment reliably occur when threat is perceived. These shifts from a regulated state to survival-in-the-moment occur with typical changes in awareness (or consciousness), affect (or emotion), and action (or behavior). You have already learned to assess all of these factors by examining the episodes of problematic emotion and/or behavior. You know how to determine if the episodes are related to survival-in-the-moment. You've also learned to assess the impact of these episodes. You know how to determine if the episodes impact the child's functioning. If you've determined that an episode in question represents survival-in-the-moment *and* the episode impacts a child's functioning, then you know the child fits within this category—*with one exception*: the third *A*, for *action*. The shift in action, or behavior, for a child in this category does not include a risk of dangerous (e.g., self-destructive, aggressive, substance-abusing, risky eating, or sexual) behavior. If the child engages in dangerous behavior during survival-in-the-moment, he or she fits into the next category, not this one.

 The child with survival states:

- Displays episodes of survival-in-the-moment (shifts in *awareness, affect, and action*) when threat is perceived in the present environment.
- Displays shifts in *action* during such episodes that do *not* include potentially dangerous (e.g., self-destructive, aggressive, substance-abusing, risky eating, or sexual acting out) behaviors.
- Experiences resulting in problems with functioning as a consequence of such episodes or their anticipation.

Dangerous Survival States

The child in this category, like the child in the previous category, displays episodes of survival-in-the-moment when threat is perceived in the present environment, and these shifts have problematic consequences for the child's functioning. Although this child may spend most of the time in a regulated emotional state, shifts to survival-in-the-moment will reliably occur when threat is perceived. These shifts from a regulated state occur with typical changes in awareness (or consciousness), affect (or emotion), and action (or behavior). Again: Your Moment-by-Moment Assessments and your determination of functional impact will help here. If an episode in question represents survival-in-the-moment and it impacted the child's functioning, then the child fits into this category—*if the child's action is risky/potentially dangerous* (e.g., self-destructive, aggressive, substance-abusing, risky eating, or sexual) *behavior.*

> Although this child may spend most of the time in a regulated emotional state, shifts to survival-in-the-moment will reliably occur when threat is perceived.

The child with dangerous survival states:

- Displays episodes of survival-in-the-moment (shifts in *awareness, affect, and action*) when threat is perceived in the present environment.
- Displays shifts in *action* during such episodes that include potentially dangerous (e.g., self-destructive, aggressive, substance-abusing, risky eating, or sexual) behaviors.
- Experiences resulting in problems with functioning as a consequence of such episodes or their anticipation.

One caution before moving to the second part of the trauma system—a caution that is discussed in detail in the next section but is also critical for assessment of the first part of the trauma system: the distinction between *perceived* threats and *real* threats. As discussed in Chapters 2 and 3, and earlier in this chapter, a core element of the problem of child traumatic stress is the child's shift to survival-in-the-moment when there is no actual threat in the present environment. The child perceives threat because his or her brain has become wired to respond to signals, no matter how subtle, that are reminders of past traumatic experience. Sometimes, tragically, children continue to be exposed to actual threats and their survival-in-the-moment responses are adaptive. This is the distinction between "cat hair" and "cats." Our definitions of the three categories described in this section are relevant for cat hair—that is, for trauma reminders—and not for cats—that is, for true threats of harm. Survival-in-the-moment, in the face of a cat, is *literally* about survival. Children should never be left in a moment when they truly need to fight for their lives. Never leave them in such a moment. Never categorize it as part of psychopathology. G-E-T R-I-D O-F T-H-E C-A-T!

> Our definitions of the three categories described in this section are relevant for cat hair—that is, for trauma reminders—and not cats—that is, for true threats of harm. Survival-in-the-moment, in the face of a cat, is *literally* about survival. Children should never be left in a moment when they truly need to fight for their lives.

Dimension 2: The Ability of the Social Environment to Help and Protect the Child

We concluded the previous section with the distinction between cat hair and cats. This distinction is one of the central ideas employed in this section, as we detail how to assess the child's social environment. In Chapter 4, we discussed the importance of the social environment and the services system. We described how children with traumatic stress may live in environments riddled with cat hair and cats, and the adults in their lives, including providers within the services system, may be ill-equipped to protect them or to help them to regulate emotion. As the social environment (e.g., family, school, peer group, neighborhood) ordinarily has core functions of helping and protecting children, it is assumed that a child's ongoing shifts into survival-in-the-moment means there is a problem with these core functions within one or more levels of the social environment. Similarly, this problem also implies an insufficiency in child service systems' provision of these functions, either because the child is "falling through the cracks" and has not yet accessed the system of care, or because the services the child is receiving are in some way ineffective. Using these ideas, the social environment can be described on a continuum characterized by one of these:

> As the social environment ordinarily has core functions of helping and protecting children, it is assumed that a child's ongoing shifts into survival-in-the-moment means there is a problem with these core functions within one or more levels of the social environment.

1. Helpful and protective
2. Insufficiently helpful and protective
3. Harmful

The distinctions among these three categories of the social environment are based on the constructs of *help* and *protect*. We define these pivotal constructs next.

- *Help.* The capacity of caregivers (including providers within the services system) to *help* the child with his or her vulnerability to switch into survival states. This capacity is defined by caregivers' and/or providers' availability and application of competence to:
  - Support the child to stay regulated, even in situations that contain age-appropriate stressors.
  - Support the child to return to a regulated state, once survival-in-the-moment occurs.
- *Protect.* The capacity of caregivers (including providers within the services system) to *protect* the child from stimuli that he or she perceives as threats and, especially, from actual threats. This capacity is defined by the caregivers' and/or providers' availability and application of competence to:
  - Decrease the likelihood the child will be exposed to a stimulus that he or she perceives as threatening (within environments over which the caregiver or provider has sufficient control).
  - Eliminate (by any reasonable standard) the likelihood the child will be exposed to a stimulus that is a true threat of harm (within environments over which the caregiver or provider has sufficient control).

A Helpful and Protective Social Environment

The child's social environment is *helpful* and *protective* when those around the child are available to apply sufficient competence to support the child's maintenance of regulation and to support the child's return to regulation when survival-in-the-moment occurs. This category is also defined by caregivers' and by service system providers' application of sufficient competence in reducing the likelihood of the child's exposure to cat hair and eliminating exposure to cats. Often, if the child's family is not able to *help* and *protect*, others in the social environment, such as extended family, friends, and neighbors, might serve to *help* and *protect* the child. The child service systems, such as school, social services, or mental health systems, are designed to support the child, his or her family, and extended social network in the service of the child's optimal functioning.

> The child's social environment is *helpful and protective* when those around the child are available to apply sufficient competence to support the child's maintenance of regulation and to support the child's return to regulation when survival-in-the-moment occurs.

A helpful and protective social environment is defined by the following:

- The child's immediate caregivers are sufficiently available and apply sufficient competence to *help* with the child's vulnerability to switch into survival states and to *protect* the child from perceived and actual threats, *or*

- Other adults in the child's life are sufficiently available and apply sufficient competence to *help* and *protect* the child, *or*

- The appropriate child service system is sufficiently available and applies sufficient competence to *help* and *protect* the child.

An Insufficiently Helpful and Protective Social Environment

> The child's social environment is considered insufficiently *helpful and protective* when those around the child are either not sufficiently available or not sufficiently competent to support the child's maintenance of regulation, and to support the child's return to regulation when survival-in-the-moment occurs.

The child's social environment is considered insufficiently *helpful and protective* when those around the child are either not sufficiently available or not sufficiently competent to support the child's maintenance of regulation, and to support the child's return to regulation when survival-in-the-moment occurs. This category is also defined by the availability and application of competence by caregivers and service system providers to reduce the likelihood of the child's exposure to cat hair and to eliminate exposure to cats. This category of *insufficient help and protection* also means that others in the child's wider social environment, and service system, are either not sufficiently available or are not sufficiently competent to help and to protect. It is important to note that in this category our definition of protection is about perceived threats and not actual threats (*cat hair* and not the *cat* itself). If a cat is in the child's environment, the environment is, by definition, considered harmful. The main distinction between this category of an insufficiently helpful and protective social environment and the next one concerns the distinction between cat hair and cats.

Examples of a distressed social environment include:

- A father who calls his 13-year-old son "weak" because the son is too anxious to attend physical education (PE) class. The boy panics before PE class because the PE teacher reminds him of a camp counselor who sexually abused him the past summer. The father declines to participate in any effort to help his son because he believes that doing so would be "indulging him."

- A soccer coach who allows other boys to make demeaning comments to a 10-year-old boy, resulting in flashbacks of physical abuse.

- A family that previously experienced homelessness and is under severe financial stress; as a result of the parents' anxious and sometimes angry discussions about finances, their daughter has nightmares and intrusive thoughts about past homeless experience.

- A foster parent who insists on a lights-out-at-bedtime rule, despite a child's extreme anxiety regarding sleeping in the dark, related to a history of abuse during the nighttime.

In each of these examples, we wish the child would receive better help and protection from caregivers. Although at some level we could reasonably say the child's environments are harmful to the child. Within TST, we reserve the category of "harmful" for only those situations when a child may be physically harmed or his or her basic needs are so neglected that it could lead to physical harm. There are several reasons for sticking to this distinction. Most importantly, it will matter a lot for knowing what to do to help.

> We reserve the category of "harmful" for only those situations when a child may be physically harmed or his or her basic needs are so neglected that it could lead to physical harm.

 An insufficiently helpful and protective social environment is defined by the following:

- The child's immediate caregivers are insufficiently available and/or apply insufficient competence to *help* with the child's vulnerability to switch into survival states or to *protect* the child from perceived threats, *and*

- Other adults in the child's life are insufficiently available and/or apply insufficient competence to *help* and *protect* the child, *and*

- The appropriate child service system is insufficiently available and/or applies insufficient competence to *help* and *protect* the child.

The Harmful Social Environment

The child's social environment is considered *harmful* when those around the child are not available enough or have not applied sufficient competence toward protecting the child from exposure to a *true threat* of harm. In this worrisome category, no one around the child is sufficiently available or able to protect the child from harm, including (tragically) the child protective system. When the environment is considered harmful, definitive, immediate intervention is needed. There is a cat that can reach the child.

> The child's social environment is considered *harmful* when those around the child are not available enough or have not applied sufficient competence toward protecting the child from exposure to a *true threat* of harm.

Examples of a harmful social environment include the following:

- An uncle who has sexually abused a 14-year-old girl either lives in the same home or can visit at any time. No efforts have been made to limit the uncle's access to the child.
- A father is violent toward his wife and two teenage sons when he abuses alcohol. He is abusing alcohol again.
- A mother frequently stays out all night and leaves her 12-year-old daughter with her 18-year-old son. The son has sexually abused his sister three times in the last year.

Among the most difficult instances of a threatening environment occur when the threat is at the hands of professional caregivers. We wish we did not have to include such situations but, unfortunately, this sad reality may occasionally occur: Examples of threat from professional caregivers include the following:

- Violence at school for which the school does not intervene.
- Sexual boundary violation by a professional caregiver.
- Lack of intervention from a social services agency following an investigation for child abuse when abuse is, in fact, occurring (think of what this means for an abused child).
- Use of mechanical restraint in a mental health/medical/educational setting with a child who has been physically or sexually abused. (We understand that this notion can be controversial, and, in some limited cases, restraint is needed to prevent significant harm. It's important to note the potential meaning of restraint to a physically or sexually abused child. Accordingly, if restraint is used in situations other than as a last resort, without reasonable and proactive efforts to prevent the use of restraint, and without consideration of the child's trauma history and the potential impact of the restraint, we would consider such a clinical social environment to be harmful.)

 A harmful social environment is defined by the following:

- The child's immediate caregivers are insufficiently available and/or apply insufficient competence to *protect* the child from actual threats, *and*
- Other adults in the child's life are insufficiently available and/or apply insufficient competence to *protect* the child from actual threats, *and*
- The appropriate child service system is insufficiently available and/or applies insufficient competence to *protect* the child from actual threats.

Four Questions for When the Reality Is Hard to See

At one level, a harmful environment may appear to be the easiest to see—a cat is there or it is not; a child is being harmed, or not. But at another level a harmful environment can be the hardest to see. Recall our discussion of the treatment principles in Chapter 6, specifically Principle 7: *Align with reality*. In the trauma system there are huge pressures *not* to align with reality. Such pressures may come from others who don't want to see what is happening or don't want to take responsibility for it. Such pressures may also be internal to providers and their organizations. It's hard to really see the horror of harm to a child. It is much easier to look the other way. However, if we see it, we need to take responsibility for doing something about it.

Accordingly, we have developed four very basic and practical questions that providers should ask themselves, their teams, and relevant members of the child's environment and service system when questions about a possible harmful environment arise. Remember: We use the category of "harmful social environment" sparingly. We reserve it for situations that require immediate, definitive interventions to protect a child from a true threat. Here are the four questions to help you know if you are in such a situation:

1. **What is the minimum this child needs for his or her help and protection?** It is important to be very careful answering this question because it will define the minimum standard for providing help and protection. The answer should not be based on what you might see as the average standard or, in any way, what you might wish would happen. It's a cold, sober look at the *minimum*. A good way of knowing whether you've reached this minimal standard is by considering the following reality: Any reasonable person should say something like "Oh my G-d!" in response to hearing about the situation in which the child is living. It's also important to make sure this minimum standard is specific to the child in question and not made generically. For example: A social environment in which a child repeatedly runs out of the house and into traffic in a dissociated state following specific interactions with her father will have a different minimum standard for help and protection than another child who does not have this vulnerability.

   > A good way of knowing whether you've reached this minimal standard is by considering the following reality: Any reasonable person should say something like "Oh my G-d!" in response to hearing about the situation in which the child is living.

2. **What care is the child receiving now and how is it related to this minimal standard for his or her help and protection?** Let's look at the reality. Is it above the standard or is it below the standard? Would a reasonable person say "Oh my G-d!" or something like "That poor kid, I wish things were a little better for her." As we describe in the treatment

planning chapter and safety-focused treatment chapter (Chapters 10 and 12, respectively), when you determine that help and protection are below the minimum standard, all efforts and all resources go to managing the risk so that safety can be established. Accordingly, it is a mistake to set the minimum standard bar higher than it should be set.

3. **Is it plausible that the child will be able to receive this minimum standard of help and protection in a time frame appropriate to the level of risk for harm?** When you've made the call that what the child is receiving is below the minimum standard, you've made the call that there is a clear and present danger. Accordingly, any foreseeable change in the environment (including any intervention you might provide) needs to plausibly lead to a level of change that is appropriate to the level of risk within an appropriate time frame.

4. **Would anyone in this room be surprised to read about this child on the front page of tomorrow's newspaper?** Sometimes there are situations involving clear and present risks of harm, and no appropriate changes are forthcoming within a reasonable time frame—and, still, providers are processing information through the dangerous "wishful thinking" lens. In such circumstances it is helpful to ask this fourth question. In our experience, it usually enlightens the necessary reality. When a child is receiving less than the minimum standard, events can plausibly unfold that will find the child described in such a tragic forum.

Handling Multiple Social Environments

All children live in multiple social environments (unless they are not allowed to leave their home). How should assessment of the social environment work in relation to the multiple environments in which children routinely interact (e.g., home, school, sports team, grandparents' home)? The rule is this: *Rate the social environment based on the more/most problematic setting.* If the school is considered harmful, for example, but the home environment is considered insufficiently or sufficiently helpful and protective, the social environment is considered harmful. Similarly, if the child's foster home is considered sufficiently helpful and protective but the child's home with his or her biological family is considered harmful—and he or she continues to visit this home unsupervised—the social

> The rule is this: Rate the social environment based on the more/most problematic setting.

environment is considered harmful. The child is unlikely to benefit from *any* modality of intervention if the child is routinely delivered to a cat by those he or she is supposed to be able to trust.

Closing Thoughts on Assessing and Defining the Trauma System

Assessing and defining the trauma system is one of the most important processes within TST (perhaps why we have called it *trauma systems* therapy). Use Section 3 of the TST Assessment Form in Appendix 2 to record your assessment of the child's vulnerability to survival-in-the-moment states and the degree of help and protection in the child's social environment, according to the definitions outlined in this section (please, *please* use these definitions). In Chapter 10, we review how to use this information to decide which phase of treatment to implement, with the help of the TST Treatment Planning Grid. In essence, the information you gather on the two dimensions of the trauma system will actually form two dimensions of a 3 × 3 grid to determine the child's treatment phase. Much more on this in the next chapter.

Section 4: What Strengths Will Be Used to Address the Child's Problems?

Remember our ninth treatment principle: *Build from strength*. It's not a platitude. It's a call to search for all the assets that can help because you'll really need them. The trauma system may be fraught with problems—but, to be sure, strengths can be found if you look for them. And the strengths you find may make the difference between an effective and an ineffective intervention. Searching for these strengths is also part of our fifth principle: *Put scare resources where they will work*. We all know that resources within the child service system are hard to find. Maybe we've been looking in the wrong places. The needed resources are not only found within providers and the organizations for which they work.

Strengths can be present in several different areas: within the child, the family or caregiver system, or within the broader social environment. The goal of this part of the assessment is to look for sources of strength present in these areas that might be used in treatment. The process of your searching for, asking about, and recording strengths may be therapeutic in itself for both the child and family members. Sad to say but many people (children and adults) who come for treatment feel like a bundle of problems and believe that other people see them that way. In fact, one of the chronic maladaptations that can take place in the wake of trauma is a negative view of oneself and world (this is why we assess for enduring, trauma-related cognitions). The process of identifying strengths simultaneously begins the process of challenging and changing these negative views.

> The process of your searching for, asking about, and recording strengths may be therapeutic in itself for both the child and family members.

Areas of strengths to consider include:

- *Child strengths.* May include intellectual strengths, such as an ability to solve problems or quickly understand new ideas; social-emotional strengths, such as being likeable, highly motivated, or insightful about him- or herself; or specific talents and skills, such as being a good artist or athlete.
- *Parent strengths.* May include their motivation to help their child and the skills they bring to the process, such as parenting knowledge or a high degree of organization, flexibility to try new things, emotional attunement, or a willingness to accept help.
- *Social-environmental strengths.* May include important other people in a child's life (e.g., friends, neighbors), aspects of culture or religion that could be a source of strength and guidance, service systems that are working well in a child's life (e.g., school), or other aspects (formal or informal) of the broader social environment that constructively support the child.

What strengths do the child and family members identify in themselves and their world? What strengths can you identify and share? How will these strengths be critically useful to helping family members meet their goals? Strengths are the platforms on which all of the ensuing intervention activities will stand. If you build on platforms that aren't really there, or that have holes, the interventions may fail. If, on the other hand, you spend the time to figure out what resources comprise this child's and family's platforms, then you can build interventions to suit them—and they will stand.

Section 5: What Can Interfere with Addressing the Child's Problems?

We once heard about a project designed to determine what might improve the likelihood that people would donate blood. A number of hypotheses were tested: What if we shared more information about how the blood could help people in desperate need? What if we appealed to one's sense of duty to community? What if we shared information about how many other people were doing it? On and on, nothing worked. Finally, some genius tried something new. He stood on a street corner and handed out directions to the nearest place to donate. *Tah-dah*, people gave blood. They just needed practical information and a practical barrier to be removed.

As we describe in the treatment engagement chapter, Ready–Set–Go (Chapter 11), even when a family's goals and pain points are carefully attended to and everyone is eager to participate in treatment, there are still some obstacles that can get in the way. Within TST, we focus on two categories of factors that can interfere with treatment:

1. The child and family's basic misunderstanding of trauma and its impact in combination with what mental health intervention entails.
2. The practical barriers in the way of treatment engagement.

Let's discuss each in turn.

The Child and Family's Basic Misunderstanding of Trauma and Its Impact in Combination with What Mental Health Intervention Entails

Most readers of this book will know a lot about these topics (and hopefully even more after reading this book). You may have taken courses on these topics. You may have received advanced training. Helping traumatized children and families may be a core part of your job. You know an awful lot about the basics, at least. What do the children and families know about the basics? What do they need to know? Again: We never presume anything. Let's assess this knowledge here. For many people, our world of mental health intervention—whether trauma-informed or not—is foreign territory. This is particularly true for families from non-Western cultures or for recent immigrants to Western nations. What do the people we work with understand about trauma, its impact, and mental health intervention? Let's record this information in the appropriate space in Section 5 of the TST Assessment Form. This information will become very important for our strategy to engage children and families, detailed in Chapter 11.

The Practical Barriers in the Way of Treatment Engagement

What might get in the way? Let's make sure not to miss this. Don't wait until the third appointment cancellation to find out the answer! Asking about potential challenges to making and keeping appointments—transportation, child care, scheduling concerns, language differences, financial concerns, or other personal reasons—allows for a frank conversation early on about potential trouble spots and a chance to problem-solve. In addition, acknowledging the challenge of making appointments work in the midst of all else that goes on in a family's world communicates respect for the many other concerns a parent faces. Record your knowledge of these practical barriers in the appropriate space in Section 5 of your TST Assessment Form.

Putting It into Practice: Using the TST Assessment Form

The TST Assessment Form provides a guide to gather all the basic information you need to be able to put together a TST Treatment Plan and engage the family.

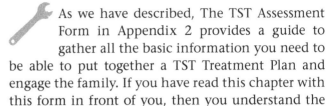 As we have described, The TST Assessment Form in Appendix 2 provides a guide to gather all the basic information you need to be able to put together a TST Treatment Plan and engage the family. If you have read this chapter with this form in front of you, then you understand the purpose of each section of the form and how to complete it. To build your knowledge about this critical tool, we present some details about a child, Tanisha, next. Think about Tanisha and how you might fill out a TST Assessment Form about her. In Appendix 3, we provide a completed copy of Tanisha's TST Assessment Form. We return to the case of Tanisha at many points throughout the rest of this book. Let's start to get to know her here.

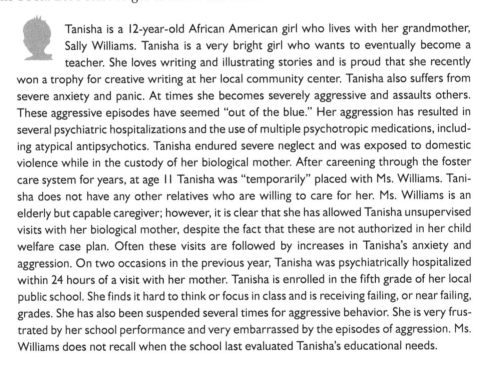 Tanisha is a 12-year-old African American girl who lives with her grandmother, Sally Williams. Tanisha is a very bright girl who wants to eventually become a teacher. She loves writing and illustrating stories and is proud that she recently won a trophy for creative writing at her local community center. Tanisha also suffers from severe anxiety and panic. At times she becomes severely aggressive and assaults others. These aggressive episodes have seemed "out of the blue." Her aggression has resulted in several psychiatric hospitalizations and the use of multiple psychotropic medications, including atypical antipsychotics. Tanisha endured severe neglect and was exposed to domestic violence while in the custody of her biological mother. After careening through the foster care system for years, at age 11 Tanisha was "temporarily" placed with Ms. Williams. Tanisha does not have any other relatives who are willing to care for her. Ms. Williams is an elderly but capable caregiver; however, it is clear that she has allowed Tanisha unsupervised visits with her biological mother, despite the fact that these are not authorized in her child welfare case plan. Often these visits are followed by increases in Tanisha's anxiety and aggression. On two occasions in the previous year, Tanisha was psychiatrically hospitalized within 24 hours of a visit with her mother. Tanisha is enrolled in the fifth grade of her local public school. She finds it hard to think or focus in class and is receiving failing, or near failing, grades. She has also been suspended several times for aggressive behavior. She is very frustrated by her school performance and very embarrassed by the episodes of aggression. Ms. Williams does not recall when the school last evaluated Tanisha's educational needs.

We return to the case of Tanisha in the next chapter. Before we turn to that chapter, we conclude this one with a difficult issue that must be addressed.

Assessment in the Context of Crisis and Risk

You are asked to gather a lot of information to complete a TST assessment. This information is important and will ultimately determine how you will focus the treatment and engage children and families in the treatment. What if you need to manage a lot of crises within your first visits with the child and family? What if it seems that you can never get to the work of completing the TST Assessment Form because of the crises that need to be managed? This is a common, and complex, problem. You need to strike a tough balance in what may seem like a Catch-22 situation:

1. If you spend your time primarily responding to crises such that you can never gather the information you need for TST assessment, you will never understand the main drivers of the crises, and children and families will continue to cycle through crisis after crisis.
2. You must respond to crises in order to prevent someone from being harmed.

Here are guidelines to manage this difficult balance:

- Make sure the situation to which you think you need to respond is really a crisis that needs a response *right now*. Sometimes family members may present a need that they believe is immediate, but with a little discussion and redirection, the need can wait. Remember: If you are continually responding to crises such that you can't complete the assessment, you will never really get a handle on preventing the crises.
- Have a frank discussion with the family at the beginning of the assessment process about the information you will need to gather during this phase. Set a rough timeline for gathering this information and explain why it is so important to gather it. Hopefully you can complete your assessment within two or three sessions. This may facilitate the discussion with the family members about using the session to respond to something they regard as urgent. They may be able to wait a short period of time if they see that you will be much better prepared to help them after completing the assessment (also within a short period of time).
- If you see there is acute risk, drop everything and respond to the risk.
- If it's hard to engage the child and family in the assessment process, use every means at your disposal to gather the needed information. If during a session, for example, there is a crisis from a child's escalating behavior, use it as an opportunity to gather information for a moment-by-moment assessment through your observations. You will probably be able to fill in any blanks to this assessment at some later point. Prioritize the gathering of information from other observers (e.g., extended family, teachers, coaches).
- The time between first contact, initial visit, and the initiation of treatment (i.e., safety-focused, regulation-focused, or beyond trauma phases) must be very short. In order to initiate treatment you must be very efficient as

you go through assessment (this chapter), treatment planning (Chapter 10), and ready–set–go (Chapter 11). Delaying the initiation of treatment for a child at risk can increase risk. How long should this take? We provide time guidelines in Chapter 11 (Table 11.1, p. 226). Here's the gist of these guidelines. The details will become clearer as you proceed through the next two chapters:

- You should establish if there is a significant risk within, at most, 1 week of first contact and/or visit. This means that you have concluded that either the environment is harmful, or the child switches to dangerous survival states and the environment is insufficiently helpful and protective, within 1 week, at most. By definition, this means the child needs safety-focused treatment.

- If you have decided the child needs safety-focused treatment, then you need to initiate treatment very soon to manage the level of risk. You may decide to spend a little more time gathering information before initiating treatment, but this time can't be too long—no more than 1 more week.

- You will therefore need to initiate safety-focused treatment for some children without fully completing assessment, treatment planning, and ready–set–go. In these cases you will not have all the information you need to make decisions on a focused treatment plan that can fully engage the family, and you will not have completed the process of engaging the family in the focused treatment plan. **This is a big compromise**, but it is necessary to preserve safety. Bottom line: Do your best to gather as much information as you can for the assessment within the time that you have. If you initiate safety-focused treatment with missing information, do your best to fill in the blanks as you go. *We strongly recommend that you do everything you can to determine at least one priority problem (with moment-by-moment assessments) before you initiate safety-focused treatment.*

- If you have decided (after 1 week of first visit/contact) that the child does not need safety-focused treatment, and therefore needs either regulation-focused or beyond trauma treatment, then you have a bit more time. The situation is not risky. It's also less complex, and you don't have the problem of crises interfering with the process of assessment, treatment planning, and ready–set–go. You should be able to complete ready–set–go within 2 weeks of this decision (at most, 3 weeks from first visit/contact).

Closing Thoughts on Assessment

This chapter began with the sentence: *"Assessment* is about how to know; it is about gathering the type of information that will give us the knowledge required to decide what to do." What if we are not supposed to know? John Bowlby (1979), the father of attachment theory, wrote a paper titled "On Knowing What You Are Not Supposed to Know and on Feeling What You Are Not Supposed to Feel." In this article, Bowlby described the terrible dilemma faced by children who live in traumatic environments and the messages they receive indicating that the reality right before their eyes is untrue. How do children process the message—whether delivered overtly or covertly—that what they think they are experiencing as trauma is something other than trauma? Bowlby described the impact and power of these reality-undermining messages. He could have extended his analysis to all who enter the trauma system, including providers. What if we are not supposed to know? What if the desire of some of the families with which we work is that we look away? What if the desire of the organizations we work for or the service systems we work within is to look away: to not see the trauma because of what we would need to do if we acknowledged it? What if a part of us, consciously or unconsciously, wants to look away because of this same burden of knowledge?

As described in Chapter 1, becoming a TST provider entails a certain type of commitment. It's the commitment to *not* avert our eyes and to squarely face the reality of the information we must gather, no matter the consequences. To look away is to walk by the drowning child. TST assessment is about gathering the facts. *We acknowledge here the courage required to gather these facts.* In the next chapter we discuss the decisions you will need to make based on the facts you have gathered—decisions that will require at least as much courage as the gathering of the facts.

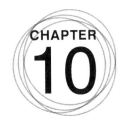

Treatment Planning

*How to Use the Information You've Gathered
to Plan What You Will Do*

LEARNING OBJECTIVES

- To learn how to use the information you have gathered to answer the five TST treatment planning questions
- To learn how to complete a TST Treatment Plan
- To understand how a well-constructed treatment plan will set the stage for an effective treatment

---

ICONS USED IN THIS CHAPTER

Essential Point	Useful Tool	Danger	Case Discussion

We began the previous chapter with the distinction between assessment, treatment planning, and treatment engagement. If assessment is about knowing how to know, treatment planning is about deciding what to do. So, now that you know how to know, how do you decide what to do? That's what this chapter is all about.

In Chapter 9, we had you go through all the trouble of gathering the information that will help to answer five treatment planning questions. In this chapter, we describe how you will answer these questions with the information you have gathered. What's so important about answering those questions? The answers become your TST Treatment Plan!

Here, again, are those five questions, with the decisions you will need to make to answer them:

Section 1: What problem(s) will be the focus of the child's treatment?
The decisions we need to make:
a. The child's TST priority problems and their relation to the child's trauma history.
b. Other problems that will be addressed in treatment, including:
    i.   Comorbid psychiatric and developmental disorders
    ii. Enduring trauma-related cognitions
    iii. Social problems that impact the child's health and development

Section 2: Why are these problems important and to whom are they important?
The decisions we need to make:
a. The order of priority of the TST priority problems and any other identified problem(s)
b. The strategy to engage the child and family to address the identified problems
c. The strategy to engage others to address the identified problems

Section 3: What interventions will be used to address the child's problems?
The decisions we need to make:
a. The phase of treatment to initiate
b. The statement about how the treatment will be directed to address the identified problems
c. The role and expectations of each member of the team in implementing the treatment
d. The role and expectations of the child and the family members in implementing treatment

Section 4: What strengths will be used to address the child's problems?

The decisions we need to make:

a. The child's strengths that will be used in the treatment

b. The family members' strengths that will be used in the treatment

c. The strengths in the social environment that will be used in treatment

Section 5: What will interfere with addressing the child's problems?

The decisions we need to make:

a. The approach to address the psychoeducational needs of the child and family

b. The approach to surmount practical barriers

The TST Assessment Form (in Appendix 2) anchored the previous chapter and provides the information you will need to make the treatment planning decisions in this chapter. The TST Treatment Plan anchors the present chapter and is the form you will use to record all of your treatment planning decisions. We recommend that you use the TST Treatment Plan, included in Appendix 4, as you proceed through this chapter.

 TOOL: TST Treatment Plan

What it is: A form that records decisions about how providers and teams will work with children and families to help alleviate their trauma-related problems.

When to use it: Once the assessment process is completed, by using the information from the TST Assessment Form to answer the five questions that will establish the TST Treatment Plan. To be revisited as new information emerges, if treatment is not progressing, or if a child is transitioning to a new phase of treatment.

Target goals: To ensure that treatment is guided by a sound treatment plan that will remediate a set of defined problems and engage children and families in their solution.

Optimally, the process of answering the five treatment planning questions to arrive at the TST Treatment Plan will be done as a team. It is so important to get it right! As detailed in Chapter 7, the treatment team getting it right can be complex. Participating on a team in which the members will wrestle with the facts together—to get it right—is very helpful. The TST team is charged with constructing a treatment plan that is very focused, clear, engaging, and—most importantly—addresses the practical realities of the child and family's problems. Before we dive into this treatment planning decision making, team-wise or otherwise, we briefly digress (yet again) to discuss the importance of facts.

> The TST team is charged with constructing a treatment plan that is very focused, clear, engaging, and—most importantly—addresses the practical realities of the child and family's problems.

Beware: Jumping to the Explanation before Knowing the Facts

Before we get into the details of treatment planning, we want to describe what we see as the single most important *trap* of treatment planning: jumping to an explanation about a child's problem before methodically gathering the facts that would support the explanation. We introduced this critical issue in the previous chapter. When a child is referred for treatment for episodes of problematic emotion and/or behavior, there is frequently a lot of pressure to explain the episodes in question, especially if danger is involved. Parents, children, schools, funding agencies, among others, want to know why the child feels and behaves the way he or she does. And we are the experts. We are paid to know, aren't we? So we feel pressure to provide an explanation. But what if our explanation only serves to make people feel better because an expert can use words to share an understanding of the problem—without really understanding it! This is what we are trying to avoid: using words that seem to convey understanding, without really understanding. A real explanation will provide an understanding of the child's problems that is sufficiently *specific* and *actionable*: It will tell us what we need to do to solve the problem. How do we get there? By identifying what we call the *TST priority problem*. When you identify the TST priority problem, you have your explanation about what is wrong and what therefore needs to be addressed. If you are able to develop such an explanation, strongly supported by the facts, a lot of good things can happen. If you are not able to develop such an explanation grounded in facts, you will not be effective (and that's a fact!).

> The single most important *trap* of treatment planning: jumping to an explanation about a child's problem before methodically gathering the facts that would support the explanation.

In order to get there, always keep two of the TST principles front and center:

1. Create clear, focused plans that are based on facts (Principle 3).
2. Align with reality (Principle 7).

Remember how we described the importance of facts and practical reality in Chapter 6 on treatment principles? We all have ways of explaining what is going on with a child and family. We all have explanations about the nature of the problem. But we should *never* jump to an explanation before looking carefully at the facts. When the facts are carefully gathered and the definitions provided in Chapter 9 are used to classify regulation, the social environment, moment-by-moment reactions, and trauma history, they will point directly to the nature of the problem and what must be done to help. When you skip the facts and jump right to your explanation, you are very likely to get it wrong.

> When you skip the facts and jump right to your explanation, you are very likely to get it wrong.

How can you tell fact from explanation? Facts are pieces of information that answer questions such as:

What happened? *He punched his brother.*

Who was there? *His brother and his mother.*

Where did it occur? *In the kitchen.*

When did it occur? *At breakfast.*

What was happening before he punched his brother? *His brother poured the last of the Cap'n Crunch.*

If you jump right to an explanation, you will be substituting "why" for a "who," "what," "when," or "where." Compare the following answers to those just above:

What happened? *He has poor impulse control and couldn't manage frustration.*

What happened? *He felt deprived based on the family history of poverty.*

What happened? *He was competing for his mother's attention.*

What happened? *He was enacting an episode in which he saw his father beat his mother.*

What happened? *HE PUNCHED HIS BROTHER.*

In the previous chapter, we detailed how we solve the mystery of *why*. We described the detective work required to make a *trauma inference*. This is our ability to understand the episodes in question, and their patterns, so well that we can clearly see why certain features of the child's trauma history have set up the child to respond in the way he or she responds. We need to arrive at this level of understanding and explanation. We get there by having the facts we need about the child's episodes and about his or her trauma history. And we've already gathered exactly these facts and recorded them in our TST Assessment Form: Haven't we? Yes we have! Now we are in position to offer real explanations, anchored by the facts. Can we do it? Yes we can!

Always remember . . . *"Just the facts, ma'am."*

How to Answer the Five Treatment Planning Questions: Everything Follows from Gathering the Right Type of Facts and Properly Using TST Definitions

If you can keep to this idea stated above (stick to the facts), then everything will line up (we promise). If your team's treatment planning process does not closely follow this idea, then things will not line up (we promise).

Let's consider each of the five questions one at a time. Take out your TST Assessment Form (Appendix 2) as we go through each. The information contained within this form, detailed in Chapter 9, will provide the facts used for treatment planning. Now take out your TST Treatment Plan (Appendix 4). This form guides you through the decisions you need to make in answer to those five questions. Now . . . to those five questions.

Section I: What Problems Will Be the Focus of the Child's Treatment?

In Chapter 9, we detailed the importance of using Moment-by-Moment Assessments to gather the facts about a child's episodes of problematic emotion and/or behavior. We described how the information from these Moment-by-Moment Assessments would eventually be used to define the problems that will be addressed in treatment. We also gave you a peak ahead: The problems that will be addressed in TST are defined from the patterns you can see through the Moment-by-Moment Assessments. The problems are also informed by knowledge of the child's trauma history so that we may be able to understand why a child would be so reactive in a given situation. In this chapter, we use all this information to answer the question: *What problem(s) should be the focus of the child's treatment?*

The Child's TST Priority Problems and Their Relation to the Child's Trauma History

As we've discussed in Chapters 3 and 9, we seek to define problems that provide good-enough explanations about what flips the switch to a child's transition from his or her usual, regulated state to a survival-in-the-moment reaction. We know the switch flips when the child perceives a threat in the present environment—cat hair. But we also know

> We seek to define problems that provide good-enough explanations about what flips the switch to a child's transition from their usual, regulating state to survival-in-the-moment.

that the cat hair can be very subtle, even hardly detectable. As *TST detectives* we have to discover what it is that flips this switch. This discovery comes from recognizing the patterns. These patterns become visible when we examine several different episodes using Moment-by-Moment Assessments. Why do we need several different episodes and their Moment-by-Moment Assessments? Why can't we define a priority problem with only one? A child's episodes of survival-in-the-moment may overtly appear to be completely disconnected. A child's expression of problematic behavior in one situation may look very different in another. The child, and those around him or her (including providers), may not see any connection between the episodes until the facts are gathered that reveals their similarity.

The case of Briana, described in Chapter 9, provides a good illustration. The episodes of cutting her arms after a school field trip to an art museum and 1 month later after going to the movies with friends seemed completely random, unrelated, and therefore unpredictable—until separate Moment-by-Moment Assessments revealed their connection through Briana's exposure to stimuli that reminded her of her uncle's body. The problems are defined through the patterns. It's a bit like playing "connect the dots." The picture/pattern only becomes clear when you have connected enough dots. Episodes are like dots. We need at least three dots (episodes of problematic emotion or behavior) to see the pattern (TST priority problem). That is why we want at least three Moment-by-Moment Assessments for each problem we might define.

The pattern we see points to our focus in treatment—the TST priority problems—always defined in one way:

TST priority problems are patterns of links between a traumatized child's perception of threat in the present environment and the child's transition to a survival-in-the-moment state.

The TST Pattern Recognition (Priority Problem) Game

To get you in the frame of mind to define your priority problems, we introduce a game. It's like playing "connect the dots." We provide basic information about three episodes from children we introduced in the previous chapter. You connect the dots to see the pattern. Ready . . .

Referral Concern	A teacher is concerned about Jason, a 7-year-old boy who repeatedly yells and pushes other children.
Episode 1	Jason pushed another boy in the locker room before swim class. The boy put his hands on Jason's shoulders as Jason was changing.
Episode 2	Jason pushed another boy in the bathroom. The other boy was standing beside Jason at the urinal and commented on Jason's "private parts."
Episode 3	Jason pushed another boy when he was on a sleepover. Jason was very anxious about the sleepover. He said he wanted to change into his pajamas in the bathroom. The boy blocked his way and called him a girl.
What is the pattern?	

Referral Concern	A foster parent is concerned about Emily, a 10-year-old girl who repeatedly states that she wants to die and bangs her head against the wall in this context.
Episode 1	Emily bangs her head against her bedroom wall and says she wants to die after a phone call with her biological mother. On the phone call her mother said to her, "How can you be so sure that Jerry did it? He's been so nice

	to you." (Jerry, the mother's boyfriend, was arrested after Emily told her teacher that he had sexually abused her.)
Episode 2	Emily bangs her head against a car window on the way home from being interviewed by police about her sexual abuse allegation.
Episode 3	Emily runs to her bedroom in tears after watching a movie on TV and was found punching herself and saying she wants to die. A woman in the movie expressed the importance of family loyalty. Emily was particularly upset by a sentence spoken by the woman: "Families first, no matter what."
What is the pattern?	

Referral Concern	**A guidance counselor is concerned about Briana, a 15-year-old girl who repeatedly cuts her arms and legs.**
Episode 1	Briana cut her arms after she returned from a school field trip to an art museum. She kept returning to look at a statue of a male torso.
Episode 2	Briana cut her arms and legs after returning from an evening when she saw a movie with friends. One scene in the movie particularly affected her, a scene in which a man removed his shirt.
Episode 3	Briana cut her arms after returning from her friend's house. Her friend was showing her photographs from a recent vacation and commented on a teenage boy's "ripped" body, seen in one of the photographs.
What is the pattern?	

Did any of the patterns become clear? Remember, the facts from the episodes are your clues, and the pattern you recognize provides the solution. When you first read about these children in Chapter 9, you could only guess at the solution for each of them. You hardly had any facts. Now you have the facts to help you see the pattern that forms your solution.

In the case of Jason, each episode is related to a situation with other boys where he is required to remove his clothes. You might begin to speculate why he becomes so dysregulated in this context—but that is getting ahead of yourself (we discuss how we use the facts gathered about a child's trauma history in the next section). For now you know that situations that require Jason to expose his body and possibly involve even minor physical contact with other boys in such a context constitute Jason's cat hair. You can also see that the more episodes you assess, the clearer the pattern and picture becomes. Clarity has tremendous value here. It will ultimately relate to the precision you will use to intervene. In the case of Emily, the context of a criminal case arising from her allegation of sexual abuse by her mother's boyfriend is very important. You also have much more specific information to go on. The suicidal/self-destructive behavior in each episode appears to

You can see that the more episodes you will assess, the clearer the pattern and picture will become.

follow situations where Emily believes she has been disloyal to her family. You can see how important this understanding will become for your plan to help Emily. We've already had a lot to say about Briana. We've added a new dot for her episodes that appears to confirm our understanding that her reaction pattern is related to images that remind her of her uncle's body.

Now you are ready for a new tool: The TST Priority Problem Worksheet (shown in Appendix 4 and reproduced in Figure 10.1).

This is the worksheet you should use to arrive at your priority problems.

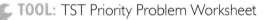

TOOL: TST Priority Problem Worksheet

What it is: A form that records information from Moment-by-Moment Assessments to facilitate decisions about the TST priority problems.

When to use it: During the treatment planning process to arrive at a decision about the TST priority problems that will be addressed in treatment. To be revisited as new moment-by-moment assessments are conducted to refine understandings of the priority problems or to add new ones.

Target goals: To facilitate providers' and teams' ability to see the patterns that point to the priority problems.

The data you use to complete your TST Priority Problem Worksheet are your Moment-by-Moment Assessment sheets. If you have completed at least three, then you are ready to complete a TST Priority Problem Worksheet using that data. Look at the TST Priority Problem Worksheet in Figure 10.1. Notice that it has three rounded boxes on the left and three rounded boxes on the right. Use the boxes on the left (labeled *Perceived Threat in Present Environment*) to record information about *the threat the child perceives in the present environment.* For the three children we have just discussed, we would record the distinguishing environmental stimuli in each of the episodes. Use the boxes on the right (labeled *Shift to Survival State*) to record the characteristics of the child's reactions in each of the episodes, using the three A's. The sets of three boxes on the left and the right each point to a box that is meant to record the pattern you see of present environmental threat and survival-in-the-moment response, respectively. You should examine your data from each of these three episodes and record the pattern you see in those two central boxes. As you can see, we are playing the TST Pattern Recognition Game here. Those two central boxes are your place to play this game. Record the pattern, or the central theme, you see between the episodes for the present environmental threat and the survival-in-the-moment reaction, respectively. What should also be clear to you by now is that the contents of these two central boxes will determine how you formulate your priority problem.

TST Priority Problem Worksheet

Perceived Threat in Present Environment

Episode 1

Episode 2

Episode 3

Shift to Survival State

Episode 1

Episode 2

Episode 3

Past Trauma Environment

Pattern of Perceived Threat

Pattern of Survival-in-the-Moment

TST Priority Problem Statement

When _____ is exposed to _____
Child's name   Description of perceived threat

She/he responds by _____
                          Description of Survival State

This pattern can be understood through past experience(s) of:

_____
Description of past trauma to inform Survival State

FIGURE 10.1. TST Priority Problem Worksheet.

You'll notice two additional boxes in this worksheet:

- A box labeled *Past Trauma Environment* (at the top of worksheet)
- A box labeled *TST Priority Problem Statement* (at the bottom of worksheet)

That *Past Trauma Environment* box is where you record the features of the child's past experience of trauma that will inform how he or she responds with survival-in-the-moment in the present environment. The *TST Priority Problem Statement* box is where you put it all together with a statement of the main problem or problems you will address in treatment. Embedded in this statement is your explanation for why the child expresses the problematic emotions and/or behaviors that have led to his or her need for treatment: Your answer to the mystery of *why*. Next we describe each of these boxes and the information they should contain.

Past Trauma Environment

You have already assessed the child's trauma history and recorded it in your TST Assessment Form. We introduced the notion of trauma inference in Chapter 9. Here's where you will make your inference. Examine all you know about the child's traumatic experiences and decide what of these experiences most informs your understanding of his or her survival-in-the-moment response within the present environment. As described in Chapter 9, a child's experience of trauma is complex, especially when it occurs over long periods of time and is of multiple types of trauma. Not all features of the child's trauma experience are equally related to the child's specific pattern of survival-in-the-moment responses. As usual, we cannot presume anything. We must examine the facts we have gathered about the child's trauma history to see how they may relate to the child's expression of survival-in-the moment. By gathering the facts described in the previous chapter and looking at the patterns, we have a terrific vantage point to determine how, exactly, the child's experience of trauma may relate to his or her survival-in-the-moment responses. When we are able to determine what, exactly, it is about the trauma that sets up the child to respond in the way he or she responds, it will help us determine how to best work with the child about his or her experience of trauma.

> Not all features of the child's trauma experience are equally related to the child's specific pattern of survival-in-the-moment responses.

In the case of Tanisha, introduced in Chapter 9, her past experience of witnessing domestic violence, being put in the position of choosing between her parents, and then being taken out of their custody to live with her grandmother set her up to switch to survival states whenever her mother requested statements of loyalty. With the cases of Jason, Emily, and Briana, discussed earlier, we can surmise how their experiences of trauma may have related to their pattern of shifting to survival-in-the-moment in response to specific signals of threat. The information contained in their TST Assessment Forms will allow us to make these inferences on what features of their trauma experience are most important for understanding these patterns.

TST Priority Problems

The TST Priority Problem Worksheet in Figure 10.1 is where you put it all together. It's how you integrate the information from those two middle boxes—with the trauma history—for your *inference* about why the child shifts into survival-in-the-moment in specific contexts. In order to help you get this right (because it's *so* important), we've created a script for you to fill in the blank spaces in order to put it all together. This is the script found at the bottom TST Priority Problem Worksheet.

Let's see how we could fill in the priority problem blank spaces for Jason, Emily, and Briana. Although we have not discussed details of their trauma histories, we will give examples of how that should be completed.

Here's the blank priority problem script.

When _____ is exposed to _____ ,
Child's name   Description of perceived threat
She/he responds by _____ .
Description of Survival State
This pattern can be understood through past experience(s) of:
_____ .
Description of past trauma to inform Survival State

 Here's Jason's priority problem script . . .

When *Jason* is exposed to *Situations with other boys where Jason is expected to change clothes* ,
Child's name   Description of perceived threat
She/he responds by *Becoming terrified he will be attacked. Pushes and yells to protect himself* .
Description of Survival State
This pattern can be understood through past experience(s) of:
Sexual assault from counselor at camp. Usually initiated after boys' changing of clothes. .
Description of past trauma to inform Survival State

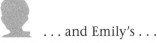

... and Emily's ...

When **Emily** _____ is exposed to *Situations where she feels disloyal to family for disclosing sexual abuse* ,
          Child's name   Description of perceived threat

She/he responds by *Feeling like she needs to be punished and die. She bangs head and punches self* .
                                       Description of Survival State

This pattern can be understood through past experience(s) of:

Sexual assault from mother's boyfriend. Then disclosure and removal from family. Told she "destroyed" her family.
                       Description of past trauma to inform Survival State

... and Briana's.

When **Briana** _____ is exposed to *Sexual images. Images of a muscular male body.* ,
          Child's name   Description of perceived threat

She/he responds by *Feeling nauseous, then terrified, then cuts arms and/or legs.* .
                                       Description of Survival State

This pattern can be understood through past experience(s) of:

Sexual assault from uncle. Always began when he entered the bedroom and removed his shirt.
                       Description of past trauma to inform Survival State

Now you have the information you need to define the problems that will be your foci of treatment, and these definitions serve as your explanation for why the traumatized children you work with have the problems that they have. You will notice that the first section of the TST Treatment Plan consists of three priority problem scripts (in case there is more than one priority problem). You should complete these scripts exactly as we have just described.

A child may, of course, have more than one priority problem. For a child who assaults others in an enraged state and who cuts him- or herself in a frightened/ashamed state, you need enough Moment-by-Moment Assessments to be confident about the nature of these two priority problems (at least three "dots" or Moment-by-Moment Assessments per priority problem).

We've included a completed TST Priority Problem Worksheet for Tanisha in Appendix 5 and Figure 10.2.

TST Priority Problem Worksheet

Perceived Threat in Present Environment

Episode 1

Mother arrived unannounced. Asked for hug. Whispered that grandmother can't love her because she is not her mother.

Episode 2

Grandmother asked her to spend time with other kids when she wanted to do something else.

Episode 3

Girl told her not to be friends with other girl. Asked if she was "best friend."

Past Trauma Environment

History of neglect and witnessing family violence. Multiple foster home placements. Coercive communication about love and loyalty.

Shift to Survival State

Episode 1

Became enraged. Ran at grandmother. Tried to punch and kick her.

Episode 2

Became enraged, yelled at grandmother. Broke furniture. Threw glass.

Episode 3

Became enraged and knocked girl to ground, kicking her.

Pattern of Perceived Threat

Put in loyalty conflict by others where she must choose between people.

Pattern of Survival-in-the-Moment

Becomes enraged related to loyalty bind and responds with aggressive behavior and some dissociation.

TST Priority Problem Statement

When ___Tanisha___ is exposed to ___loyalty binds/choosing between people___,
    Child's name   Description of perceived threat

She/he responds by ___becoming enraged, aggressive, and dissociative___.
                             Description of Survival State

This pattern can be understood through past experience(s) of:

___neglect, witness to violence, coercive communication re. loyalty___.
             Description of past trauma to inform Survival State

FIGURE 10.2. Completed TST Priority Problem Worksheet for Tanisha.

199

Other Problems That Will Be Addressed in Treatment

We've spent a lot of time defining the TST priority problem and detailing how you arrive at it. If you get this right, your treatment is set up to be very effective. You will know the patterns of how a traumatized child shifts to survival-in-the-moment in specific types of situations. In many cases you will be the first to understand how and why this child feels and behaves the way he or she feels and behaves. You also may have clarified the mystery of *why*. This understanding brings the possibility of helping the child escape from being perpetually haunted by his or her past. You may now have an understanding about exactly what it was about the child's trauma history that leads him or her to respond with survival-laden emotion and behavior in situations that other children tolerate very well. As we will describe in other sections of this chapter, all of this information becomes critically important to set up an effective treatment. As we've said before: If you have this information, a lot of good things can happen. And if you don't have this information . . . we don't know how you can help the child.

> Any problem that you choose to address will take your time and focus away from the priority problem(s) you have defined. Are you sure you have the time and energy to focus on these other problems?

Are we now done with defining the problem(s)? Maybe. There may, however, be other problems that could be addressed in treatment. In the previous chapter, we defined the categories of "other" problems as (1) comorbid psychiatric and developmental disorders, (2) enduring trauma-related cognitions, and (3) social problems. Remember, if any of these are integrally related to the TST priority problem, then they are not "other" problems; they should be addressed with the priority problem. In this section, we are focused on problems that are present but are not directly related to the priority problem. Should they be addressed? Only if they are believed to be really important. Any problem that you choose to address will take your time and focus away from the priority problem(s) you have defined. Are you sure you have the time and energy to focus on these other problems? Don't underestimate what it will take to be successful in addressing a priority problem.

> Don't underestimate what it will take to be successful in addressing a priority problem.

We also have a way out for you, if you feel you really must put other problems into your treatment plan: the beyond trauma phase of TST. As we briefly outline in another section of this chapter, and detail in Chapter 14, *beyond trauma* is the phase where the child is no longer shifting into survival-in-the-moment and the environment is helpful and protective enough. In this phase, we do focus on the enduring trauma-related cognitions. We also focus on problems that could not be addressed, given the immediacy of other problems that were prioritized. In this phase, for example, other comorbid psychiatric problems may become more salient. If you have identified other problems that might be addressed, see if they can wait until the beyond trauma phase. If you have identified a problem that is important enough and cannot wait for the beyond trauma phase to be addressed, you should put it in your treatment plan for focus in whatever phase the child needs. Just don't put too many other problems here. Record your decision in Section 1.b of your TST Treatment Plan.

One last item before moving to the next section: Sometimes a child is referred who is pretty well regulated and his or her environment is helpful and protective enough. In such children, the reason for referral often relates to their enduring trauma-related cognitions. These children will start TST in the beyond trauma phase and these enduring trauma-related cognitions will be the focus of their treatment.

Section 2: Why Are the Child's Problems Important and to Whom Are They Important?

In the previous section, we detailed the critical process of defining the TST priority problem(s) that will become our treatment focus. We also described the process for deciding whether to address other problems in treatment. In this section, we decide on the relative priority of the problems we have chosen to address (if more than one), based on the observed impact on the child, and others, if the problem is left untreated.

Arriving at clarity on the impact of the selected problems is important for reasons other than to assign priority to the problems. The effort we expend to advocate for services for the child will be optimized by a high degree of clarity in relating the impact of the problem on the child. Clarity about level of impact is also an important component when appraising the level of concern experienced by the child, and those around him or her, about the problem in question. Any difference between our degree of concern and the concern felt by others is very important to recognize and understand. It is critical to reconcile such a disconnection in the process of treatment engagement. All the information needed to make these decisions has been gathered and recorded in the TST Assessment Form. As usual, use the information in that form to make your decisions (and record your decisions in the right place in Section 2 of your TST Treatment Plan).

> Any difference between our degree of concern and the concern felt by others is very important to recognize and understand. It is critical to reconcile such a disconnection in the process of treatment engagement.

The Order of Priority of the TST Priority Problem(s) and Any Other Identified Problem(s)

The priority of the problems you have identified should be based on your appraisal of the impact of the problems on the child and others. Use the information you have gathered during the assessment process and decide the priority here. Record your decision in Section 2.a of the TST Treatment Plan.

The Strategy to Engage the Child and Family to Address the Identified Problem(s)

Here's where you will see if it will be easy or hard to engage the child and family. Do you and they see the impact of the problem the same or differently? If you and they see it differently, what is your strategy to reconcile this difference? Without such reconciliation, there will be no possibility of treatment engagement. Of course, the child and family members may see things very differently among themselves—which is why any engagement strategy will need to be defined in relation to each of the individuals you need to engage.

In this section of the TST Treatment Plan, record the level of concern expressed by the individuals you need to engage about the problems you have defined as the focus of treatment and your strategy to reconcile any differences in concern. Hopefully, everyone is on the same page. If someone is not on the same page, you need to decide: What's the problem and its fix? Perhaps the problem is simply missing information. Maybe the child and or/family member doesn't have enough information to know why you are so concerned about the problem. The effort to reconcile the differences in levels of concern may then be simple: Communicate better! Let them know more about why you are so concerned. If that's what you see as the problem, record your plan to communicate with the relevant individuals here.

While we are discussing the matter of communication, we have to acknowledge that it is a two-way street. Maybe the reason you and a key player do not share the level of concern is because *you* are missing information. Your strategy may then include ways to help the child or family member say what is on his or her mind. Differences in level of concern about a problem will often have a more complex cause than simply a lack of sufficient understanding. The differences often relate to what are more immediate and tangible concerns, *to them*, the child and family members, than are the problems we say need to be addressed in treatment.

Remember Edward's mother, introduced in Chapter 9? Her pain over being alone, without a partner, may be so immediate and tangible that anything we say about Edward's priority problem will not receive her attention because it is unrelated to her overriding concern. But what if we helped her make a clear connection between her pain and Edward's priority problem? If we are successful here, we open the possibility for real treatment engagement. Recall an important reason that Edward's mother could not establish a stable relationship with a man: because, as she stated, any man she brings home "runs for the hills" when he sees Edward's "disrespect." If we successfully address Edward's priority problem, it is possible that he will be in better behavioral control when his mother brings a man home. From Edward's mother's perspective, the only problem she has the capacity to focus on is her loneliness. That's fine. That will be our main focus, with her, too.

The best way to establish a successful engagement strategy is to align the problems we see with whatever the people we work with see as most important. If the child and family tangibly see that our effort to address the problem we believe is most important will also address the problem *they* see as most important, we will have our treatment alliance. Our strategy in this section must successfully make this connection.

The best way to establish a successful engagement strategy is to align the problems we see with whatever the people we work with see as most important.

Fortunately, we have already assessed what is most important to the child and family and recorded it in Section 2 of the TST Assessment Form in Appendix 2. Let's examine what we have recorded—what we see as the child's main problems—and see if our effort to improve that problem could result in improvements in what the child and family see as most important. If we can see this possibility, let's record it in Section 2.c of the TST Treatment Plan. In the next chapter, on treatment engagement, we detail how to turn this *plan* to engage the child and family into a treatment that *actually* engages the child and family.

The Strategy to Engage Others Concerned about the Child's Problems

Of course, do your best to engage the child and family. It is critically important. What about other people? During the assessment process, have you identified anyone else who is very concerned about the child's problem(s) and who might be able to help? Who are these people, and how can they help? You've gathered this information already. Record your decisions about this in Section 2.c of your TST Treatment Plan.

Section 3: What Interventions Will Be Used to Address the Child's Problem(s)?

You've made your decisions about the problems that will be the focus for TST treatment, so now you need to decide *how* to treat those problems. This section is about making those decisions. The first part of making these decisions involves deciding with which of the three phases of TST treatment the child should start. Once that is decided, a lot about what you will do in treatment becomes clear. In Chapters 12, 13, and 14 we describe the three treatment phases of safety-focused treatment, regulation-focused treatment, and beyond trauma treatment, respectively. Once you have decided on the treatment phase to initiate, you will then draft an overall strategy for how you will address the child's problems. This is a statement that broadly states your plan for reducing the *cat hair* and helping the child build regulation skills in the face of the cat hair. Finally, your treatment plan will include a statement of roles and expectation. Who on the team will do what? You also should be clear about the roles and expectations of the child and family members in treatment. Let's take these one at a time.

The Phase of Treatment to Initiate

We are about to describe what may be the easiest decision to make in TST: the treatment phase to initiate. Recall your effort in assessment to categorize the child's trauma system. You needed to decide whether the child you assessed fits within one of three categories of *vulnerability to switching into survival states*. Then you decided whether the child's social environment fit within one of three categories of *ability to help and protect* the child. If you forget all this, here's a reminder: You recorded all this in Section 3.a of the TST Assessment Form. Take a look to remind yourself. Remember? Good. Now the really easy part: Open your TST Treatment Plan to Section 3.a. Look at a tool called the TST Treatment Planning Grid. Now allow the magic to happen . . .

The TST Treatment Planning Grid, shown in Figure 10.3 (and Section 3.a of the Treatment Plan), puts the information together about the trauma system to indicate which phase to use. Simply put your assessment of shifting into survival states on the vertical axis and your assessment of available social-environmental help and protection on the horizontal axis. Look for their point of intersection and—*presto*—you have your TST phase! Nothing more complicated than this. If, for example, you assessed the child as switching into survival states and the environment to have insufficient ability to help and protect, you look for the point of intersection on the grid—it's *regulation-focused*—and that's your phase! Alternatively, if you assessed the child as switching into dangerous survival states and the environment as harmful, the treatment phase is . . . *safety-focused*!

TST Treatment Planning Grid		The Environment's Help and Protection		
		Helpful and Protective	Insufficiently Helpful and Protective	Harmful
The Child's Survival States	No Survival States	Beyond trauma	Beyond trauma	Safety-focused
	Survival States	Regulation-focused	Regulation-focused	Safety-focused
	Dangerous Survival States	Regulation-focused	Safety-focused	Safety-focused

FIGURE 10.3. TST Treatment Planning Grid.

Now that you know the phases, what do they mean? The treatment phase is a primary way that we orient interventions within TST. Each phase connotes a set of interventions appropriate to the needs of the child, within his or her social environment. Your experience tells you that a child who switches into *survival states* and lives within an environment that is *insufficiently helpful and protective* will need something very different than a child who shifts into *dangerous survival states* and lives in a *harmful environment*. Our treatment implementation chapters (Chapters 12, 13, and 14) describe the interventions delivered within each of these three phases. We briefly summarize these phases next.

> The treatment phase is a primary way that we orient interventions within TST. Each phase connotes a set of interventions appropriate to the needs of the child, within his or her social environment.

Safety-Focused Treatment

The primary goal of the safety-focused phase of TST is to establish and maintain safety and stability in the child's social environment and to minimize risk to the child and to others, based on his or her difficulty with survival-in-the-moment states. This intensive home- and community-based phase of treatment is always offered if the social environment is considered harmful, or if the child is at risk to switch into a dangerous survival state and those in the child's environment are not sufficiently helpful and protective. This phase of treatment is organized around activities that build the capacity of those around the child to help and protect.

> The primary goal of the safety-focused phase of TST is to establish and maintain safety and stability in the child's social environment and to minimize risk to the child and to others, based on his or her difficulty with survival-in-the-moment states.

Regulation-Focused Treatment

> The primary goal of the regulation-focused phase is to give the child sufficient skills to manage emotional states when triggered by perceived threats.

The primary goal of the regulation-focused phase is to give the child sufficient skills to manage emotional states when triggered by perceived threats. Unlike treatment delivered in the safety-focused phase, treatment delivered in the regulation-focused phase may occur in the clinic or office. Regulation-focused treatment phase is offered when the child continues to have difficulties due to shifting to survival states (and given that the environment is considered safe). If the child shifts into dangerous survival states, the environment must be sufficiently helpful and protective for this phase of treatment to apply. This phase of treatment is organized around activities that build the child's capacity to regulate emotional states, and the capacity of those around the child to help him or her with this self-regulation.

Beyond Trauma Treatment

> The primary goal of the beyond trauma phase is to work with the child and family to gain sufficient perspective on the trauma experience so that the trauma no longer defines the child's view of the self, world, and future.

The primary goal of the beyond trauma phase is to work with the child and family to gain sufficient perspective on the trauma experience so that the trauma no longer defines the child's view of the self, world, and future. We are primarily working with those enduring trauma-related cognitions in this phase. Learning cognitive skills and processing the trauma characterize this phase, which is typically offered when the social environment is stable and the child is sufficiently able to regulate emotional states.

The Overall Strategy to Address the Identified TST Priority Problems and Other Identified Problems

In the previous section you decided which of the three treatment phases you would offer the child at the start of TST treatment. In this section you should note the overall strategy you will use to address the problems you have identified, within that first phase of treatment. You don't need to provide a large amount of detail here: just the basics. What will be your overall approach to addressing the child's problems within that first treatment phase? How will you address the threats you have identified in the environment? How will you enhance the child's capacity to regulate his or her emotional states? Using the examples of Jason, Emily, and Briana, whose TST priority problems were described in a previous section of this chapter, we show their overall treatment strategy statement next. This is the statement written in Section 3.b of the child's TST Treatment Plan.

Here's Jason's treatment strategy:

> Jason shifts into survival-in-the-moment in situations when he is required to remove his clothes when other boys are present. This vulnerability can be understood through his experience of sexual abuse by a camp counselor. In these situations he feels panicked and then yells and pushes other boys so that adults will respond and help him. Let's create the situation that he doesn't feel he has to push for protection and yell for help. We'll create an atmosphere of safety to talk about this situation with Jason and his parents. They will help him anticipate and manage this problem at sleepovers and trouble spots like locker rooms, swimming pools, and public restrooms. We will also share this information (with Jason and his family's permission) with the school to help him in these trouble spots in that context. We'll also try to build Jason's emotional regulation skills so that he can manage these situations without getting aggressive.

Here's Emily's . . .

> Emily is in a crisis situation. She has recently disclosed sexual abuse by her mother's partner, Jerry. Jerry has been arrested and Emily's mother blames her. Emily feels she has "destroyed her family" because that is what she was told after she disclosed the abuse, and her mother's statements to her continue to reinforce this idea. Emily shifts to survival-in-the-moment with suicidal thoughts and head banging in situations that remind her of what she believes her disclosure of the abuse did to her family. These situations include discussions with her mother, making police statements, and recently seeing a television show with family loyalty as a theme. We need to protect her now. She has recently been placed in foster care. We need to establish clear expectations about communications from the mother as part of Emily's child welfare service plan. All calls with the mother should be monitored. We should work with Emily to anticipate all police interviews and, if possible, to accompany her. We need to build her emotional regulation skills for these interviews and for any other situations when she would need to talk about the abuse. We also should talk with her about her notion that saying something to her teacher that led to the abuse being stopped was an act of disloyalty to her family.

And now to Briana's . . .

> Briana shifts into survival-in-the-moment in situations where she sees sexually provocative images, particularly related to images that remind her of her uncle's body. In such situations she feels nauseous, and then terrified, and she cuts her arms and sometimes legs to manage those emotions. As a teenager, it will be hard to protect her from all such images. But now that we recognize their impact, we can work with her to anticipate them. We can help her to be more careful of the movies she goes to and the TV shows she watches. Perhaps she can talk with trusted friends about being more careful of the images she is exposed to and to identify a friend to whom she can go for help if she notices that a shift is underway, with feelings of nausea on the rise. We should talk with her about letting her mother and school know about her vulnerability. We should definitely work to build her emotional regulation skills when she is exposed to these types of images.

The fact that nausea is a signal for her that survival-in-the-moment may be occurring will be helpful for treatment.

The Roles and Expectations of Each Member of the Team (Including the Child and Family Members)

The clearer we are about everyone's roles and expectations, the more effective we will be in delivering our treatment. How do we decide who is going to do what? We've more or less already done this with our treatment strategy statements.

In this section of the treatment plan, we decide who is going to do what, who is responsible for what. This includes all members of the treatment team who will be working with the child and the family. It also includes the roles and expectations of the child and family, themselves. The clearer we are about everyone's roles and expectations, the more effective we will be in delivering our treatment. How do we decide who is going to do what? We've more or less already done this with our treatment strategy statements. Take a look at the treatment strategy statements for each of the three children described above. If the statements are done well, they should take you well on your way to defining who is going to do what. Then fill in the charts in Section 3.c and 3.d of the TST Treatment Plan. In the next chapter, we discuss how you develop a solid agreement with the child and family about the items specified in this section.

Section 4: What Strengths Will Be Used to Address the Child's Problems?

 There are two important principles to keep in mind as you make decisions about how to leverage strengths to address the problems you have identified and to engage the family:

1. Build from strength (Principle 9).
2. Put scarce resources where they'll work (Principle 5).

The applicability of "build from strength" is obvious enough. What about scarce resources? In a world of scarce resources (which, yes, is what we live in) we cannot afford to try interventions that don't have a good chance of working. By "cannot afford," we don't just mean that it's too expensive and that insurance companies might get mad. We mean that *we can't afford to fail* with families. We can't afford to ask them to do something that is too hard, or not a good fit, or makes them feel demoralized because it just wasn't possible. Think of it this way. A girl joins a track team. She's tall, and runs fast, and jumps far, but has weak arms. Don't ask her to do only shot-putting on her first day out. Build her confidence, get her running and doing the long-jump. Don't lose her engagement, and don't set her up for a humiliating defeat right off the bat.

Same with treatment: Find the strengths and build your interventions *there*. The child hates to write but loves to draw? Integrate art. A parent has deep religious convictions and a strong church community? Bring those into play. Whatever the problems are, build interventions that take into

> Find the strengths and build your interventions *there*.

account the strengths of the child, family, and environment. We bring the professional resources to help solve the problem(s), but we sell everyone short if those are the only resources we will consider using. Children and families and their environments may well have strengths that could make a big difference. We've already assessed what they are and recorded them in the TST Assessment Form. Now we put that information together with everything else we have decided. We are particularly focused on the strengths that may be used to help the child regulate emotion.

The job here is to answer the following question: Given the problems I have decided are most important to address in treatment, and the strengths I have identified in the child, family, and environment, what strengths will be most important for helping with the problem(s)?

> Given the problems I have decided are most important to address in treatment, and the strengths I have identified in the child, family, and environment, what strengths will be most important for helping with the problem(s)?

Here's one more question you can ask (and then write the answer in Section 4 of the treatment plan):

What is the best way to use the strengths I have just identified, for helping with the problem(s) that need to be addressed?

Section 5: What Will Interfere with Addressing the Child's Problems?

We don't have a magical answer for what to do about poor mass transit systems, busy schedules, or any of the other multitudinous reasons a family might not be able to engage in treatment. But we do know that unless you start with a clear understanding of what the issues are, you won't solve them. We also don't have a simple answer for how to address families' psychoeducational needs. It all depends on how much they understand about trauma, its impact, and mental health intervention. You've assessed all of this and recorded the information in Section 5 of the TST Assessment Form. Take all that information out. Here is where you begin to develop your approach to addressing these issues. In the next chapter, on treatment engagement, we talk about these concerns in a lot more detail. In that chapter, we describe the kinds of practical barriers families typically face and possible ways around them. Time to get creative! Figuring out how to help a family get the right bus might not seem like the most important intervention you'll ever do, but if you don't do it . . . you won't ever get to those important interventions.

Closing Thoughts on TST Treatment Planning

We began this chapter by describing the importance of taking the information you have gathered in assessment and making decisions in five categories that will answer the five TST treatment planning questions. As we have described, the answers to these questions form the TST Treatment Plan, and the purpose of this chapter was to help you learn how to complete one. A well-constructed treatment plan will make the difference between a treatment that engages children and families, focuses on the right problems, and successfully addresses these problems, from a treatment that will not succeed in these critical functions. Once your treatment is set up, you will spend a great deal of time and energy with a child and family to try to help them. You will also ask children and families to expend a great deal of their time and energy—and they will dedicate this time and energy if they have hope that you can help them. This is a great responsibility. Please make sure you have dedicated sufficient time and energy to setting up your treatment plan in the way we have described. It's very important. To give you a little more help, we've included a copy of Tanisha's completed TST Treatment Plan in Appendix 6.

> A well-constructed treatment plan will make the difference between a treatment that engages children and families, focuses on the right problems, and successfully addresses these problems, from a treatment that will not succeed in these critical functions.

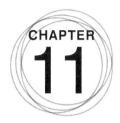

Ready–Set–Go

Treatment Engagement

LEARNING OBJECTIVES

- To learn how to form a treatment agreement with the child and family members
- To learn how to create a treatment agreement letter from the TST Treatment Plan
- To learn how you can "go" to treatment implementation

ICONS USED IN THIS CHAPTER

Essential Point	Case Illustration	Key tool

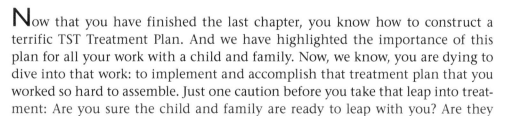

Now that you have finished the last chapter, you know how to construct a terrific TST Treatment Plan. And we have highlighted the importance of this plan for all your work with a child and family. Now, we know, you are dying to dive into that work: to implement and accomplish that treatment plan that you worked so hard to assemble. Just one caution before you take that leap into treatment: Are you sure the child and family are ready to leap with you? Are they (and you) ready to go? Do you have time for a parable before you take that leap? Please don't leap quite yet . . .

Imagine, for a moment, that you are deeply concerned about Problem A. You journey to a mountaintop to seek counsel with a wiseman. After listening to your problem, the wiseman nods knowingly and tells you he knows the solution to Problem B. You are a bit confused, since you sought counsel regarding Problem A, but you listen. The wiseman then proceeds to list a series of arduous, painful, and seemingly irrelevant tasks that you must perform in order to solve Problem B. He tells you not to expect Problem B to disappear right away even if you do perform these tasks, but to trust that this is the answer to Problem B. He then sends you on your way and requests that you return to his mountaintop next week.

Would you do it? Would you put your own concerns about Problem A aside to focus on Problem B, and put your effort into tasks that you had little faith would make a difference? Probably not. And we wouldn't blame you for it.

The point of the parable is the need to make sure that we understand what is most important and concerning to the child and family before we design a treatment to address anything else. If a person comes to us for help with Problem A and we design a treatment for Problem B, we should not be surprised about that person's hesitancy to leap into treatment with us. Fortunately, the information you have already collected in your assessment and the decisions you have already made in your treatment plan give you a great vantage point from which to join with the family in a treatment that will address *their* Problem A. You already know what is most concerning to the child and family, whether your conception of the problem is concerning to them, and have thought through how the treatment you plan will be directed to their Problem A.

This chapter is called Ready–Set–Go because it is about what you need to make sure is in place in order to move forward with treatment implementation. What needs to be in place?: a child and family who are fully engaged in what you plan. Once what we review in this chapter is in place . . . you are ready to go! And so are they! Together with you!

This chapter is divided into three parts:

1. The treatment agreement
2. The treatment agreement letter from the TST Treatment Plan
3. Finalizing the treatment agreement (so that you can—finally—*go!*)

In the first part, we expand on our discussion from Chapters 9 and 10 on the importance of understanding what is most concerning to the child and family so that you can develop a strong-enough agreement about what the treatment will address and the expectations of all parties.

In the second part, we take the TST Treatment Plan you have assembled and translate it into a format that is clear and tangible to the family, so that you may reach an agreement. This format is a letter written from the TST team to the family that, in a language tangible to them, specifies the treatment elements and what agreeing to participate in it would entail. This letter will specify the role of every member of the team who will work with the family, and what the family should expect of each team member based on their respective roles. This letter also specifies what is expected of the child and family. We call this letter the *treatment agreement letter* and it is a way of implementing the engagement strategy that you drafted in Section 2 of your TST Treatment Plan.

In the third part, we describe the process of sharing the treatment agreement letter with the family so that an agreement will be reached. This process includes our effort to troubleshoot practical barriers to treatment engagement, and to make sure the child and family have sufficient knowledge about trauma, its impact, and mental health treatment to make an informed agreement. *Ready–set–go* begins with our drafting of this treatment agreement letter and ends when we have reached a good-enough agreement with the child and family on the "terms" of this letter. Reaching this agreement means that you never will implement an intervention for Problem B, when the family came to you for help with Problem A.

The Treatment Agreement: What It Is

Let's start with a *thorny* discussion. Remember when we reviewed organizational planning in Chapter 8 and described the challenge that Susan, the clinical director of a busy mental health clinic, faced in trying to engage her boss, Linda, in decision making to support her planned TST program? The only way for Susan to have that type of conversation was if the conversation, in some way, addressed what we described as Linda's major source of pain. We used the example of Androcles, who pulled the thorn out of the lion's paw. Linda would not be engaged until Susan figured out what the thorn in Linda's paw looked like and developed a strategy for removing it. When you think of engaging people in treatment, the example of Androcles and the lion is relevant. What are the thorns in the paws of the individuals we need to engage?

Why start a discussion on the treatment agreement with a description of thorns and paws? A real agreement can *only* address thorns in paws. Agreements require engagement. They require people to keep their word with another person, and keeping their word usually entails doing something that they would not ordinarily do. And why should they do it? Why should they expend the time and effort to keep agreements, which usually means doing things they would not ordinarily do? They will do these things to keep their agreement because they have hope that it will result in the removal of that thorn from their paw. This is how we all work. We will only expend time and effort to do things that we would not ordinarily do, if we have some hope it would result in a benefit we desire. In this regard, we are no different from the children and families who are in our care. We all have our thorns. We will only make and keep agreements if we have a hope that the agreements will result in the thorn's removal. Our treatment agreements, therefore, must *only* be about thorn removal.

Remember Edward's mother. We faced a challenge engaging her because she was so overwhelmed and so distraught by her loneliness and the absence of a male partner, that we were not able to get her attention unless we could figure out how Edward's problem and her sources of pain fit together. This loneliness due to the lack of a partner was Edward's mother's thorn in the paw. Helping Edward contain his behavior when his mother brought a man home was a part of pulling the thorn out of her paw. Once we determined this integral relationship between her thorn and what we saw as Edward's priority problem, then we were able to engage her enough to form a real treatment agreement. And that is how we constructed our engagement strategy in Section 2 of the TST Treatment Plan. We need to go through this process with all the children and families who come to us for help; this is exactly the process of achieving a treatment agreement.

We need to engage Edward as well. Remember from Chapter 9 how we identified that Edward has wanted all his life to become a police officer, to "get that badge." Our strategy for engaging with him centers on this goal. Edward may not believe he can achieve his goal, or may not see how he can overcome the barriers. Our job is to help him see the pattern between his behaviors (skipping school, fighting, smoking marijuana, getting arrested) and what is triggering these behaviors, and how this pattern is a barrier to becoming a police officer. If we can help him to believe that working with us can help to overcome these barriers, we have a chance of getting him to sign on as a member of the team.

The Treatment Alliance and the Treatment Agreement

The treatment agreement is very much the same as the treatment alliance. What does it mean to have a strong treatment alliance? Some believe that a strong treatment alliance simply means that we share positive regard with the people we work with; that is, we like each other and want to work together. The treatment alliance in TST is much more specific. It involves the provider, child, and family *agreeing on the specific problem* that must be worked on and also *agreeing on a plan for how to solve this problem*. Since agreements are so central to the treatment alliance, we simply use the term *treatment agreement*. In order for these types of agreements to occur, they must first be based on a shared understanding of thorns and their removal. The provider needs to communicate clearly—and with a great deal of respect and genuineness—with the child and family. For children and families to be able to do the work that we will ask them to do, they need to know clearly, up front, what this work will entail, how this work might plausibly address their greatest concerns, and that they are being asked to do this work by a real person who cares about them and respects them. Anything less will not work.

Agreeing on the Problem, the Solution, and the Central Role of Hope

Parents bring children to treatment for a lot of different reasons. Sometimes they come because they are worried about their child. Sometimes they come because their child is driving them crazy. And sometimes they come because someone else is making them. What the parents see as the problem might look really different depending on why they are coming for treatment. Is the problem that their child is sad a lot? Or that the furniture in the house keeps getting broken? Or that DSS won't get off the family's back?

You have already assessed the problems that you believe are most important to the child and family. During ready–set–go, you will make sure you've gotten this right. You, of course, know that you are not likely to get too far if you are heading down the road in search of a solution to a problem that the parent doesn't see, and meanwhile are ignoring all the red flags the parent is waving to get help for what he or she does see as the real problem. So the first step is to come to some agreement on the problem.

> The first step is to come to some agreement on the problem.

You have also already drafted your ideas about the solution. This is your strategy for intervening. How, exactly, will the treatment you propose serve to remove the thorns that the child and family have told you about? Remember, this undertaking requires *hope*. When you communicate your ideas about the solution, the child and family will agree to participate only if they have hope that your solution will lead to the removal of their thorns. Sometimes children and families seek mental health treatment as a last resort—they've tried everything, and nothing has worked. Will this be any different?

Hope can be offered to families in different ways. Of course, no one can predict the future of any given child. But we *do* know a lot about kids generally, and about how they can recover from trauma more specifically. We know that, with enough time and energy and support, treatment really works! Part of the education you provide to the parent about TST will help to spark this hope.

Once the parent has a sense of hope that you and TST may be able to do something to help, you can get more specific about *how* you will be working together to fix things. Parents need to know, and agree to up front about, whatever goes into the treatment. If home-based care will be involved, spend some time talking with the parent about how this might help. If you are making a psychopharmacology referral, share your rationale and learn what the parent's attitude toward medication is.

Let's review another child and family:

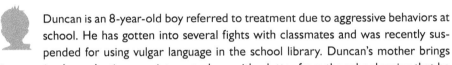 Duncan is an 8-year-old boy referred to treatment due to aggressive behaviors at school. He has gotten into several fights with classmates and was recently suspended for using vulgar language in the school library. Duncan's mother brings him to an intake evaluation appointment, along with a letter from the school saying that he cannot return to school until he receives a psychological evaluation. In the course of this first meeting, she becomes tearful as she describes the violent relationship she has had with Duncan's father, the financial difficulties she has faced since she moved out on her own 2 months ago, and her feelings of being overwhelmed by "having to handle Duncan" all on her own. She works at an office in the filing department, but has had to leave work so many times to get Duncan from school when he misbehaves that she is afraid that she will be fired. In fact, she says that she missed work again to come to this appointment today.

Following the intake appointment, the therapist schedules a weekly meeting. They miss the first appointment. After a phone call from the therapist, they reschedule for the following week. They again miss the appointment.

When a family repeatedly misses appointments or doesn't come back after an evaluation, it's easy to dismiss it as "They're being resistant" or "They're not ready for treatment." Unfortunately, however, often the very families that are not able to commit to regular treatment are the ones that are in the greatest distress.

> Often the very families that are not able to commit to regular treatment are the ones that are in the greatest distress.

In the case of Duncan, his mother is clearly overwhelmed—in part because of Duncan's behavior problems. Duncan himself is dealing with a history of witnessing serious violence at home, the recent transition of having moved out from living with his dad, and significant stressors in the financial and emotional environment at home. From this vantage point, safely behind this book we're reading, it seems pretty clear that TST could really help this family. But what does it look like from Mom's point of view? One more meeting (or more!) a week, missing more work, paying money to get the bus to the clinic. Basically a lot of stress and hassle and work, and it's all for Duncan—who she's pretty angry with anyway ("Why can't you just *behave* at school??!").

Until Mom shares an understanding of why treatment could help, and until some of her very real problems are solved (how *can* she get her kid to appointments without losing her job?), she will never *really* agree to treatment (she may *say* she agrees, but that's a very different issue). Or, more to the point, addressing these issues *is* the way to reach a real agreement.

Pulling the Thorn Out of Duncan's Mom's Paw

What are the thorns in Duncan's mother's paw? She clearly has several thorns, but there are one or two with which your treatment can directly help her. She is continually called from school about Duncan's behavior and needs to leave work so much that she worries she will lose her job. This problem is real, and meaningful, and it will be hard for Duncan's mother to focus on anything else with this type of pain in her paw. Therefore, Duncan's mother must clearly and tangibly see that, should she engage in treatment, there is a real possibility that this thorn will be removed from her paw. She must have enough hope to agree.

The Treatment Agreement Letter from the TST Treatment Plan

In the previous section, we reviewed the treatment agreement. Filter every request you make to a child and family member through the following question: Do I have a strong-enough treatment agreement to reasonably make this request? If you are not sure that your agreement is strong enough, seek consultation. Ask your team. Ask your supervisor. You don't want to move forward with treatment if you are not confident about this. How to best build this confidence? Draft a treatment agreement letter (and *get agreement* from the child and parent).

> The treatment alliance is very specific. It involves the provider, child, and family *agreeing on the specific problem* that must be worked on and also *agreeing on a plan for how to solve this problem*.

What is this *treatment agreement letter*? This is your effort to translate your TST Treatment Plan into a language and format that will be most tangible to the child and family, so that they may reach an agreement with you. Your treatment plan is written in a format that fits for you, your team, and your organization. It is written in a relatively technical language. The *treatment agreement letter* takes the content of your treatment plan and translates key components of it into a language and format that are most immediate and tangible to the child and family. This letter will eventually become a living, breathing document. It will guide your work in each encounter with the child and family. *Ready–set–go* ends when you reach a good-enough agreement with the child and family that they will "sign off" on this agreement letter.

A blank copy of this treatment agreement letter is provided in Appendix 6. In this section we describe its various components. We recommend that you read this section with a copy of this agreement letter and the treatment plan in front of you. You need to understand the crosswalk between them. As you see, the treatment agreement letter has eight sections. We will go through each.

What Is Most Important to the Child and Family?

1. **Our work will be about helping you achieve what is most important to you. We understand that what is most important to you is:**

This part of the agreement letter comes from Section 2 of the TST Treatment Plan. We have already assessed what you believe is most important to the child and family and decided which of these will be most important to anchor the treatment. What you put here could fit within categories of sources of pain, concerns, or life goals and priorities—it doesn't matter. What does matter is that whatever you cite in this letter is *very* important to the child and family. Your agreement must be based on *thorns*—make sure this section is filled with them. Put whatever you think is most important for the child and family members separately. Remember our discussion in the previous chapter. Whatever we put down here should be specific enough and achievable. Of course, make sure that you write in a language that is most tangible for the child and family.

Noting the Strengths

2. **We believe you have several strengths that will really help you to achieve what is most important to you. These strengths are:**

> It powerfully supports our relationships if we show the people we work with that we know what their strengths are and we have thought through how these strengths can help in their treatment.

As detailed in the previous chapter, strengths are very important for many reasons. Leading with problems interferes with engagement. Who wants to spend time with someone who thinks they are a bundle of problems? We lead with strengths here. It powerfully supports our relationships if we show the people we work with that we know what their strengths are and we have thought through how these strengths can help in their treatment. You have already collected this information and recorded it in Section 4 of the TST Treatment Plan. Write about the strengths here, in the best way you know how, to engage the child and family member(s).

Noting the Problems

3. **We have identified a number of problems that we believe should be the focus of the treatment. These problems are:**

Here is the place to list the problems that you have spent so much time defining. These are the priority problems, and any other problems, that you have decided are important enough to address. You have also thought through the impact of these problems on the child's functioning and healthy development. Here's the place to clearly state what you see as the problem or problems and why you think they are so important. You've developed an understanding of the episodes of problematic emotion and/or behavior. In many cases the child and family believe there is no explanation or ability to predict these painful episodes. Or, the explanations they give may completely stigmatize the child (e.g., he or she is "crazy," "chemically imbalanced," "possessed," or "manipulative"). Here's your chance to communicate an understanding that may give them some hope. If appropriate at this point, you can also communicate your understanding of how the child's trauma history is related to the way he or she feels or behaves. Of course, this information comes from Section 1 of the TST Treatment Plan.

Impact of Identified Problems

4. **These problems make what is most important to you worse. The way these problems can make what is most important to you worse, is:**

In this section, write how you believe the problems you have identified can impact what you understand is most important to the child and family. You have already considered this matter and recorded it in Section 2 of the TST Treatment Plan. This is the space where you will communicate your intention to *pull out thorns*. Your treatment alliance will depend on what you write here.

Presenting the Intervention Plans

5. **Here is what we will do to help:**

You have recorded how you will address the problems in Section 3 of the treatment plan. You've put together an overall treatment strategy and decided which team member will be responsible for what. Here's where you write all of this, clearly. You want to make sure this is written in a user-friendly language so that the family truly knows what to expect from the treatment team. If there are other providers/agencies that you have engaged in the treatment plan, because their work is essential to address the defined problem(s) (e.g., child welfare case worker, teacher), list them here and make sure they sign off on what is expected.

Expectations for Child and Family's Participation

6. Here is what you will do to help:

You have also recorded what you expect from the child and family in terms of the treatment in Section 3 of the treatment plan. It is very important to be clear about your expectations. This clarity strongly supports trust. No hidden agendas here. Write your expectations of the child and family here in a user-friendly language so that they will know what is expected of them.

Expected Tangible Treatment Benefits

7. If our treatment helps, you will know it in the following way:

In this section, make the benefit the family will receive from participating in treatment as tangible as you can. State it in a way that you understand will be most meaningful to the child and family, given your knowledge of what is most important to them. Of course, use the language of thorns.

 For Edward's mother, you might say:

> I expect Edward to be able to control his emotions and behavior in a much better way at school and at home. He has lost his temper with you on several occasions when you have brought a man home, and was very disrespectful to you and your friend. I expect Edward will be able to control himself in this type of situation so that you don't feel so embarrassed and you don't worry so much about men not wanting to be with you.

For Edward you might say:

> I expect you to be able to become a good candidate for the Police Academy. This will require a lot of work for you to go to school, keep control of your temper, and to stay off marijuana. I know you can do this, with my help. Together we'll work to make you a great candidate, when it's time to apply to the Police Academy.

For Duncan's mother you might write:

> I expect that you will be called less from the school to pick Duncan up. He really needs treatment to help him control his behavior at school. I am confident that if he attends treatment regularly, and with your participation, he will be able to be in better control and you will be called less. I've arranged my schedule to meet with you, outside of your work hours.

Impact of Not Participating in Treatment

8. **If our treatment does not help, you will know it in the following way:**

You should be clear on the implications for the child and family, if they do not participate in treatment. You have already considered this and written about it in Section 2 of the treatment plan. Write what you believe about the impact on the child's functioning and development if he or she does not receive treatment.

Documenting Accountability

9. **Here is everyone's agreement:**

Remember TST Principle 6: *Insist on accountability, particularly your own*. This section is all about accountability. It documents the roles and expectations of everyone. And when everyone signs on this section, ready–set–go ends, and treatment implementation begins.

We provide an example of Tanisha's treatment agreement letter in Appendix 6. You can also look at her TST Assessment Form and TST Treatment Plan, shown in Appendices 3 and 5, respectively.

Finalizing the Treatment Agreement (So That You Can— Finally—Go!)

At this point, you have fully translated the treatment plan into a format that will maximize your chance of reaching a real treatment agreement, by putting together a strong treatment agreement letter. In this section we discuss getting to that real agreement. Remember: Ready–set–go ends when everyone signs off on the treatment agreement letter. Here are some steps to consider to help you get there:

- As soon as you finish your TST Treatment Plan, begin to draft the treatment agreement letter.
- Share it with your team and your supervisors. Do your best to get it right. When you think you've got it right, check "Draft" in the first section of the Treatment Agreement Letter. The letter is always considered a draft until it is finalized with the child and family. How do you know if it is finalized? They sign off on it! You can then check the box that says "Final"!

- Share the first draft of the treatment agreement letter with the family, as soon as you can. Use a session to go through each of the items. Make sure everything is well understood. Express your openness to answer any of their questions as well as disagreements. You want to know if anyone believes you've gotten something wrong. If someone believes you've gotten something wrong—and doesn't feel comfortable to tell you—you will find out soon enough—through missed appointments and other evidence of poor engagement.

- After you have gone through the treatment agreement letter, answered questions, and discussed any possible disagreements, you need to decide if you are all on the same page. If you believe you are all on the same page, don't necessarily rush to get a signature on the treatment agreement letter. You may want the child and family to take the letter home and think about it before they sign. You want to give them every opportunity to let you know if there is anything about which they feel uncomfortable.

- If there is a disagreement, it needs to be reconciled. Do everything you can to understand their point of view. If the child or family raises a point you have missed or gotten wrong, acknowledge your mistake and then update your treatment plan and agreement letter. If there is a disagreement over something you are confident you did not miss or get wrong, figure out the best way to discuss the matter with the child and/or family. Remember Principle 7: *Align with reality.* Never deviate from this type of alliance in the hope another tack will result in a better alliance with the family. That is always a mistake.

- When you are confident there is a good-enough agreement, go for the signatures. Congratulations! You are ready to go!

Usually, it will take you several sessions to get to an agreement. Those sessions are very important. They may be the first time a child and family member have worked with someone who tried so hard to get it right, to understand their perspectives, and to create something that *truly* addresses their needs. Although we say that *ready–set–go* comes before treatment implementation, it may represent the most therapeutic process the children and families have ever experienced.

What If the People You Need Cannot Serve as Partners?

We raise an uncomfortable issue with this question: What if the people you need to have as partners in order to implement the treatment plan are not able or willing to do what is needed? As described, the treatment agreement is based on coming to a shared understanding of the problems and solutions and forming a workable agreement regarding what everyone must do. In order to reach such an agreement, we put great effort into understanding everyone's perspective, and to making sure the treatment addresses what is most important to everyone.

If we think that a caregiver or anyone else may not be the partner we need—that is, may not be able or willing to do what is needed to implement the treatment plan—the first question we must ask ourselves is: What have we missed? Have we missed information that may indicate our perspective is not as well grounded as we think it is? Let's make sure we are appropriately vigilant about this possibility. It is, of course, a serious conclusion to draw that someone we need is not able to be a partner in our efforts to help and protect a child. On the other hand, this sometimes is the case, and there is a great cost to missing this reality. We never want to be in such a situation but sometimes the facts simply point to this sad reality. And, again, there are tremendous consequences for proceeding as if this were not the reality. What does such an unfortunate situation look like? It looks like this:

You define a problem that concerns you. You gather the facts and decide the problem has significant consequences for the child. You decide what the caregiver (or anyone else) must do to address the problem and seek an agreement with him or her to do this. You know—for sure—that this concerning problem cannot be sufficiently addressed without this agreement. You make every reasonable effort to integrate the caregiver (or anyone else's) perspective to make sure there are no misunderstandings and to address practical barriers. In response, the person you need:

- Will not make the agreement, within an appropriate time frame, given the nature of the problem.
- Will make the agreement, but shows through his or her behavior that he or she cannot keep it.

What do you do?

You are, clearly, in a difficult situation. You've identified an important problem. It concerns you for good reason. You've identified the partners you need, and you know the problem will not be impacted unless you can count on them—and you know you cannot count on at least one of them. If you find yourself in such a situation, the main piece of information that guides what you need to do is what you already know: the level of the child's risk, defined by the phase of treatment—specifically, whether the child needs the safety-focused phase or a more advanced phase (regulation-focused or beyond trauma).

When You Don't Have a Partner You Need and the Child Needs Safety-Focused Treatment

You are in a dangerous situation here. Recall, there are only two reasons a child needs safety-focused treatment:

- The environment is harmful.
- The child switches into dangerous survival states and the environment is insufficiently helpful or protective.

You have already decided that the situation is such that the child, or someone else, can be hurt. Therefore, every day you wait in the hope of reaching the agreement adds another day to the child's staying in an environment where he or she may be hurt, or others may be hurt. In such a situation you must act very quickly and decisively. Do you have the partner you need, or not? If you are not sure, set a very short period of time to find out. The instant you decide that you do not have the partner you need, ready–set–go ends, and safety-focused treatment begins. And safety-focused treatment begins by providing you with what you need to manage the unfortunate situation in which you find yourself.

When You Don't Have a Partner You Need and the Child Needs Regulation-Focused or Beyond Trauma Treatment

This situation is unfortunate, but not nearly as concerning. You have a larger window of time to potentially reach an agreement or even to reconsider your intervention strategy. By definition, no one is at risk to be hurt if you are not in safety-focused treatment. If you find yourself in such a situation, you should ask yourself the following two questions:

- Is the problem really as concerning as I thought?
- Is the person that I need as a partner really the only person available to help address the problem?

What do the answers to these two questions mean?

- If the answer to the first question (is it really concerning?) is "no," then you should reconsider whether the problem is important enough to address in TST.
- If the answer to the first question is "yes," and the answer to the second question (do I really need this partner?) is "no," you should find another partner and do everything you can to reach agreements with him or her.
- If the answers to both questions are "yes," you are a bit stuck. Do your best to reach the agreements within the time frame you have for ready–set–go.

Start regulation-focused or beyond trauma treatment and do your best. The impact of your work will be more limited than if you had a partner, but you can still do a lot of good.

Partnerships, Risk, and Time Frames

The discussion in the previous section about partnerships points to another important issue that we introduced in Chapter 9. How long should this all take? The child comes for treatment for an important problem. How long should assessment, treatment planning, and ready–set–go take before treatment can begin? As we described in the previous section, a lot depends on the level of risk. If a child needs safety-focused treatment, the situation is, by definition, dangerous. You have already decided, through your ratings of the level of potential harm in the social environment and the level of danger in the survival states, that the child or someone else could be hurt. You have used the TST Treatment Planning Grid to decide that safety-focused treatment is needed based on this information. If this is the case, how long does it make sense to wait to achieve a good-enough treatment agreement, or to decide that such an agreement cannot be reached within a time frame appropriate to the level of risk? Obviously, if the child does not need safety-focused treatment, you have more time to get to the treatment agreement and to initiate either regulation-focused or beyond trauma treatment. With all this in mind, we offer the following guidelines for the time frame to complete assessment, treatment planning, and ready–set–go based on the level of risk and the quality of partnerships. These guidelines are shown in Table 11.1.

What Else Can Interfere with Treatment Engagement?

In the previous section we reviewed the most important item that can interfere with treatment engagement: a lack of partnership on what is needed. In this section we review two additional factors that can interfere: *psychoeducational gaps* and *practical barriers*. Information was gathered and decisions made about each of these factors and recorded in Section 5 of the TST Assessment Form (Appendix 2) and the TST Treatment Plan (Appendix 4), respectively. Next, we expand on how you can best use this information, in the process of reaching your treatment agreement.

Psychoeducational Gaps

In Chapters 9 and 10, we reviewed the importance of understanding what the child and family understands about trauma, its impact, and about what mental health intervention entails. In Section 5 of the treatment plan, you recorded what you planned to do about these psychoeducational gaps. In this section,

TABLE 11.1. Guidelines for Initiating TST Treatment

Time from first visit/contact	Milestone	Guidelines
At most, 1 week	Decide on the required treatment phase	You need to know the level of risk you are dealing with very quickly. A prolonged assessment, treatment planning, and treatment engagement process that does not arrive at this level of risk in a very short period of time can place the child, and others, at risk. You should use the definitions of treatment phases given in Chapter 9, Section 3, to decide whether the child needs safety-focused treatment or either of the other treatment phases.

If the Child Needs Safety-Focused Treatment

At most, 1 *more* week	Complete ready–set–go by signing the final treatment agreement letter	You have decided that the child or others are at high risk with the child in his or her current environment. You must initiate treatment very soon by either reaching the agreements for the environment to become safe enough, or by getting the child to a safe-enough environment. You should set the maximal time it is appropriate to continue to work to reach the treatment agreement as soon as you decide the child needs safety-focused treatment. Ready–set–go ends and safety-focused treatment begins as soon as this period expires. The longest period of time should be 1 week. Ready–set–go also ends at the point you decide that caregivers cannot be partners in the needed agreements (as detailed in the previous section). For children who need to start safety-focused treatment before the assessment and treatment plan are completed, do your best to complete all of this in conjunction with the work you will do to *establish safety* in safety-focused treatment. It is *strongly recommended* that you do everything you can to determine at least one priority problem before safety-focused treatment begins.

If the Child Needs Regulation-Focused or Beyond Trauma Treatment

At most, 1 *more* week	Complete ready–set–go by signing the final treatment agreement letter	You need to move the child into treatment, but there is not nearly the urgency as in safety-focused treatment. There is also not nearly the complexity of problems or the need to respond to crises that often interfere with the process of assessment, treatment planning, and engagement. You should be able to have this all completed by 3 weeks after the first visit/contact.

we detail what we believe is a good approach. It's important to find out what a family knows about trauma, the effects of trauma, and what to expect from TST. Chances are there will be at least a few, if not many, gaps in the family's knowledge about these areas. After all, it's *your* job to know all that stuff. But it's also your job to share that knowledge with family members so that they can be empowered to understand what's going on with, and what will help, their kid.

The basic areas of psychoeducation that should be covered are as follows:

1. How trauma can affect a child's emotional nervous system (the survival circuit detailed in Chapter 2).
2. How the social environment can help or hinder a child's emotional regulation.
3. What TST looks like.

These three areas are covered in detail earlier in this book. But even though we think Chapters 1–4 are great, we don't think parents should have to read them. Instead, below is the Cliffs Notes™ version of what you might want to share with parents.

1. Trauma affects a child's ability to regulate emotions.
   - Sometimes emotional responses can feel more intense, and be harder to regulate, for kids who have been traumatized.
   - Sometimes their behaviors are attempts to handle these intense feelings, and they need help learning other ways of handling those feelings.
2. The social environment is a big part of what leads kids to have these intense emotions.
   - Traumatic reminders can quickly put the child in a different emotional state, where emotions are more intense and harder to manage.
   - Traumatic reminders can lead to changes in awareness, affect, and actions.
3. TST helps by simultaneously giving kids and families ways to better regulate emotions as well as to decrease traumatic reminders in the social environment. TST involves a whole treatment team, including the family, working together and really committing to helping the child.

Providing this type of information to children and families can be very helpful for building the treatment alliance. As parents learn more about how trauma affects kids, and what they can do to help, they are likely to feel more empowered. Have you

As parents learn more about how trauma affects kids, and what they can do to help, they are likely to feel more empowered.

ever heard a parent say "I don't know what happens—it's like somebody flips a switch and then suddenly Gregory is out of control!"? As parents begin to get a sense of how and why traumatic reminders "flip the switch," this kind of reaction will feel less out of the blue and more predictable. And once something is predictable, you're on your way to preempting it, or at least being able to prepare for it. *Whew.* As a parent, that feels better already.

Let's think about Duncan's mom for a minute. She's talked about Duncan being "difficult to handle." She's also talked about some traumatic events in his life, such as witnessing violence. Is she connecting these two areas? If not, it will be helpful to educate her about how trauma affects kids. She has mentioned a lot of life stressors and continuing stressors that could potentially be exacerbating the situation. We know she's aware of how her financial stress has made her feel pretty overwhelmed, but how is it affecting Duncan? And what about Mom being less available because she has to work—did his social environment just get less supportive, and is this affecting his ability to regulate emotions? If Mom begins to see the connections between trauma, social environment, and Duncan's behavior, this new understanding could help with a lot of situations. She may get less angry at Duncan and blame him less. She may realize that there are concrete ways in which she can help him. In brief, she may be able to become Duncan's ally in helping their family to survive and move beyond the trauma they've been through.

Troubleshooting Practical Barriers

Like the psychoeducational needs detailed previously, practical barriers were also assessed and decisions were made about how you might handle them, recorded in Section 5 of the treatment plan. In this section, we describe how to work on these practical barriers as we form the treatment agreement. No matter how committed a family may be to treatment, there still can be very real, practical barriers to engaging in treatment. If we, as providers, don't recognize and deal with these real-life barriers, then we send a message that we don't really care. Not only that, but we lose our shot at providing good, consistent treatment for the family.

We can't solve all of the barriers. But we *can* find out what they are and brainstorm with the family about how to solve them. Or we can make compromises in our own ways of doing things that make it easier for the family.

We'll talk about some specific situations here. Solutions will vary depending on the resources of your agency, the family, and the community. The key is to pick up at least part of the responsibility of recognizing, and trying to diminish, barriers to treatment.

Transportation: "I'd love to have my kid in treatment, but how do I get her there?"

Good question, and not as simple as "Go straight down Mass Avenue and turn left at the light." Cars and public transportation take money. Single parents with three kids might have to take *everyone* to the appointment. Throw in the fact that Susie's school is on the other side of town, and you've got a real pickle. What to do?

- Ask parents if they have a way to get here. Acknowledge the problem if there is one.
- Brainstorm about other transportation. Have they tried public transit? Will the school bus drop the child off at the clinic? Does the clinic provide any transportation? Is there a godfather or someone else invested in the child's care who could help?
- Identify any related barriers, such as finances or social phobia. If the family doesn't have money for public transit, can you initiate advocacy to get the family more financial resources? If social phobia is preventing the parent from bringing the child out, work on getting him or her treatment.
- Consider other modalities/locations of treatment. Could your clinic do home-based individual therapy? School-based?

Scheduling: "I have to be at work until 5:00, so there's no way to get here in time."

Sometimes scheduling conflicts are a reflection of the fact that other things hold higher priority than treatment. If you find that the child's favorite TV program is bumping therapy from the schedule, it might be time to revisit "agreeing on the solution" in the first part of this chapter. But other times scheduling conflicts are very real, such as the mother in our heading who has to work until 5:00.

> Sometimes scheduling conflicts are a reflection of the fact that other things hold higher priority than treatment.

Let's take Duncan's case again. Mom is working hard to make ends meet so that they can be independent from the abusive father. This endeavor is obviously important. And it could very well be that if she left work early once a week to take Duncan to therapy, she would lose her job. This would be bad for everyone involved. So what can you do?

- Examine your appointment hours. Could you shift your schedule a half hour later to accommodate the family? Is there a better day of the week for them? A little flexibility sometimes is a big gesture, and a big help. (On the other hand, being late for your *own* child care commitments or coming in on a Saturday could quickly lead to resentment, so be careful that you don't make concessions that are going to tax you.)

- Brainstorm about other people in the child's life who might be able to help. Could Grandma Jane bring Duncan to therapy some days? Is Grandma Jane willing to be a part of the treatment team?

- Try to double-up appointments. If the child needs to come for psycho-pharmacology appointments and therapy appointments, and Mom needs to meet with a legal advocate, that's a lot of meetings! One trip with back-to-back meetings cuts down on the time for the family.

- Encourage creative problem solving. Could Mom go to work early on Thursdays so she could leave early? Does Mom feel comfortable talking to the boss so that he or she is aware of the situation and doesn't penalize Mom for leaving early on appointment days?

- Initiate advocacy so that the parent can fulfill his or her obligation to care for the child. If a child is in serious need of care, such that a parent needs to be able to go to multiple appointments during the week and/or provide constant supervision, the Family Medical Leave Act of 1993 protects a parent from being fired.

Child Care: "That's great that you'll meet with Jan—what should I do with the rest of the Brady bunch?"

Particularly if you want the parent to be involved in the treatment, this issue of child care for other children is a thorny problem. We've seen our waiting room ripped to shreds by siblings while the mother is in the room with the therapist and client. Here are some possible ways of addressing this issue:

- Initiate a volunteer program, or glom onto an existing volunteer agency, and get someone to staff your busiest waiting room hours.

- Brainstorm other community or family support services that could help out.

- Schedule appointments at a time when some of the kids are in after-school programs, or Dad is home, or . . .

Language: "Estoy tan contento finalmente haber encontrado alguien que entiende realmente!"

Huh? Right! Now try saying "The declarative memory system is largely mediated by the hippocampus. . . ."

We are an incredibly diverse country, with the proportion of non-English speakers increasing daily. Immigrants and refugees are going to be part of the clientele we serve no matter where we are and what languages we do (or don't) speak. So what do you do if the parent, child, or both who are seeking treatment don't speak the same language as you do?

- Work toward systemic change in your clinic; advocate for hiring multilingual staff.
- Build partnerships with community agencies that *do* provide some types of services in different languages.
- Work with an interpreter. *Don't* use the child as the interpreter. In a pinch, you can use a nationwide phone-based interpreter system.
- Remember that body language is very communicative. Maybe you don't learn until the first appointment that the family speaks Somali, and you just can't get a translator on such short notice—you can still communicate respect and caring for a family. Make eye contact, speak sincerely, and then do everything you can to get an interpreter there next time.

Parent Limitations: "Sure, I'll bring Tony to treatment (unless, of course, it means I have to leave the house)."

Trauma often affects a whole family. Parents may themselves have significant mental health needs or other problems that make it difficult to follow through with treatment for their child—despite their best intentions. Parental PTSD might lead to avoidance of talking about past traumas—and, naturally, avoidance of their child's appointment. Drug or alcohol use might render the parent incapable of getting the child to appointments. Depression might affect a parent so deeply that he or she doesn't get out of bed. Cognitive limitations or disorganization might lead to habitual forgetting of the appointment.

> Parents may themselves have significant mental health needs or other problems that make it difficult to follow through with treatment for their child—despite their best intentions.

All of these problems not only prevent the child from getting treatment, but also are shades of a distressed social environment. They are big red flags that the family really does need help. Here are some suggestions:

- Work to get the parent into his or her own treatment.
- Try to have the parent see you as a supporter in this undertaking, not as someone who is critical and shaming because Mom or Dad is (yet again) failing his or her child.
- Consider home-based care as a way to get treatment started for a family that can't make it to the office.

Stigma of Mental Health Services: "*I don't want my child*
to be branded as crazy!"

The stigmatization of mental illness is an unfortunately prevalent phenomenon. Find out if the family is worried about this, and do your best via psychoeducation to whittle away at the myth that mental health services means they're crazy, weak, or otherwise less than someone else.

Fear of Social Services: "*If I bring my child here,*
you're just going to file a report to the social services agency.
I don't want anything to do with you!"

This barrier would be a lot easier to handle if we could just say "No, I promise, I won't file!" But we can't. We're mandated reporters. And we have a duty to protect kids.

But we can do a lot to help parents understand exactly when and why we would report child abuse to the authorities. And if we have to make a report, we can do our best to work *with* the parents while doing it. You can certainly emphasize the strengths: for example, "The family is engaging in treatment, is here with me in the office, and we agreed to call this in together. Mom is open to support around parenting. . . ." And hopefully if social service personnel get involved, you can bring them into the treatment team, so that they are part of the integrated system of care under TST.

Closing Thoughts on Ready–Set–Go

Finally, we show you a beautiful picture to give you a sense of the bliss you will experience when you are successful at ready–set–go. Savor the picture for a few minutes. Let it sink in. Let it anticipate the feeling you will have when you are truly ready to *go*. If you respond to the picture in the way we think you will, your days as a wise man or wise woman are over. Now . . . *go*!

Treatment Agreement Letter

☐ Draft (team's ideas)   ☑ Final (by discussion and agreement with family)

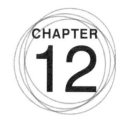

CHAPTER
12

Safety-Focused Treatment

Establishing and Maintaining Safe Environments for Children

LEARNING OBJECTIVES

- To learn how to establish and maintain safety in the child's current environment
- To learn how to determine if safety can be established in the child's current environment, and what to do if this is not the case
- To learn how to support caregivers through this difficult work

---

ICONS USED IN THIS CHAPTER

Essential Point	Key Tool	Case Illustration	Academic Point

When a child needs the safety-focused phase of treatment, there is high risk that someone can be hurt. Caregivers may hurt the child. The child may hurt him- or herself or others. Accordingly, treatment must be conducted most carefully, intensively, and decisively. We enter the safety-focused phase making sure we leave all traces of wishful thinking at the door. The work is stressful and difficult. The

> We enter the safety-focused phase making sure we leave all traces of wishful thinking at the door. The work is stressful and difficult. The risks are high. The possible benefits are also very high.

risks are high. The possible benefits are also very high. This is a phase of treatment when you are in a position to dramatically improve a child's life and hope for a better future by helping to create a safe-enough environment for him or her to grow into that future. How might you do this? First, we focus on the basics.

Children need safety-focused treatment for only two reasons, and therefore you only have to accomplish two things. What reasons and which things? Here are the only two reasons that a child will need safety-focused treatment:

- The child lives in a *harmful* environment.
- The caregivers are *insufficiently helpful and protective* for the child who shifts into *dangerous* survival states.

Here are the two things you must accomplish:

- Improve the child's environment so it is no longer harmful (or get the child out of the harmful environment).
- Diminish the likelihood a child will shift into a dangerous survival state by improving his or her regulation capacity, and/or by improving the caregiver's capacity to be helpful and protective, or help get the child to an environment that has the capacity to be sufficiently helpful and protective with a child who demonstrates dangerous survival states.

All you have to accomplish in safety-focused treatment are these two things for those two reasons. Simple, right?? We anticipate what you are now thinking. How will we accomplish those two things for whatever reason?? And that is why we wrote the rest of this chapter.

What You Already Have in Place to Support Your Work

 It's important to recognize that you don't enter safety-focused treatment from "scratch." You already have three supports in place that will help you accomplish what you need to accomplish:

- An *organizational plan* that enables you to conduct the work.
- A definition of a *safe-enough environment*, which is the marker for the completion of the work.
- An *agreement* with all relevant parties about what they will do so that a *safe-enough environment* can be reached.

It's important to acknowledge, before we detail each of these supports, that some children arrive in safety-focused treatment without these supports fully in place. In Chapters 9 and 11, we described the situation when a child and family need intervention—given the level of risk—but there is not enough time to fully complete the assessment, treatment planning, and ready–set–go processes. In such cases, you may not have defined a safe-enough environment as clearly as you might, or reached the needed agreements to establish safety. We provide details for handling this problem later in this chapter. For now, we simply want to acknowledge that some of you will be proceeding with the safety-focused phase of treatment on stronger foundations than others.

An Organizational Plan That Enables You to Conduct the Work

The safety-focused phase of treatment requires intensive work close to the source of the problem. Accordingly, safety-focused treatment is primarily implemented in the home, community, or residential treatment milieu. The work in safety-focused treatment is crucial. It involves risk. It must be planned carefully. Accordingly, resolving all necessary organizational planning issues is paramount to ensure that the team implementing safety-focused treatment has sufficient support from the organization within which they work. These organizational planning issues are the focus of Chapter 8. We remind the reader of these issues here because they are so important. Before providers and teams embark on this difficult work, the details of how this work will be supported must be thoroughly vetted and appropriate organizational decisions made. In short: Make sure the organizational plan you struck for your TST program truly supports safety-focused treatment. Make sure that home- and community-based care are well integrated and properly supported in the plan. If you find yourself, as a TST provider, expected to implement care services for a child and family in the safety-focused phase of treatment, and you have no means of offering this care except from your office, then you are likely to embark upon an exercise in frustration. Additionally, this organizational plan should also account for the psychopharmacology services and legal advocacy expertise that may be needed. Finally, because this is a phase of treatment in which things can go wrong, it requires constant vigilance and the support of a supervisor and team. Threat is real. Stakes are high. This is also a phase of treatment that saves lives. If these organizational structures are in place, you are in a position to have a major impact on the life and future of a child.

> This is a phase of treatment in which things can go wrong. Threat is real. Stakes are high. This is also a phase of treatment that saves lives. If these organizational structures are in place, you are in a position to have a major impact on the life and future of a child.

A Definition of a Safe-Enough Environment

In Chapter 9, we reviewed several questions to ask yourself if you are having difficulty discerning the level of threat and danger in the trauma system of a particular child and family. The first question concerns defining the minimum that would need to be in place to ensure a child's safety. The second question concerns a realistic appraisal of what the child needs in order to be safe is in place: Does the environment fall above or below the minimal standard? The third question concerns whether, given the risk, safety can be achieved within a reasonable time frame. These questions all relate to the minimal standard of a *safe-enough environment.* The only reason the child needs safety-focused treatment is because his or her environment falls below this minimal standard. A harmful environment is obviously below this standard. An insufficiently helpful and protective environment, for a child who expresses dangerous survival states, also falls below this standard.

 A safe-enough environment is one in which:

- Caregivers are able to *protect* their child from actual threats, and
- Caregivers are able to *help* their child regulate dangerous survival states and *protect* their child from stimuli that provoke those dangerous survival states.

Does the child's trauma system reach that threshold or fall below it? Your work will be very much guided by the answer to this question.

An Agreement with All Relevant Parties about What They Will Do So That a Safe-Enough Environment Can Be Reached

You've done a lot of work to get here. You've assessed the child and the environment and developed a clear vision about the problems and solutions, reflected in your treatment plan. You've translated the treatment plan into a treatment agreement letter, and then spent the time with the child and family—and anyone else you might need—reaching agreements on the terms of that letter. Most important for safety-focused treatment, the agreements you've reached were mainly about what the child and family need to do to ensure a safe-enough environment. The bulk of the work in safety-focused treatment is about helping everyone involved to successfully keep these agreements.

> For safety-focused treatment, the agreements you've reached were mainly about what the child and family need to do to ensure a safe-enough environment. The bulk of the work in safety-focused treatment is about helping everyone involved to successfully keep these agreements.

Treatment Structure

Safety-focused treatment requires the capacity to provide intervention on site, where survival-in-the-moment occurs, and with sufficient intensity to manage high-risk cases. As detailed in Chapter 8 on organizations, different communities have different ways of providing and financing this kind of care. From the vantage point of TST, safety-focused treatment requires that services can be provided:

- In the home, community, or residential facility where the child spends most of his or her time and, accordingly, experiences most of his or her survival moments.
- With sufficient safety for the providers; home-based care is optimally delivered by teams of two.
- With sufficient intensity to allow for close monitoring of safety and rapid implementation of changes (typically, two or three visits/week).
- By, or with, close involvement from mental health provider(s).
- By someone with knowledge of how to advocate effectively.

Safety-focused treatment has three related components. They are:

- Establishing safety
  - Activities that will ensure the environment becomes safe enough in a time frame that is appropriate for the level of risk, or gets the child to a safe-enough environment if the current environment cannot become safe enough in the time frame required.
- Maintaining safety
  - Activities that support the continuation of the safe-enough environment until providers are confident the changes are real and can last.
- Caring for caregivers
  - Activities that support caregivers for what they need to do to establish and maintain a safe-enough environment.

When Is the Work Done?

The work of safety-focused treatment is accomplished, as we have described, when a safe-enough environment is established and when providers and their teams are confident enough that this safety is real and can last. Once that happens, the child can safely transition to regulation-focused treatment. Safety-focused treatment, like all treatment phases of TST, is about developing two capacities:

1. Developing the *capacity of those around the child to help and protect* so the child can best navigate his or her world without switching into survival states.
2. Developing a *child's emotional regulation capacity* so the child can best navigate his or her world without switching into survival states.

Notice that these two capacities are exactly those required to address the trauma system. The emphasis in safety-focused treatment is to develop the caregiver's capacity to help and protect the child. Of course, building a child's capacity to regulate emotion is also critically important within TST and is strongly emphasized in the next treatment phase: regulation-focused treatment. This type of work will be initiated in the present, safety-focused phase. The focus in the safety phase is the social environment. How can it be stabilized enough so that the child can safely live within it? And if it can't be stabilized enough in a time frame commensurate with the level of risk, how can we get the child to a stable-enough, or therapeutic-enough, environment—also in a time frame commensurate with the level of risk? When a child needs safety-focused treatment, there are a great many things we might choose as the focus of treatment. It is important to choose carefully, given the level of risk. Our priority is to build the capacity of those around the child to help and protect him or her. This especially involves immediate caregivers. It also extends to anyone in the social environment whose help and protection are needed, including the providers and organizations within the service system that can help and protect the child.

Navigating Your Way through Safety-Focused Treatment

Navigating through safety-focused treatment can often seem like you are steering a ship in a storm, through treacherous waters. TST has some navigational tools to help you. Soon we will introduce you to the Safety-Focused Guide (SFG). This guide contains several tools that will help you navigate the treacherous waters of the trauma system during the safety-focused phase of treatment. Before we detail the nuts and bolts of the SFG, we want you to consider several navigational ideas, upon which the SFG was based. These ideas should be familiar to you from various places in the book. We repeat them here so you have them in the forefront of your mind as we walk you through the SFG.

The Importance of Standards

Standards are milestones that tell you about your destination and how close you are to reaching it. It is very important that these standards are defined clearly and tangibly, and that they relate to meaningful achievements. It is especially important that these standards are defined proactively and not "as you go along." We defined one standard earlier in this chapter, the minimal safe-enough environment standard. This is the most important standard we use in this chapter, but there are others.

The Importance of Time

Standards, without time limits, quickly become meaningless. What does a standard for a safe-enough environment mean if you may not reach it until the distant future? If you set such a standard, it will almost certainly matter whether it is reached in 3 days, 3 months, or 3 years. If you are not able to set reasonable time limits for reaching standards, you will not be able to grapple with the critical tradeoff between the cost of waiting with hope that the standard can be reached versus the cost of acting because you think the meeting of the standard is not possible. Children in unsafe environments usually bear the cost of this waiting.

Standards, without time limits, quickly become meaningless. What does a standard for a safe-enough environment mean if you may not reach it until the distant future?

The Importance of Agreements

We've introduced the importance of agreements earlier in this chapter. Certainly, your work in ready–set–go was instrumental to reaching the agreements that will anchor the work in safety-focused treatment. You will begin the work by taking a careful look at the agreements that have been made to make sure they are strong enough for what is needed in this phase of treatment. A primary way that we work to establish and maintain a safe-enough environment is through helping all relevant parties successfully implement these agreements. The monitoring of agreements is all about accountability, and we insist on it (especially our own). Remember TST Principle 8.

The Importance of Decisive Action

We have lined up all of these navigational tools to help you act effectively within the trauma system. A compass and a map serve no purpose if the ship's captain does not use this information to decisively steer the ship through the treacherous waters. If the information you have gathered suggests that a child will not be safe unless he or she moves to a different setting, the job becomes doing whatever you need to do to make that happen. This might involve advocating for the child to be accepted into a higher-level-care facility (e.g., inpatient unit) or working with child protective services to move the child out of a dangerous home. Advocating to remove a child from the parent's home is, of course, a very serious decision, never to be made casually. Taking this stance may lead to a lot of anger from those we are charged with helping. No one likes to be in this situation, but we must be prepared to act if the reality indicates that the child is not safe. We stand with you to make the right decision. The purpose of much of this chapter is to help you feel confident about these sorts of decisions.

The Importance of You

> Take care of yourself. Use your team, supervisors, spouse, partner, friends, and family. Do everything you can to stay human in the trauma system. You are *really* important. The work cannot happen without you.

This is tough stuff—among the toughest. Navigating these waters can affect us deeply, because we are human. As we described in Chapters 5 and 7, there can be an important cost to you for this work. Take care of yourself. Use your team, supervisors, spouse, partner, friends, and family. Do everything you can to stay human in the trauma system. You are *really* important. The work cannot happen without you.

The Safety-Focused Guide

 As described, treatment in the safety-focused phase is guided by a central document: the Safety-Focused Guide (SFG), located in Appendix 7.

TOOL: Safety-Focused Guide

What it is: A treatment guide for TST providers that describes concrete steps related to three components of safety-focused treatment: Establish safety, maintain safety, and care for caregivers.

When to use it: From the initiation of treatment for children in the safety-focused phase until the family has safely transitioned into regulation-focused treatment. Some elements of the guide may continue to be used in the regulation-focused treatment phase.

Target goals: To ensure that the environment is safe enough for a child and to guide providers through the central activities of safety-focused treatment in order to get there.

The SFG is organized around the three components of safety-focused treatment, described previously: Establish safety, maintain safety, and care for caregivers. The SFG walks you through sets of activities to accomplish each of these three components. The SFG is a dynamic document that changes as a provider's understanding of what is needed changes. The SFG is intended for providers, to help guide care and adherence to the TST model. It is not meant to be given to a family; other tools have been developed with families in mind and are presented later. The SFG should accompany the TST providers throughout the safety-focused phase of treatment, and sections of it may continue to be helpful as a child transitions into the regulation-focused phase of treatment. The rest of this chapter walks you through implementing the SFG. Take it out. Let's walk through it together.

Anchoring Safety-Focused Treatment

Anchoring safety-focused treatment involves writing a simple statement that adapts the overall treatment strategy to the aims of this phase of treatment.

Safety-Focused Guide: anchoring safety-focused treatment

Through the assessment process you will have completed the TST Assessment Form (Appendix 3), drafted a TST Treatment Plan (Appendix 5) and reached an agreement with the child and family that is documented in the Treatment Agreement Letter (Appendix 6). You've already drafted an overall treatment strategy and recorded it in Section 3.b of your TST Treatment Plan. The process of anchoring the treatment is to make that overall strategy a little more specific to the goals of safety-focused treatment. For children who needed to start safety-focused treatment before you had the opportunity to draft your overall treatment strategy, here is your opportunity to draft one, specific for the requirements of safety-focused treatment. We provide an example of Emily's anchor for safety-focused treatment, based on her overall treatment strategy statement (shown in Chapter 9). A version of this statement is also adapted for Items 5 and 6 of the treatment agreement letter. Throughout treatment in TST, that letter is referenced continually, including in the safety-focused phase. Obviously, if safety-focused treatment needed to be started without a full treatment agreement letter in place, it should be a big priority to complete one. As we noted in Chapter 11, this letter provides the best possible chance of engaging children and families in a focused treatment that directly addresses the most important problems.

Here is Emily's safety-focused anchor:

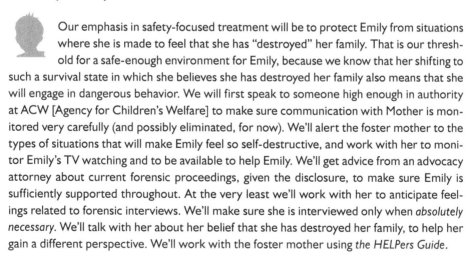

Our emphasis in safety-focused treatment will be to protect Emily from situations where she is made to feel that she has "destroyed" her family. That is our threshold for a safe-enough environment for Emily, because we know that her shifting to such a survival state in which she believes she has destroyed her family also means that she will engage in dangerous behavior. We will first speak to someone high enough in authority at ACW [Agency for Children's Welfare] to make sure communication with Mother is monitored very carefully (and possibly eliminated, for now). We'll alert the foster mother to the types of situations that will make Emily feel so self-destructive, and work with her to monitor Emily's TV watching and to be available to help Emily. We'll get advice from an advocacy attorney about current forensic proceedings, given the disclosure, to make sure Emily is sufficiently supported throughout. At the very least we'll work with her to anticipate feelings related to forensic interviews. We'll make sure she is interviewed only when *absolutely necessary*. We'll talk with her about her belief that she has destroyed her family, to help her gain a different perspective. We'll work with the foster mother using *the HELPers Guide*.

Implementing Safety-Focused Treatment

The logic of safety-focused treatment is pretty simple. First, we must make sure the environment is safe enough (*establish safety*). Then we make sure the changes made to the environment to establish safety are real and will last (*maintain safety*). And while we are establishing and maintaining safety, we make sure the caregivers are supported for the difficult work they must accomplish to work with us (*care for caregivers*). And that's about it.

Establish Safety

This component of safety-focused treatment is most critical. Children only need safety-focused treatment, by definition, if the environment they are in is not safe enough, given their vulnerability to shifting into survival states. The *establish safety* component of this phase of treatment is about how to make sure the environment improves such that it can be considered safe enough—or work to move the child to an environment that is safe and can effectively manage the child's dysregulation. You only have two choices for your work in establishing safety. Your appraisals will very much help you make your choice:

> Children only need safety-focused treatment, by definition, if the environment they are in is not safe enough, given their vulnerability to shifting into survival states.

1. You will establish safety in the child's current environment, *or*
2. You will work to move the child to a different, safe-enough environment.

The establish safety part of the SFG (Section 1) provides a set of tools that will enable you to make these decisions to carry out the appropriate action. It's important to note that this guide is written to address the needs of both the children who arrive in safety-focused treatment with assessment, treatment planning, and ready–set–go fully completed, and those for whom these processes could not be fully completed, given the level of risk.

Section 1 of the SFG on establishing safety includes these five steps:

1. Appraise whether the current environment is safe enough.
2. Develop the plan to establish a safe-enough environment (the safety plan).
3. Determine the risk to establishing safety in the current environment (with the safety plan).
4. Reach the decision on whether to keep the child within the current environment, based on the risk.
5. Reach the decision on whether (and under what conditions) to return the child to the environment, based on the risk (for children who have been placed in a new environment).

Step 1: Appraising Whether the Current Environment Is Safe Enough

In this section, we take information gathered through the assessment, treatment planning, and treatment agreement processes of TST and we make sure we have the most realistic appraisal of risk that is possible. We cannot possibly establish safety without a realistic appraisal of risk.

THE SAFE-ENOUGH ENVIRONMENT STANDARD

As we've discussed, you've already defined this standard previously. Here's where you put it together. We define the safe-enough environment as one in which:

> Safety-Focused Guide:
> Establishing Safety Step 1A:
> safe-enough standard

- Caregivers are able to *protect* their child from actual threats, and
- Caregivers are able to *help* their child regulate dangerous survival states and *protect* their child from stimuli that provoke those dangerous survival states.

The safe-enough standard is that which needs to be in place—at a minimum—for the child to be safe. If the child does not shift to dangerous survival states, don't worry about the second part of the definition. You have enough work to do addressing the first. In this case, your work in safety-focused treatment is *only* about protecting the child from actual threats.

THE CURRENT EVIDENCE

You've defined the minimum, based on your understanding of the child and his or her vulnerabilities. What, actually, is in place? You have the facts—you've already gathered them. Put them here

> Safety-Focused Guide:
> Establishing Safety Step 1B:
> the current evidence

because you will use these facts to help improve the situation. Again: If the child does not shift into dangerous survival states, don't worry about that part here. Focus only on the first part: protecting the child from actual threats. Make sure you get these facts down accurately. If important facts are still unclear, gather some more evidence to clarify. Then record it.

We also have a section to describe what caregivers are relying on to create safety in the environment. This might be support from friends or family members. It might be help from a mental health or child welfare provider. It might be a support written into the child welfare case plan or the child's educational plan. It's important to record these supports and determine their reliability and sustainability. A safe-enough environment that is dependent on, for example, a

> A safe-enough environment that is dependent on, for example, a grandparent, will quickly fall below the safe-enough standard if the grandparent becomes sick or moves to another region.

grandparent, will quickly fall below the safe-enough standard if the grandparent becomes sick or moves to another region.

THE REALISTIC APPRAISAL

Safety-Focused Guide:
Establishing Safety Step 1C:
the realistic appraisal

Here is where you make your judgment, based on the evidence about whether the environment is above or below the safe-enough standard. Do the facts indicate that the environment is above the minimum standard or below it? Make sure you get it right because the activities that follow will depend on your decision. If the environment is below the safe-enough standard, your activities will be dedicated to reaching the standard (*establish safety*). If the environment is at, or above, the standard, your activities will be directed toward making sure the environment will stay safe enough (*maintain safety*). If you have decided the environment is above the safe-enough standard, you can skip to the *maintain safety* section of the SFG.

Step 2: Developing the Plan to Establish a Safe-Enough Environment (the Safety Plan)

Safety-Focused Guide:
Establishing Safety Step 2:
developing the safety plan

You are in a situation where you know the environment is below the safe-enough standard. You know the situation is very risky. You may want to intervene to get the child to a safe-enough place. You may want to give it one more chance to see if safety can be established in the child's current environment. In this section you put together the best plan you can manage to help the environment reach your defined safe-enough standard in a timely way. Of course you want to support caregivers in every way you can to help them to reach the safe-enough environment. Your assessment of their vulnerabilities and needs pointed to decisions about what you would do to support them. This is your (and your team's) part of the treatment agreement letter. Your agreements should be front and center in this safety plan. And if you are not able to keep your agreements for supporting people to reach the safe-enough standard, then you cannot reasonably hold them accountable for their agreements. (Remember our Principle 8: *Insist on accountability, particularly your own.*)

Your safety plan should include the specifics about what you and your team will do, what caregivers will do, what the child will do, what those in caregivers' extended network will do, and what providers in the service system will do to make the environment safe enough. Again, many of these agreements were reached during the ready–set–go phase and recorded in the treatment agreement letter. Make sure the agreements recorded are still the right ones for establishing safety. If a treatment agreement letter was not fully drafted, this is the time to make sure it is completed and focused on the agreements you need to establish safety. Remember, the whole point of your work here is to get the environment to the safe-enough standard. Record only the relevant agreements for reaching this point on the safety plan.

In the case of Emily, you wrote in your anchor for safety-focused treatment that your safety plan will include her foster mother's agreement to stop contact with Emily's mother, the social services case workers' support of this agreement within the case plan, and the court's agreement to wait until Emily is out of safety-focused treatment for her to be interviewed forensically (assuming this delay will not unduly interfere with the legal case). In order for all this to work, you need the engagement and agreement of both the child welfare system and the court system. In the best of all possible worlds, you would get full engagement and agreement from the relevant parties within these systems. Sometimes such engagement and agreement are not forthcoming. What do you do? If you need specific forms of engagement and agreements to create a safe-enough environment, then—by definition—what you need is a matter of life and death. You will need to advocate in order to reach these agreements. (We provide greater detail about advocacy in later sections of this chapter.)

Step 3: Determining the Risk to Establish Safety in the Current Environment (with the Safety Plan)

This part of the SFG is intended to provide you with an additional checkpoint to make sure you've gotten it right. Let's call it the *align-with-reality* checkpoint. As we discussed in Chapter 6, it's easy to lose track of reality in the trauma system. In no context is this more relevant than when you are working with a child and family who are below the safe-enough standard. Accordingly, we've included this section to help keep you as aligned with reality as possible.

You've put together a safety plan: Is it practical? Is it realistic? Can it be accomplished within an acceptable time frame? What will you do if the answers to any of these questions are "no"? You are already working in a situation that is high risk, so you must be very cautious about proceeding with a safety plan if it is not realistic. In this section of the SFG we include a set of tools to help you. They are:

THE SAFETY PLAN TIME LIMIT

The safety plan time limit is your realistic appraisal of the time limit for establishing safety in the child's current environment, given the appraised level of risk. You have drafted a safety plan in the previous

Safety-Focused Guide:
Establishing Safety Step 3A:
safety plan time limit

section. How long can you wait for this safety plan to work (i.e., to bring the environment to the safe-enough standard) before the risk is too high? Of course, the safety plan time limit is used if you have decided the environment is below the safe-enough standard. Accordingly, time is not on your side. A child can be hurt. A child can hurt others. And there are not the needed supports in the environment to mitigate the risk. How long can you wait until you must intervene to get the child to a safe-enough place? Here is where you define the length of time it makes sense to wait before the risk is intolerable. There are, of course, a range of risk levels and corresponding time frames that you will encounter in safety-focused treatment. A 7-year-old boy who punches classmates and a 17-year-old boy who assaults classmates with baseball bats pose different levels of risk and require very different responses from their environments to be sufficiently helpful and protective. Presumably, you would set a much shorter period of time to work with the child and the environment in the case of the 17-year-old than the 7-year-old.

SAFETY PLAN CONFIDENCE LEVEL

Safety-Focused Guide:
Establishing Safety Step 3B:
safety plan confidence level

You've assembled a safety plan. You also know the child and caregivers, their strengths and vulnerabilities, and the support that will be needed from others to implement the plan. Consider carefully the track record of everyone you believe is needed to succeed at this plan in relation to what you are asking of them. Is it realistic? Can this be accomplished? The *safety plan confidence level* is the rating of your degree of confidence that the safety plan can be accomplished within the *safety plan time limit*. Be brutally honest with yourself and others. Get advice, if you need it. You don't want to be overly optimistic with your rating. The stakes are too high. Of course, we understand that you are not a fortune-teller. There is always uncertainty about predicting the future. Nevertheless, you have a lot of information to use to make your estimate. In particular, make sure to use the following information in your rating of all those whom you need to implement the safety plan:

- Their understanding of what is expected.
- Their motivation to do what is expected.
- Their ability to do what is expected.
- Their track record of following through on other expectations.
- Their taking of responsibility for problems they have caused, related to safety in the environment.

It's critically important to make sure those with whom you are working to establish safety can be real partners with you, for what is needed. Obviously, if you have decided that someone is not able to be a partner for an agreement that is really important, you will not have much confidence in his or her part of the safety plan. We reviewed details of determining partnerships in Chapter 11. As we reviewed, determining that someone is not able to be a partner is a serious decision. Before you make such a decision, ask yourself the following two questions:

1. Is there anything I may have missed?
2. Have I kept my agreements?

Here is our Safety Plan Confidence Level Scale, included in the SFG.

Instructions: Consider the strengths and limitations of all those caregivers/ providers who are needed to successfully implement the safety plan. Based on this consideration, please rate your level of confidence that the safety plan will achieve the safe-enough standard within the defined time limit:

1. *Very confident*: I am very confident that the safety plan will be implemented so successfully that it will result in the environment reaching the safe-enough standard within the defined time limit.
2. *Somewhat confident*: I am somewhat confident that the safety plan will be implemented so successfully that it will result in the environment reaching the safe-enough standard within the defined time limit.
3. *Hardly confident*: I am hardly confident that the safety plan will be implemented so successfully that it will result in the environment reaching the safe-enough standard within the defined time limit.
4. *Not at all confident*: I am not at all confident that the safety plan will be implemented so successfully that it will result in the environment reaching the safe-enough standard within the defined time limit.

Here are two examples of why this rating is important:

You believe a child's suicidal behavior is very much related to her mother's substance abuse. Given the acuity of the child's impulses, you believe the maximum time to have the substance abuse addressed is 3 days (*safety plan time limit*). The mother says she finally understands the impact of her substance abuse on her daughter's suicidal behavior and will stop drinking immediately. You know from her track record that her ability to keep this agreement is extremely unlikely. At the very least she will need to enter a substance abuse program that you may be able to help her access in 3 or 4 days—at the earliest—and then you would need to be confident that the substance abuse is under control. The earliest you can imagine this occurring would be a few weeks after the program starts. You record the safety plan confidence level as 4 (*not at all confident*).

You believe a child is at high risk to be exposed to violent behavior from his mother's boyfriend. This man pushed the mother down and almost struck her in the face, in front of the child, 2 nights ago. The man does not live at the home, but there is a history of violence at least monthly, over the last year. You believe the longest it makes sense for the child to stay in the home without the risk being definitively addressed is 3 days (*safety plan time limit*). The mother says she can take her son to live with her sister in another neighborhood today, and also take out a restraining order against her boyfriend. Her level of concern about safety in the home impresses you. You have also met with the mother's sister on a previous occasion and were impressed with her ability to help. You call her on the phone with the mother present (after she agrees) and confirm this plan as viable. You record the safety plan confidence level as 1 (*very confident*).

Remember: Your confidence level is not a matter of your subjective impressions. It is based on *specific activities* that need to be accomplished within a *specified time frame*. These activities are specified in the safety plan. The time frame is specified as the safety plan time limit. Your safety plan confidence level indicates the level of risk entailed by attempting to implement the safety plan while the child is staying in the current environment. If you proceed with this plan to establish safety while the child is in this environment, it is important to be clear about the level of risk you are taking. The SFG includes a table to translate your confidence level to this level of risk. This table is shown below.

> Your safety plan confidence level indicates the level of risk entailed by attempting to implement the safety plan while the child is staying in the current environment. If you proceed with this plan to establish safety while the child is in this environment, it is important to be clear about the level of risk you are taking.

Confidence Level	Risk to Establish Safety in the Current Environment
1	Manageable Risk The risk is manageable. Stick with the plan, but monitor the keeping of agreements and safety information carefully.
2	Marginally Manageable Risk You may not need to intervene immediately, but the situation poses a level of risk that is marginally manageable. If you are not able to devote a high level of vigilance to monitoring safety over the period of the safety plan time limit, you should bring the child to a safe-enough environment.
3	Unmanageable Risk The risk is unmanageable. You should work to engage systems that will move the child to a safe-enough environment. In unusual circumstances, the child could stay in his or her current environment for a very brief period of time while awaiting placement, as long as safety can be monitored very carefully within this time frame.
4	Critical Risk The child must be brought to a safe-enough environment immediately.

Step 4: Reaching the Decision on Whether to Keep the Child in the Current Environment, Based on the Risk

It's decision time: Is the risk manageable for you and your organization? If not, you need to bring the child to a safe-enough/therapeutic-enough environment.

Safety-Focused Guide: Establishing Safety Step 4: reaching the decision on whether to keep the child within the current environment

Use the authority that you and your organization have to engage child protective services or the emergency psychiatric system, depending on the nature of the problem. If the risk is manageable, then implement the safety plan within the time limit specified. What do you do if the safety plan does not result in the environment reaching the safe-enough standard within this time frame? You make sure that the child is brought to a safe-enough environment by the end of this time frame, because you have already decided it was too risky to go beyond that time frame. Obviously, if you see information that suggests the safety plan will not work—at any time—you should get the child to a safe-enough environment.

A NOTE ABOUT MEDICAL–LEGAL RISK

You may have some concern about documenting events when the clinical picture falls below the safe-enough standard and you don't immediately intervene to bring the child to a safer environment. What type of medical–legal risk are you taking in such a situation? Do you need to immediately complete a mandated child protection report as soon as you've made this determination? Do you need to immediately hospitalize the child—and if the caregivers will not comply with your decision—fill out a mandated child protection report? Sometimes, but not all the time. We support thoughtful, prudent, timely decision making and clear, definitive action based on those decisions. We believe the legal system supports this approach, too. That is why we organized the establishing safety section in the SFG to help you to be as systematic as possible with your decision making and actions. The safety plan time limit is especially important here. Once you've decided that the environment is below the standard, you have a correspondingly short window of time to work with the child and caregivers in the child's current environment—if you decide the child should stay there. Even though the situation falls below a safe-enough standard for a given child, there are variants of risk and corresponding actions. These variables can be seen in the following examples, each of which falls bellow the safe-enough standard.

A 15-year-old girl reports to you that her father is sexually abusing her. This report seems credible. You believe her. You talk to her mother. Her mother responds with rage, yelling at her daughter and blaming her. She tells her daughter that she will be punished when she comes home. Her father lives at home.

Action: File a mandated child protection report and strongly advocate for immediate removal from the home.

A 15-year-old girl reports to you that her mother's boyfriend is sexually abusing her. This report seems credible. You believe her. You talk to her mother, and her mother responds empathically. She shows strong evidence of wanting to support her daughter. She is very angry with her boyfriend and says she can make him stop abusing her daughter. She wants to confront him that evening, with her daughter present. She responds well to your concern about this plan, and agrees to make sure to keep her boyfriend away from her daughter.

Action: File mandated child protection report. Work with mother, child, and child protection caseworker intensively over the next 3 days to make sure the child is safe and that a plan to keep her safe is enacted.

A 15-year-old girl reports to you that she has strong impulses to slash her neck with a knife. Last night, after a fight with her mother, she took a kitchen knife to her neck and made a superficial cut. She has cut her arms and wrists previously, on one occasion leading to significant blood loss. She does not know if she can withstand the impulse to cut her neck if she has another fight with her mother. Mother responds defensively and says her daughter is "dramatic" and only interested in making her "look bad." She shows no willingness to help her daughter or to avoid the type of arguments that lead to this dangerous behavior.

Action: Arrange for immediate emergency psychiatric evaluation with likely inpatient psychiatric hospital admission. If mother declines to agree with the plan, then file a mandated child protection report, with urgent response required.

A 15-year-old girl reports to you that she cuts her arms and wrists. Last night after a fight with her mother, she took a kitchen knife to her wrist and made a superficial cut. The intensity of her cutting has increased over the last few weeks, related to fights with her mother. She does not know if she can withstand the impulse to cut her wrist if she has another fight with her mother. Her mother initially responds defensively but acknowledges her own problem with her temper. She also acknowledges that she can say "really mean things" to her daughter. Her mother expresses remorse and pledges to do everything she can to avoid fights with her daughter, including accepting your suggestions for avoiding such fights. The girl feels safe enough to go home, and the mother agrees with this plan. They agree to call you immediately if the girl has impulses to cut and the mother has impulses to fight with her daughter.

Action: Continue with safety plan for daughter staying at home. See them again in 2 days to monitor the plan. Arrange mother's own treatment. Consider hospitalization if the safety plan cannot be followed.

The best way to manage the medical–legal risk related to your work in establishing safety is to follow the guidelines offered in this section and make sure you document your thoughtful, prudent, timely decision making and your clear, definitive action based on those decisions.

ADVOCACY FOR GETTING CHILD TO A SAFE ENVIRONMENT

Getting the child to a safer environment will often require others as partners. Depending on the problem, these partners frequently are the child welfare system and/or the emergency/inpatient psychiatry system. What if you are in a situation where you believe the child is not safe in his or her current environment and those partners do not agree? What happens if they do not believe they need to work with you to get the child to a safe-enough environment? This is, obviously, a terrible situation to be in, but you have already lined up things as well as you possibly can to get the people you need moving. Here is what you have:

- A defined minimal level of safety that any reasonable person would agree is required (the safe-enough standard).
- Strong evidence that what the child is receiving falls below that standard.
- Strong evidence that efforts to try to establish safety within a reasonable time frame were not successful.
- Justification of your confidence level indicating that more effort to establish safety cannot be accomplished within a reasonable time frame.

We will talk more about how you get the right thing to happen when we review advocacy in a later section. Now, you should see that everything you have done gives you the best chance of getting the child to a safe place. If a person from whom you need help keeps turning from reality, despite all the evidence you have presented, we recommend asking him or her the question we introduced in Chapter 9, for just this situation. In our experience, people don't often say "no" when you ask them this question:

> *Would you be surprised to read about this child on the front page of tomorrow morning's newspaper?*

Let's now consider your job *after* you successfully get the child to a safe-enough environment.

Step 5: Reaching the Decision on Whether (and under What Conditions) to Return the Child to the Previous Environment, Based on the Risk (for Children Who Have Been Placed in a New Environment)

You've helped the child get to a new, safe-enough environment. We are sure the work to accomplish this was very difficult and stressful—but it was absolutely necessary. Now what do you do? First, take a few breaths. Relax a little. Maybe even celebrate the fact that the child is no longer in immediate danger because of your work. Second, refocus your work on making sure the child stays safe. How do you do this?

> It's important to acknowledge that there may be significant variations and limitations to what a TST team can do once a child has been brought to a different environment.

It's important to acknowledge that there may be significant variations and limitations to what a TST team can do once a child has been brought to a different environment. In some cases, the child is placed out of his or her geographic region. In other cases, insurance can no longer pay for the work. Sometimes the plan is for the child to return to the team within a relatively brief period of time. In other cases, a decision is made that the child's care will be managed by another agency or service system, and the TST team will no longer be directly responsible for the care. Sometimes the child will be brought into foster care. Sometimes the child will be brought to residential or inpatient psychiatric care. Sometimes the child will live temporarily with neighbors or extended family. Of course, we cannot account for all of these variants in this discussion of what the TST team should do in these sorts of situations. We do know one thing for certain: The work you have done and the information you have gathered to bring the child to this point will be critically important for whatever happens next. We present the following material understanding that, in many cases, it will be an ideal situation. Nevertheless, within the limitations that you may face, do your best to reach this ideal. This next material is intended for providers and teams with TST programs that are not based in structured therapeutic settings (e.g., residential and inpatient programs). We provide some guidelines related to these issues for providers and teams based in these structured settings in the section on maintaining safety.

First: Find out how long the child is able to stay in this new environment, so you know how much time you have to answer the question about returning him or her to the previous environment. If the child was admitted to an acute psychiatric unit, you may only have a few days. Make sure you know how long you have to figure this all out. If the plan is less than you need, you will need to advocate with the appropriate authorities for the delay in the return to the previous environment. If you've lined up the facts in the way we have suggested in the previous section, you will have plenty of evidence to justify the danger of returning the child until you are able to do your work. Such evidence will usually make someone in authority very cautious about returning a child to such an environment.

OK. You've bought yourself a little time. What can you do with it? You have two things to do:

1. Work with those in the child's previous environment to bring it to the safe-enough standard, while the child is in the new environment (or to determine that a return to the previous environment is too risky).

2. Work with those in the child's new environment to make sure it is safe enough, given the child's vulnerabilities.

In this section we focus on the first activity; we review the second in the section on maintaining safety because the child is in an environment that is now considered safe enough. The activities of maintaining safety are all about making sure the environment can *stay* safe enough for the transition to regulation-focused treatment. We are still *establishing* safety in this section. The question about returning a child to an environment that is below the safe-enough standard is very much within the domain of this present section.

How do we know whether a child can be returned to his or her previous environment, and what needs to be in place for such a return to be safe enough?

WORKING WITH THE PREVIOUS ENVIRONMENT
TO REACH THE SAFE-ENOUGH STANDARD

You have a critical role here. You know a lot about the environment from which the child was removed. You know a lot about the child's dangerous survival states and what is needed from those around the child to keep him or her safe. You know why the environment was determined to be below the safe-enough standard and its impact on the child. You may have worked with the child, caregivers, and others on a safety plan that was unsuccessful. With all your experience, you likely have a very good sense of what needs to be in place for a child's safe return to the previous environment, and of what you might do to support those in the environment to put in place what is needed. Your work here follows a similar logic that you used to help get the child to the new environment. We recommend that you follow this logic here in a way that is adapted for this context. To be most successful, your decisions should be based on answers to the following questions, and your plan should implement activities that correspond to those decisions:

1. Based on your work with this child and all those around him or her, what is the minimum that needs to be in place for the child to safely return to the previous environment?

2. What do caregivers, and others in the previous environment, need to do to make sure the requirements of #1 are in place?

3. How can you best support caregivers, and others in the previous environment, to do what is needed for #2?

4. What is the plan for the child to be returned to the previous environment (and when)?

5. What is the likelihood that #1 will be accomplished in time for #4?

6. Who in the new environment needs to know all of this and what is your plan to make sure they know?

Safety-Focused Guide: Establishing Safety Step 5: Reaching the decision on whether (and under what conditions) to return the child to the environment

Your answers to these questions will guide you to set clear expectations with caregivers, and others, for what needs to be accomplished for the child to be safely returned. Your answers will also specify your role in supporting caregivers and others to meet those expectations so that there is the best chance for the child to be able to safely return. Your answers also specify your strategy for communicating information to the right people in the new environment to help them with decisions on how to help the child and caregivers, and on the time frame for returning the child to the previous environment—if that is appropriate.

ADVOCACY FOR DECISIONS ON RETURNING THE CHILD TO THE PREVIOUS ENVIRONMENT

If you have done your best to reconcile perspectives, but there are still disagreements—*and* a plan is in place that you believe is not in the child's best interests— *you need to advocate.*

Whatever your decision about whether a return to the previous environment is safe enough, and its time frame, you will need others to agree with you. Optimally, everyone is on the same page, but what if this is not the case? In some cases you will be confident that a return to the previous environment is safe enough, and in the best interests of the child, but others in authority disagree. In other cases, you will decide that a return is not safe enough, and not in the best interests of the child, yet those in authority want a return. If you have done your best to reconcile perspectives, but there are still disagreements—*and* a plan is in place that you believe is not in the child's best interests—*you need to advocate.* We discussed a similar issue in the previous section about the partners that you need to get the child to a safe-enough environment, when you did not have the confidence that the environment could be brought to the safe-enough standard in the required time limit. You need such partners here as well. These partners will include:

• Providers/administrators on inpatient units or residential programs with plans to discharge the child home, after they believe the child no longer meets criterion for their program.

• Child welfare workers/administrators with a service plan that is directed toward reunification.

• Family court judges who have directed the child welfare service plan toward reunification.

The more typical need for advocacy is a plan to return the child to an environment that you believe is not safe enough. In such a situation you should get in touch with whomever has the authority to make this decision. Put the facts together for them. Do they dispute your assessment of the safe-enough standard (unlikely)? Do they dispute your recording of the evidence about the meeting of this standard (also unlikely)? Do they dispute your appraisal of the likelihood of caregivers meeting this standard by the time they plan to return the child to the previous environment (also unlikely)? When you present this information as a total picture in the way we know you can, it will be very hard for those in authority to find reasonable grounds to continue with the plan to return the child. And if they still decide not to do the right thing, you can, of course, ask them that recommended question:

> *Would you be surprised to read about this child on the front page of tomorrow morning's newspaper (if you send the child home, knowing what I have told you)?*

Let's not keep the child in limbo for the foreseeable future. Let's create a safe and stable plan for where he or she needs to grow up.

Maintain Safety

Establishing safety is all about making sure the child is in a safe-enough environment. *Maintaining safety* concerns what happens after that milestone is reached. If you have worked hard to bring the environment to a safe-enough standard, or to bring the child to a new, safe-enough environment, are you ready to transition to regulation-focused treatment? You need to make sure these changes are real and will last. Your work in this section on maintaining safety is to make sure the safe-enough environment is real and will last.

> You need to make sure these changes are real and will last. Your work on *maintaining safety* is to make sure the safe-enough environment is real and will last.

There are three sorts of activities to accomplish in order to maintain safety. Each of them is meant to consolidate the gains made in the establishing safety section and to build the supports that will make safety last through the remaining phases of TST and, hopefully, until the time the child becomes an adult. These activities are:

1. Cleaning out the cat hair.
2. Supporting emotional regulation.
3. Advocating for needed services.

Before we discuss each of these activities in detail, we review several general ideas that should guide all of the work involved in maintaining safety:

1. The situation is no longer urgent. The environment, by definition, is above the safe-enough standard. The work here is to make sure it stays there. In establishing safety, you had very little flexibility. You were working below the safe-enough standard and therefore all activities were focused on trying to create a safe-enough environment in a short window of time so that no one was harmed. Now you have more time. The situation is not so urgent. Take the time you need to build the supports needed to keep the environment safe in a way that is sustainable, long after safety-focused treatment ends.

2. When the child starts regulation-focused treatment, there will not be the safeguards in place to monitor and establish safety that exist in safety-focused treatment. In regulation-focused treatment, the work is done from a clinic or office and usually involves less frequent contacts than does safety-focused treatment. In the safety-focused phase we are operating within the child's social environment and therefore have tremendous opportunities to directly observe the nature of these perceived threats and their impact. We will not have nearly that vantage point once we transition into regulation-focused treatment. Let's make the most of this opportunity while we have it. Accordingly, make sure you use the limited time you have left in safety-focused treatment well. Use the opportunity of having a home- or community-based team that can provide intervention more frequently to make sure supports are in place that will last.

3. At the beginning of the maintaining safety phase, define the time you will likely need to make sure all of this happens. The most important aspect of this estimate is getting clear on the time you need in order to have confidence that the safe-enough environment will last. It may be that when you started safety-focused treatment, the family had already reached the safe-enough standard. Perhaps during the process of ready–set–go, caregivers became so concerned about the safety in the environment that they made the needed changes. Terrific! How long should they demonstrate those changes for you to feel confident they are real and will last? Similarly, when safety becomes established during safety-focused treatment, how long should it be established until you are confident enough that it is real and will last?

Activity 1: Cleaning out the Cat Hair

In this phase of maintaining safety, there are no cats that can reach the child. Your work in establishing safety addressed this problem definitively. The environment is no longer harmful. Further, any cat hair that can lead to a shift into dangerous survival states was also addressed in the establishing safety phase. The situation is now much more stable because the perceived threats that lead to dangerous survival states have been removed. What is left to do? Three things:

Safety-Focused Guide:
Maintaining Safety Activity 1:
cleaning out the cat hair

1. Make sure the cat stays away from the child.
2. Make sure the cat hair that provokes dangerous survival states also stays away.
3. Make sure other sorts of cat hair (stressors) are also removed when therapeutically indicated and when possible.

The first two are handled in a relatively straightforward manner. Agreements have been made and—so far—kept with relevant caregivers and providers about the actual threats, and about the perceived threats that lead to dangerous survival states (the safe-enough environment). Your job here is to monitor that these agreements are kept and to make proactive decisions if the agreements are not kept. If you find that an agreement responsible for establishing safety is not kept, then go right back to the protocol for establishing safety detailed in the previous section. Usually the process of monitoring the agreements and continuing to offer the support defined in the safety plan will continue to maintain the safe-enough environment. And the longer it is maintained, the longer it will last. This section of the SFG is simply a place to record your monitoring of safety, the evidence, and any adjustments you need to make, based on the evidence.

What about other sorts of cat hair—that is, stressors or perceived threats that don't lead to dangerous survival states? Should you address those in safety-focused treatment? Which ones should you choose to address?

One of the goals of safety-focused treatment is to help parents and other key people in a child's social environment protect the child from stressors or perceived threats that lead to survival states; however, at times it may be neither possible nor desirable to eliminate all perceived threats from the child's environment. Indeed, if a child is triggered by essential activities of life, such as being around other people or going out of the house, removing these triggers would reinforce avoidance strategies and hinder the child's development. Sometimes a child will purposefully avoid certain settings or situations that lead to his or her feeling distressed. Sometimes this avoidance itself becomes the first problem to treat. Unless a child begins to have the experience of facing a feared (but necessary) stressor and successfully managing the distress, it will be impossible to help him or her build regulatory skills. The provider can remind the parent that it is the process of helping the child learn to regulate his or her emotions (rather than just avoiding dysregulation) that leads to recovery.

Following is a child's hypothetical list of cat hair stressors, and a commentary on whether or not these should be removed from the child's environment:

- "When my teacher tells me I need to sit down." Learning to be a part of a classroom is essential in life. Assuming the classroom is appropriate for this child, this is a trigger that should not be eliminated. Instead, the child needs to work on skills for regulating in that moment.
- "On the bus, when all the kids are throwing things." Being able to be with other kids is essential—tolerating a rowdy bus is not. If this consistently triggers the child, consider advocating to have a bus monitor put on the bus.
- "At home when my big brother and his friends watch sexy movies." Watching movies is not only nonessential, in this case it also is inappropriate. The provider should work with the parent to provide better monitoring, or work with the whole family to help everyone understand why these movies can't be watched at home.
- "Going to school." Unless there are extraordinary circumstances, a child needs to go to school. A child who refuses to go to school may be doing so because school leads to feelings of distress. In this situation, gradually helping the child acclimate to more and more aspects of the school day again may help him or her learn that he or she can manage attending school without being overwhelmed by feelings.

 Generally speaking, cat hair (and what to do about it) falls into three categories:

1. Triggers/stressors that are unnecessary, unhelpful, or downright damaging parts of life that ideally would be reduced or eliminated.
2. Triggers/stressors that are a necessary part of life but could be temporarily reduced or eliminated until better regulation skills are learned.
3. Triggers/stressors that are a necessary part of life and cannot or should not be removed and instead must be learned to be tolerated.

Sometimes adults in a child's life may initially resist the idea that stressors should be removed: "Isn't that just part of life? Aren't we creating an artificial environment, and my child will never make it in the *real* world?" Well, yes and no. The next phase of treatment (regulation focused) is largely dedicated to building the child's emotional regulation capacity so that he or she will be able to stay regulated when exposed to such stimuli in the future. If there is too much of these stimuli in the child's environment when he or she is expected to learn to regulate emotion, it will be very difficult to benefit from emotional regulation skill training. As triggers are identified, consider which of the three categories they fall into: to be removed, to be removed temporarily, or to be tolerated. Triggers that fall into the first category—unnecessary or even damaging stressors—may require an advocacy plan (more on that below). Jot down the plan for removing that trigger.

Triggers that fall into the third category—necessary parts of life that need to be tolerated—will likely require the teaching of emotional regulation skills that can be used specifically in response to that stressor. This will be the focus of the next phase of treatment.

Triggers that fall into the middle category—those that are necessary parts of life but could be *temporarily* reduced or withdrawn—will likely require both kinds of efforts. Let's say a refugee child is triggered in gym class because the thundering feet on the floor of the echoing gym sounds a lot like when his or her hometown was carpet-bombed. An advocacy plan to work with the school to temporarily remove the child from gym class is needed, or at least an effort made to have all the kids remove their shoes! At the same time you can introduce relaxation exercises so that when the child hears the thundering sound, he or she automatically thinks "I'm in school, I'm safe, and I'm going to breathe in through my nose and out through my mouth 10 times."

Activity 2: Supporting Emotional Regulation

Here we are at the risk of contradicting ourselves. We know that, in the previous section, we stated that the next phase—regulation-focused treatment—is the time to build emotional regulation skills. Although that statement is largely correct, we do need to support a child's emotional regulation capacity prior to his or her reaching regulation-focused treatment. The primary way we support this capacity in safety-focused treatment is via our efforts to remove cats and cat hair. The reason this is such an emphasis in safety-focused treatment is because there is so much work to do to establish and maintain a safe-enough environment. We know that regulation-focused phase is pretty much dedicated to building emotional regulation skills, so we will leave a lot of that work to the next phase. Still, there are some things that can be done in safety-focused treatment to support emotional regulation. We summarize some of them in Table 12.1.

TABLE 12.1. Supporting Emotional Regulation

	Strategy	Mechanism of action	Example
Safety-Focused Guide: Maintaining Safety Activity 2A: emotional regulation skill introduction	Emotional regulation skill building	Provides child with concrete coping strategies to use when revving to prevent going into a reexperiencing state. Choose easy-to-implement strategies from Appendix 11.	Breathing exercise: "Imagine smelling a flower [take deep, slow breath in] and blowing out bubbles [let deep, slow breath out]." Repeat 10 times.
Safety-Focused Guide: Maintaining Safety Activity 2B: psychopharmacology plan	Psychopharmacology	Dampens emotional arousal and survival response.	Sertraline to help with child's state of depression
Safety-Focused Guide: Maintaining Safety Activity 2C: supporting child's basic health needs	Supporting the child's basic health needs	Reduces vulnerability to emotional dysregulation by making sure child isn't tired or hungry.	Help parents come up with a consistent bedtime routine. Take the TV out of the room. Let families know that kids and adolescents need a lot of sleep!

Activity 3: Advocating for Needed Interventions and Services

Safety-Focused Guide: Maintaining Safety Activity 3: advocating for needed interventions and services

Success in establishing and maintaining safety requires access to the right type of interventions and services. In safety-focused treatment, we must be effective in making sure the child and family receive the services they need. Some of these services are already embedded in the TST team. In safety-focused treatment the child and family will receive home-/community-based care and, sometimes, psychopharmacology, because these are services the team offers and delivers as part of TST. Some TST teams offer other services that they believe will be very important for the families they serve. The specifics of the services offered by a particular TST team are usually worked out in the organizational planning process and can be very helpful. For example, some teams include cultural brokers to facilitate engagement for families unfamiliar with Western culture. Other teams have integrated the capacity to provide treatment to caregivers, if needed. This process of expanding the interventions and services provided by the TST team can be very helpful when it appears that reliable access to a given intervention or service will be needed for a good proportion of children served by the team. Again, this is worked out in the organizational planning process and is often established through the process of interagency agreement (if the given intervention or service is not provided by the agency that establishes the TST program). Very often, the child and family will need services not provided by the TST team. Of course, you have already considered these needed interventions and services as part of your assessment and treatment planning process. If you decided that an intervention or service was needed, you engaged the relevant organization and providers as part of ready–set–go, and they signed the treatment agreement letter indicating their agreement to offer such services as part of the treatment plan. Such services may include:

- Specific educational support
- Specific medical support
- Specific child welfare support
- Specific legal support
- Specific housing support
- Specific financial support
- Specific mental health, substance abuse, developmental support for children (not found on the TST team)
- Specific mental health, substance abuse, developmental support for caregivers

ADVOCATING FOR NEEDED INTERVENTIONS AND SERVICES DURING THE ESTABLISHING SAFETY PHASE VERSUS THE MAINTAINING SAFETY PHASE

We've already discussed the process of advocating for *urgent* interventions and services in the establishing safety section. In such a situation, an intervention or a service is needed to prevent serious injury to someone. We reviewed the process of engaging such critical interventions/services as child protection and acute psychiatric hospitalization. In the establishing safety phase we had very little time and needed to systematically gather the information and decisively act within that very short window of time. In the maintaining safety phase, we have a bit more time, but we still need to be systematic and decisive. The purpose of advocating for needed interventions and services during the establishing safety phase was to prevent harm. The purpose of these activities in maintaining safety is to institute the supports the child and family need to address their identified problems throughout TST—and, if necessary, beyond. There is a common logic to this work irrespective of whether it occurs during the establishing or maintaining safety phase. This logic should be very familiar to you from previous sections of this chapter and includes:

- Clarity on the problem definition.
- Clarity on the standard of intervention/service required to address the problem.
- Clarity on the time frame needed for the problem to be addressed.
- Clarity on the results about whether the problem was actually addressed.
- Clarity on the decisions that need to be made, based on the results.

FRAMEWORK FOR ADVOCATING FOR NEEDED INTERVENTIONS AND SERVICES

We provide a framework for this type of advocacy and embed it in the SFG. This framework should be used to maximize the chance of the child and family receiving the support that they need. As described, you have already done a lot of work to define the needed interventions and services in the treatment plan and engaged the people you need in the treatment agreement letter. The framework we propose fleshes this out a bit more so that you have the best chance at success. One caution: It takes a lot of work to ensure that the child and family have access to a needed intervention and service. Make sure every intervention

> One caution: It takes a lot of work to ensure that the child and family have access to a needed intervention and service. Make sure every intervention or service that becomes a focus of your advocacy is *absolutely* needed. You don't have unlimited time or resources.

or service that becomes a focus of your advocacy is *absolutely* needed. You don't have unlimited time or resources. Any effort to access a less important intervention or service has the potential to undermine the effort to access a more important intervention or service. With this caution in mind, we recommend that you follow the steps below to successfully advocate for a needed intervention or service:

1. *Define* the problem that needs the intervention/service.
2. *Identify* the intervention/service the child needs for the defined problem.
3. *Propose* how the intervention/service should be used to address the defined problem, including:
   - The potential impact of the intervention/service on the child's functioning.
   - The potential impact on the child's functioning should the child not receive it.
   - The maximal time frame the child could wait to receive it, without significant impact on the child's functioning.
4. *Engage* the relevant organizations/providers who are responsible for delivering the intervention/service.
5. *Evaluate* the quality of this engagement, the implementation of the needed intervention/service, and the results of this implementation.
6. *Adjust* the plan based on these results.

Let's use this framework to consider the case of Jason, introduced in Chapters 9 and 10. The treatment plan specified that his teachers should monitor his activities in the locker room and bathroom—those situations where he needed to change his clothes in front of other boys. The treatment plan included, for a while, planning bathroom and locker room visits when there were no other children present. His teachers agreed to participate in this plan and to track the plan's success in helping with this defined problem.

1. *Define* the problem that needs the intervention/service.

   Jason becomes very aggressive with other children in situations where he needs to remove his clothes (such as locker room and bathroom) and feels they get too close to him. He has assaulted several classmates in this context.

2. *Identify* the intervention/service the child needs for the defined problem.

   His teachers will monitor bathroom and locker room visits.

3. *Propose* how the intervention/service should be used to address the defined problem.

   His teachers will take him to the bathroom and locker room when no other children are present and make sure he feels safe enough when he changes. The teachers will try this for 1 month. If they are successful, he will not assault other children at school.

4. *Engage* the relevant organizations/providers who are responsible for delivering the intervention/service.

   We had a good meeting with Ms. Smith. She seems very willing to try.

5. *Evaluate* the quality of this engagement, the implementation of the needed intervention/service, and the results of this implementation.

   The first week is over. Ms. Smith or her aide was able to follow the plan fully. There were no aggressive episodes this week.

6. *Adjust* the plan based on these results.

   The plan is working! Let's keep it going!

WHEN YOU NEED TO ADVOCATE MORE STRENUOUSLY

We love the situation just described. Jason's teacher rolled up her sleeves with us and fully engaged with the plan—and it achieved the desired result. Sometimes we have less success engaging a provider to do what is needed. What if Jason's teacher, Ms. Smith, would not engage with the plan? What would we do? We've already decided that the plan is important enough. In fact, we cannot imagine achieving impact on Jason's aggression in school without this plan. We must figure this out. There are several common reasons that a provider will not engage with the plan. We list these below. We also list the solution to each sort of engagement problem.

1. When the provider does not understand what is expected
   - We communicate better.

2. When the provider has practical barriers in the way of engagement
   - We troubleshoot the barrier.

3. When the provider is unwilling to engage or does not see what is expected as part of his or her job
   - We step it up.

We want to address the engagement problem with an effective solution, and such a solution requires an accurate understanding of the problem. If we believed we had an agreement with Ms. Smith about her role in helping with Jason's problems and after 1 week we saw she had never followed through, we would need to understand the reason. Let's start with the simplest problem. She didn't understand what was expected. Let's check it out. If this is true, let's make the expectation clearer. Will she engage then? If yes, let's keep going. If no, why not? Perhaps there is a practical barrier in the way. Maybe Ms. Smith is well meaning, but she is so overwhelmed with work that she just is not able to follow through. Maybe the classroom aide she counted on is not available. In this case, let's work with her. Perhaps the principal can be brought in, shown the plan, and helped to see that a small intervention, such as a reliable classroom aide to accompany Jason for bathroom and locker room trips, for the short term will make a big difference.

What if the problem is not a practical barrier? What if Ms. Smith just cannot be bothered or believes this is not part of her job? Then we step it up. We find out to whom the teacher reports and bring the problem to that person's attention. We have lined up everything to communicate clearly about the consequences for Jason if such a simple plan is not followed. We know that this small intervention is absolutely something to which Jason is entitled. If we need to, we will push to have this intervention embedded in his IEP. In these cases we often consult with our advocacy attorney to find the best strategy to get the right thing to happen. And we absolutely line up everything to maximize our chance of success.

FURTHER THOUGHTS ABOUT STEPPING UP THE ADVOCACY PLAN

We try our best not to go to the stepping-up stage. We try to make agreements with providers that are fully in the interest of helping and protecting children. If an agreement we seek is not forthcoming, our first questions are: What did we get wrong? Are we missing information? Is there a perspective to integrate that we have not yet integrated? We go through that process—always doing our best to align with reality—and at some point we say, *no*. There is *no* reason to keep working to understand another perspective. There is *no* more relevant information to integrate. There is *no* alternative way to address the problems we've identified. A child is in need. That child may be hurt. There is *no* reason *not* to do what we are proposing. And then we step up the advocacy plan. Advocacy is our process for making sure the right thing happens. It's what we do when we refuse to walk by a drowning child. And we don't stop until the right thing is achieved. It's that important. Will we choose any instance of failure to

> We always do our best to align with reality—and at some point we say, *no*. There is *no* reason to keep working to understand another perspective. There is *no* more relevant information to integrate. There is *no* alternative way to address the problems we've identified. A child is in need. That child may be hurt. There is *no* reason *not* to do what we are proposing.

reach an agreement on a priority problem as a reason to step up advocacy? No. We will be going *all in* on these situations. We have to be sure they are important enough. We have already assessed and made decisions about the importance of all problems we will be addressing in treatment, so we are poised to advocate if we need to do so.

The following are examples of common reasons to step up advocacy:

- A child protection investigation considers—or makes—a decision that fails to recognize that the child is not safe.
- A family court judge considers—or makes—a decision that the team believes is contrary to the safety needs of the child.
- An immigration court judge considers—or makes—a decision that may lead to the deportation of the child and family, and the team believes such an act will significantly jeopardize the child's physical and emotional health.
- A school considers—or makes—a decision to provide an educational plan that does not adequately address the learning needs of the child.
- The family lacks basic resources, such as adequate food, housing, or income.

Establishing and Maintaining Safety in Residential Programs and Inpatient Units

There are two ways that TST is used in structured therapeutic settings such as residential treatment programs or inpatient psychiatry units:

- When the TST program is based outside those programs/units, and the child is brought to the unit to establish safety.
- When the TST program is based within those programs/units.

WHEN A CHILD IS BROUGHT TO A RESIDENTIAL PROGRAM/INPATIENT UNIT TO ESTABLISH SAFETY

We described this situation in the establish safety section. In this context, a TST team has decided the environment is not safe enough and the child is brought to the structured therapeutic setting to establish safety. We expect the environment of the program/unit is safe enough for the child. We also know a lot about the child's vulnerabilities and the process of his or her transition into dangerous survival states. Our work is largely devoted to helping the clinical and direct-care staff of these units understand as much as possible about these vulnerabilities so that the treatment plan developed for the child on the unit effectively addresses these vulnerabilities. Ideally, the child's treatment plan on the unit is completely continuous with the TST treatment plan. A critical role for the TST team is to communicate its opinion about what needs to be in place such that the child can be safely returned, as detailed in the section on establishing safety. As described, this is the minimum standard of help and protection that would need to be in place to return the child to the environment from which he or she was removed. There are usually great pressures on these units to discharge children in a timely way. The TST team should be advocating that discharge to the home environment *not* take place until a safe-enough standard has been reached. The team should also communicate whether discharge home makes sense at all, based on the information the team has gathered about the home environment. If the TST team does not believe the child should be discharged home, the team should work closely with unit staff to find a more reasonable discharge plan, based on knowledge of the child's vulnerabilities.

While this interaction with the child's unit is occurring, the TST team is working with the child's caregivers to do everything possible to help the environment reach the safe-enough standard. Information about this effort and its results can be critically important in guiding decision making about discharge plans.

WHEN THE TST PROGRAM IS BASED WITHIN A RESIDENTIAL PROGRAM OR INPATIENT UNIT

TST has been used as a primary program model in residential programs and inpatient units. It is important to understand that, by and large, the children admitted to the TST program on these units require such admission because they switch to dangerous survival states and their home environment was insufficiently helpful and protective, given the level of dysregulation. Sometimes their home environment was harmful. In other words these children meet our criteria for safety-focused treatment, as is almost always demonstrated through the implementation of the TST assessment, treatment planning, and ready–set–go processes established on the unit. The program on the unit will usually follow an adaptation of what has been detailed in this maintaining safety section. How to implement safety-focused treatment from a program based on a structured therapeutic unit? The most successful of these programs incorporate many of the following components:

- An established TST team responsible for developing the treatment plan, engaging all stakeholders in it, and tracking its implementation and the results yielded.
- A milieu program that is fully integrated in the team and addresses perceived threats and consequential survival states on the unit.
- Psychopharmacology providers who are well integrated into the team and deliver interventions (as described in Chapter 15).

- An approach to the child's family that fully addresses the need to bring the home environment to a safe-enough standard for discharge. Such an approach integrates decisions about phone calls, family visits to the units, and visits home within this context.

- A home-based program that can work to support the family to reach the safe-to-return standard.

- A collaboration with an outpatient program and/or home-based program that can manage the transition to either regulation-focused treatment or home-based safety-focused treatment upon discharge, depending on the child's needs.

Caring for Caregivers

Throughout safety-focused treatment—indeed, throughout all of TST—we need to think about how to support caregivers to better help and protect their child. Obviously, a lot is asked of caregivers to establish and to maintain safety. What are their needs and how can we best meet them? What we describe in this section about enabling parents to HELP is very relevant for the goals of safety-focused care, but is also important for each of the other phases of TST treatment. We describe our approach to working with parents in this section and offer a tool called the TST HELPers Guide (see Appendix 8). This approach and its tool are utilized by the supporters (with our support) throughout TST treatment.

When a child is assessed to be in the safety-focused phase of treatment, it signifies that the social environment often has a long way to travel before it can be considered able to both help and protect. But the journey begins here. A major focus of treatment in the safety-focused phase is to support parents in becoming more attuned to their child's needs and better able to help him or her regulate. Primary objectives are to support parents or other caregivers in the following four areas, noted with a handy mnemonic device (HELP) to help everyone remember:

> A major focus of treatment in the safety-focused phase is to support parents in becoming more attuned to their child's needs and better able to help him or her regulate.

1. **Handling the difficult moments.** Helping caregivers stay regulated in the face of their child's dysregulation.

2. **Enjoying their child.** Reestablishing a loving relationship between caregivers and children; fostering stronger attachment.

3. **Learning parenting skills.** Helping caregivers develop parenting skills to reduce stress in the home and encourage positive child behaviors.

4. **Planning for emergencies.** Establishing a concrete plan for emergencies, and clarity around what constitutes an emergency.

Different sections of the HELPers Guide will be emphasized in different steps and phases of the work. Within establishing safety, the two most critical sections are *handling the difficult moments* and *planning for emergencies*. The safety plan will be kept by the child and family throughout treatment, and should be established at the beginning of safety-focused treatment. First, handling the difficult moments will be especially helpful for parents who struggle with maintaining a calm and helpful environment when their child is experiencing survival states. Second, enjoying their child, can be useful at any point in treatment to help build the parent's relationship with his or her child, and may be emphasized in beyond trauma as part of undoing the lingering effects of past trauma and dysregulation. During the phase of maintaining safety, learning parenting skills should be emphasized. Constructive and effective parenting strategies will help give parents the skills to safely manage their child's behavior, and are typically also an important focus during regulation-focused treatment.

The HELPers Guide is a companion guide to the SFG, and is meant for parents to use and fill out in collaboration with the therapist. Like the SFG, the HELPers guide is a dynamic document that can be filled out over time, revisited, and revised. It may be useful to pull it out at the beginning of each parent meeting to check on how things are going in the four areas.

TOOL: HELPers Guide

What it is: A clinical tool for providers to use with parents that offers concrete steps to build parents' capacity to help and protect their child. Can also be used with other caregivers, such as foster parents and residential treatment staff.

When to use it: Throughout treatment in all phases (safety-focused, regulation-focused, and beyond trauma)

We describe the four main objectives in working with parents and how to use the HELPers Guide in the following section.

Handling the Difficult Moments: Helping Caregivers Stay Regulated

HELPers Guide: Handling the difficult moments

Unfortunately, here is a simple truth: A child in a survival-in-the-moment state can be hard to be around. Consider what it must be like for Ms. Williams to manage Tanisha's severe aggression. Consider Tanisha's teachers, who believe that her aggression is completely "out of the blue." Consider the following "moments" for these other children:

Ten-year-old Peter, enraged that his little sister doesn't want to share her donut, wrenches it out of her hand and pushes her over, yelling "You stupid brat! I hate you!" His little sister looks pleadingly at her mother, tears rolling down her face.

 Eight-year-old Nina, terrified that someone is going to come through her window, calls hysterically for her mother for the fourth time that night, and then inconsolably screams until the whole family is awoken.

 Sixteen-year-old Jenna, upset that her parents had another fight earlier in the evening, sneaks out her window and takes the car. Her parents later are woken by a call from the police, telling them Jenna has been driving drunk and crashed the car.

Now consider what it is like to be around this kind of dysregulation, day in and day out. Consider what it is like to see little sisters, or whole families, suffer from the rages and behavior of the "moments." Now consider, with empathy, how the parents of Peter and Nina and Jenna might respond . . .

 Peter's mother wrenches the donut out of his hand and yells "Don't you DARE push your sister! You say you hate her, but if anyone should be hated here, it's YOU!"

 Nina's mother, exhausted from dealing with night after night of her daughter's terrors, drags herself to her bedroom to rub her daughter's back one more time and try to assure her no one is coming in the window. But when she enters the bedroom Nina screams even louder, "Get out! Get out!" Nina becomes hysterical, flailing her arms and legs and hitting at her mother. Nina's mother, desperate to quiet her so she won't wake the whole house (again) and to stop Nina from hitting her, pins Nina's arms to the bed and begins to sob, "Stop it! Stop it! You are ruining everything!"

 Jenna's father fumes all the way to the police station. When he sees Jenna, she rolls her eyes at him. Jenna's father feels a wave of anger and pushes his face into hers, yelling, "That is it! I'm done with you! You hear that? DONE!"

These are not crazy, spiteful, incompetent parents. They are exhausted. They are worn down. They are suffering from the accumulation of moments of survival that have gradually torn down their reserves, their hope, their capacity to feel love. They, themselves, now enter survival states whenever their children do. The combination is deadly. We can guess how Peter, Nina, and Jenna will respond to their dysregulated parents. It is not pretty. It is a vicious, downward spiral. And it is where many families in the safety-focused phase of treatment begin.

Helping children manage their intense emotions and behaviors is a core element of treatment throughout TST. Much of the next chapter, on the regulation-focused phase of treatment, provides a great deal of detail about how to build the skill sets to support a child's regulation. But in the safety-focused phase of treatment the work focuses on one single (but not simple) step of helping parents to stay regulated in the face of their child's dysregulation. So, how do you help parents stay regulated?

The capacity to regulate emotions is like a muscle. If you use it too much, you temporarily wear it out and it gets weaker.

The capacity to regulate emotions is like a muscle. If you use it too much, you temporarily wear it out and it gets weaker. Think of a time when you responded pleasantly and calmly to the first 30 provocations of your day, and then when the poor 31st person walked in and said something, you snapped. So it is with parents trying to remain calm in the face of a dysregulated child. So how do you strengthen that regulation muscle?

There are ways to minimize the likelihood that your "regulation muscle" will wear out on you, including taking a break, making sure you are physically healthy, getting the sleep and nutrition you need, and laughing. Really!

For some parents, the encouragement to make some changes, concrete strategies that they can use in difficult moments like the ones described above, and the persuasive fact that it will help their child are all they need to move toward better managing their own emotions. However, in many cases parents need additional support and help—particularly if they themselves have experienced trauma. In some cases, parents and children can end up being traumatic reminders for each other.

In addition to the support provided by the TST team, some parents will benefit from having their own therapist. Working with parents to recognize this need and the potential value of a therapeutic relationship, acknowledging the tremendous effort that is consistently asked of parents of traumatized children, and guiding parents to treatment that matches their needs and wishes are central to this work. Whether it is substance abuse treatment, treatment for depression, or treatment for their own traumas, helping parents to reach the most appropriate support and services is among the most helpful interventions you can offer a child.

Review the information in the "Handling the Difficult Moments" section with the parent. When a child gets upset, it is easy for a parent to get upset. When a parent gets upset, it is hard to do the things that he or she needs to do to calm the child. Once you feel that the parent is in agreement that staying calm is important, talk through the three concrete strategies in the HELPers Guide.

1. **Take a break!** There may be many barriers to parents getting the respite they need. Some parents may feel they can't be away from their child because they are needed. Others may not have someone who can step in for a brief period. Talk through the reasons why this may be a challenge and strategize around a concrete solution. Jot down the plan and when this time can be scheduled—and be sure to check in the next week to see if it happened. Taking a break is not a one-time deal; help parents structure in regular times that they can step away and recharge.

2. **Take care of yourself.** Parents often expend inordinate energy making sure their children get what they need—healthy food, enough sleep, exercise, health care. Parents need these too. Self-care may be an area that requires more than just a commitment to try things differently. If they have problems with substance use, mental health issues, or other significant ways in which their health and well-being are compromised, then this discussion may need to center on how to connect parents with the services they need. Again, there may be many barriers here, including a parent's own experience of trauma and resulting avoidance or reactivity. Try to understand what these barriers are and to think about how attaining these services might help address a parent's primary source of pain. Depending on the circumstances, it may be helpful to communicate to parents that although they have made it this far without this kind of help, their child would really benefit from the parents getting support. If parents won't seek help for their own sake, sometimes they will for the sake of their kids. Jot down specific self-care steps a parent plans to take for him- or herself. Make sure to check back the next week to see how these are going and how the parent feels.

3. **Seek support.** Parents need friends. But sometimes having a severely dysregulated child causes collateral damage: Families start withdrawing, losing friends, being difficult for others to be around. Social support is one of the most critical ways of supporting healthy, resilient families. To whom can parents turn, not just in times of crisis, but to rebuild the power and strength of community? With whom can they spend time that will make them laugh? Write down specific people or places—such as their church or a community organization—the parents plan to reach out to in the coming week. Make sure to check back the following week to see what happened.

These three areas can help build resilience and promote better regulation over time, just like exercising can get you in shape to play in a big game. But getting in shape is only part of being a great athlete; players also need to know how to perform under pressure during the big game itself. In the world of parenting, that means parents still need a concrete plan for what to do, in the moment of a child's survival state, to keep from being overwhelmed by emotion. The next part of this point on seeking support in the HELPers Guide provides just that: a survive-the-moment plan. It begins with a simple flowchart to help a parent make sound decisions in a moment of high emotion and crisis. Walk parents through the steps in this flow chart.

1. Is my child in danger (i.e., at risk to harm self or others, at risk to be harmed)?
   - Yes → Go to the emergency plan at the back of this guide.
   - No → Keep going.
2. Am I upset (e.g., angry, frightened, worried I might lose control)?
   - Yes → Walk away and take 10 deep breaths, think a calming thought, or tense and release muscles in different parts of your body. Ask yourself again, "Am I calm?" Keep taking space and deep breaths or use other coping skills until you are calm.
   - No → Keep going.
3. Offer help to your child.

The idea behind this flowchart is fairly simple, and when you are sitting with the parent, in a moment of calm, these ideas may seem moderately ridiculous. Do you really need a flowchart for this?

Yes. Because, remember, the parent's amygdala may be leading a hostile takeover of conscience by emotion (remember Chapter 2?), particularly if the parent has experienced trauma. So this little flowchart becomes a temporary stand-in for his or her higher-order reasoning. And simply knowing that they know what to do can make a moment of crisis feel less frightening for parents.

So, is the child in danger? As you will see in a minute, by the time the parent has worked with a therapist to complete the "Planning for Emergencies" section of the HELPers Guide he or she will know how to determine this. That, alone, can bring some clarity to chaos. Next, is the parent upset? This is a personal, subjective evaluation. Parents need to check in with their body responses, their heart rates, their thoughts, the way they feel. If they feel like yelling, they are upset. They need to walk away and breathe deeply until they are no longer upset. If they feel like they are "revving" toward something more serious, help them identify ways they can return to a regulated state.

Now, finally, the parents can help their child. Exactly how to help will look very different depending on the child, the parent, and the types of survival moments that occur. Whatever the particulars, the therapist can work with the parent to come up with a plan, write out some concrete to-dos, and revise this as everyone gets to know each other—and what works—better.

Enjoying Your Child: Establishing (or Reestablishing) a Loving Relationship between Parents and Child

Think back to Peter, Nina, and Jenna. Could you feel the love? No, probably not. And at times it may be hard for their parents to feel it, too. But helping parents and children to reestablish that fundamental, enduring, and essential sense of love, trust, and attachment is the foundation on which healing happens. As we reviewed in Chapter 5, if there are not enough safety signals communicated, it is very hard to improve anything. So how do we help Peter, Nina, Jenna, and their parents emit safety signals and reestablish loving relationships?

HELPers Guide: Enjoying your child

Helping parents and children to reestablish that fundamental, enduring, and essential sense of love, trust, and attachment is the foundation on which healing happens.

First, it is important to recognize that survival states cause collateral damage. *Collateral damage* occurs when injury is inflicted on something other than the intended target, such as civilian casualties in a military operation. The survival circuits in the child fire in order to "target" the perceived danger. The collateral damage occurs in the form of the harsh words, punched fists, and havoc wrought on any and everyone nearby during the survival-in-the-moment outburst. Parents often bear the brunt of this damage. Over time, the collateral damage erodes the loving relationship. Parents may feel scared, angry, or resentful of their children. They may see their lives in shambles because their child requires so much energy and causes both physical and emotional damage to the world around them.

Of course one of the most basic ways of stopping the collateral damage and allowing the relationship to heal is by helping the child heal, so that survival-in-the-moment responses do not happen. But it's a Catch-22: to help the child heal, the parent needs to be able to feel, and show, love and acceptance. Even when parents know they love their child, the feeling may be temporarily inaccessible. We also know that when parents have experienced trauma, it can make them feel negatively about themselves as parents and about their children. They may be more likely to feel that their children are intentionally doing things to upset them—whether those things occur during an episode of dysregulation or when the child is doing something age-appropriate but nevertheless difficult to handle. Being attuned to parents' negative attributions about their kids is important because those attributions can signal that their own trauma reactions are impacting their parenting—and that you need to intervene with them. So how can you help?

We also know that when parents have experienced trauma, it can make them feel negatively about themselves as parents and about their children.

The HELPers Guide includes several specific exercises to help parents reconnect to the genuine feelings of love they have for their children. There's no simple shot of oxytocin to rebuild a loving relationship, but there are ways to help parents remember and foster the genuine attachment that is possible between parents and children.

Providers and staff working with children and families can have these sorts of reactions too, and it is also important for them to stay regulated, especially when the child with whom they are working is dysregulated.

The HELPers Guide provides the parent with three activities, to be done with the support of the provider, that help caregivers *enjoy their child*—nurturing a strong attachment, rebuilding a sense of love and connection, and fostering joy:

1. **Make a "good times" album here and in your head.** In this exercise, parents write down specific times they've felt loving towards and had fun with, their child. Ask them to hold it in their head as an image, like a snapshot, in addition to writing it down. When they start to remember good times, often many more memories will come to the surface. Have them write these down too, and make more mental snapshots. It is important to have the parent state and share these memory snapshots to make them more concrete and vivid.

2. **Make a "good times" date.** Parents sometimes spend so much of their time managing the messes that they have very little time to spend on more joyful, fun activities—or they may be so angry or stressed that they don't want to. But time spent enjoying each other is fundamental to making all the other moments of the day go more smoothly, and to fostering the love and joy that are at the heart of a healthy family. Whether it is called "special time" or "child-directed play" or just plain old "good times together," help the parent strategize around how to spend time doing something with the child that they both enjoy. Encourage the parent to let the child determine the play and lead the way, and to refrain from using the time to teach, correct, direct, or otherwise take control of the play. For older children who may not eagerly opt-in to parent–child playtime, encourage the parent to observe a moment when the child is engaging in something and to join by being curious, asking questions, and showing interest. Ideally parents will find two or three times per week that they can have a "good times" date.

3. **Make a "good kid" slogan.** Imagine all the negative things parents hear about their children when children are having a difficult time managing behaviors and emotions. "Spoiled! Aggressive! A jerk! Noncompliant! Stubborn!" Helping parents hold in mind all the positive ways of seeing

their child can help to reshape underlying attitudes so that they view the child for his or her whole, valuable self—rather than just as a pile of problems. Review the "'My Kid' Adjectives" list at the end of the HELPers Guide and have parents circle all the adjectives that fit their child. Take the top three and make a sentence that parents can think to themselves, and shout out loud, when negative statements start to take over.

Learning Parenting Skills: Reducing Stress in the Home and Encouraging Positive Child Behavior

Remember Peter, who grabbed the donut and pushed his sister? He's a mean-spirited kid who seems to take pleasure out of hurting his vulnerable, sweet little sister.

> HELPers Guide: Learning parenting skills

How are you feeling toward Peter? What kind of emotions sweep through you thinking about him? If Peter saw your face, what kind of signals of care or danger would he perceive?

Now try this. Remember Peter, who grabbed the donut and pushed his sister? Ever since he was abused by his Uncle George, he has felt things more intensely, more deeply. The smallest provocation can send him into a survival state, and when he's in that state, he lashes out like a wild animal in a cage. He doesn't even seem to know he's bigger than his sister, he feels so vulnerable.

Now how are you feeling toward Peter? Would it be easier to respond calmly, and with empathy, than in the earlier scenario?

Parents carry scripts in their head that explain their children's behavior. These scripts have been shaped by experience, by well-meaning grandmas telling parents what is wrong with their children, by parenting books or past therapists, by their own hopes and fears for their children: "He's just spoiled"; "She's a brat"; "You just need to show him who's boss"; "She's an insolent, selfish, and disrespectful teen," and so on. These scripts don't help. They lead to a surge of anger. They wear down the relationship a little further. They shape the kinds of signals of care or danger the child receives . . . which shape their perceptions of themselves and the world . . . which contribute to the next survival moment, in which the script pops into the parent's head again— "See? I knew it! She *is* a spoiled brat!"

Parents of traumatized children often need new scripts. They need new, and true, ways of understanding their children's behavior. Helping parents understand the basics of trauma, of survival-in-the-moment states, and of the way cat hair works gives the parents a new script. Trauma education is not just about showing parents how science-based and knowledgeable we are. It is critical information that helps parents see their children's survival moments—their meltdown, outbursts, and other terrible moments—through a new lens. It boils down to this:

Parent thought → parent emotion and associated action

So for Peter . . .

Parent thinks, "Peter is mean" → parent feels angry and wants to punish.

Or . . .

Parent thinks, "Peter is feeling scared, vulnerable, and in a survival state" → parent feels empathy and wants to help.

> Helping parents understand trauma changes the scripts they carry with them, which in turn changes the signals of care versus danger given off day in and day out.

Helping parents understand trauma changes the scripts they carry with them, which in turn changes the signals of care versus danger given off day in and day out. Often, however, these scripts don't change overnight in parents. In the safety-focused phase of treatment clinicians can use real examples, real incidents in which the child experiences survival-in-the-moment, to gently challenge parents' scripts about their child and help them see how both the child's and their own past traumas can be related to current behavior.

In addition to a different way of *thinking* about their child's behavior, many parents also need new ways of *managing* their child's behavior. Let's go back to Peter and the donut. The first step in undoing this negative pattern was for Peter's mom to *not* react with her own anger. The skills and tips we just reviewed under "Handling the Difficult Moments" and "Enjoying Your Child" should help with that, as will changing her script from "Peter is mean" to "Peter is having a survival moment and needs help." But now what? If Peter's mother does not have concrete, constructive behavior management strategies to use, she may find herself staring, horrified, as Peter continues to beat up his little sister.

There are many models for encouraging positive behavior in children. The basic ingredients are to reinforce positive behavior; set clear, firm limits; and provide mild discipline for negative behavior. The HELPers Guide describes specific ways to work with parents to help them develop these skills.

This next section of the HELPers guide, on *learning parenting skills*, builds on the earlier skills. If parents are not able to stay regulated, they will not be able to implement parenting skills. If children do not feel loved by their parents, they will be less responsive to the praise and less likely to want to please them. So make sure the earlier parts of the HELPers Guide are implemented thoroughly before moving on to this section.

Introduce the three main parenting strategies listed in the guide (reinforcing desired behavior; setting firm, clear limits; and providing mild discipline for negative behavior) and help parents come up with concrete plans for implementing these strategies. Introduce one concept at a time and help parents gain confidence in using this new strategy before moving on.

> If parents are not able to stay regulated, they will not be able to implement parenting skills. If children do not feel loved by their parents, they will be less responsive to the praise and less likely to want to please them.

1. **Focus on the positive!** What you see is what you get—meaning, if a parent "sees" the child doing something right and comments on it, the parent will get more of that desired behavior! And the reverse is true as well. If all parents "see" are the misbehaviors, those are all they will get. Encourage parents to observe their child's behavior and comment on the positive. Many children hear far more negative comments throughout the day than positive—but really, the ratio should be reversed! Think about signals of care; helping parents to observe and comment on a child's positive behavior helps to change that balance from signals of danger to signals of care. Interestingly, recent research suggests that just commenting on the behavior in a nonjudgmental way ("I see you put your dishes in the sink!") can be more effective in promoting positive behavior than praise ("You did a great job clearing your plate!").

   Although this is one of the most important parenting skills out there, it is easy for parents to forget to keep it up. So . . . reinforce the behavior you want to see in parents, and make a point of noticing when they put this skill into practice with their child. Check in weekly about it; you are helping parents develop a new habit, which takes some reinforcement and time.

   At this same time, the therapist can introduce the concept of reward systems. Typical reward systems involve the use of sticker charts or cards with checkmarks on them that help to keep track, in a visual way, of every time a child does a specific behavior. Once the child has done something a certain number of times (e.g., brushed teeth without being told, every night of the week), he or she gets a reward. The reward does not need to be expensive; work with the parent to think of something easy to give but meaningful to the child (e.g., a special game time with the parent, extra TV time). A few tips on making reward systems work:

- Pick a behavior that is specific, observable, objective, and that the child can succeed in doing. For example: "Shower your sister with kindness" or "Be nice to kids at school" does not fit these criteria, whereas "Brush your teeth before bed" or "Finish your homework the teacher sends in your folder" does.

- Pick a behavior that you want the child to *start* doing, rather than stop doing. For example: "Don't hit your sister" does not fit this criterion, but "Use your quiet corner when you get mad at your sister" does.

- Make sure the behavior is noticed and rewarded consistently.

- After the behavior has become regular (i.e., a habit), pick a new behavior on which to focus. The new, good "habit" should continue on its own.

2. **Set clear, firm limits.** Parents' expectations of their children are not always clear to the children and, in fact, may change from day to day. This is confusing for children and encourages testing of limits and a sense that "they don't really mean it."

Work with parents to identify "trouble spots" around limits and help them define, out loud, what they would like those limits to be. Then develop a plan for communicating these limits to their child, and for helping the child respect those limits (see below—the limits will be tested, and the parents need a plan).

- Make sure the parent has reasonable expectations of the child. Better to start out successful with a small step and work up, than to start big and set the child up for failure.

- Pick just one or two limits with which to begin.

3. **Have a plan for what to do if your child does something he or she shouldn't.** More is not always better, and this is particularly true of consequences and discipline. Overuse of any form of discipline makes it less potent. The key is to help the parent introduce discipline to address behaviors that are generating strife and sometimes creating stress that then leads to survival-in-the-moment reactions. Getting a concrete behavioral management strategy in place without overdoing it is critical.

Natural and logical consequences can be particularly effective, but if it is hard for a parent to generate these "on the fly," having a standard, mild form of discipline, such as a time-out, can be used. Also, make sure that the punishment "fits the crime"; consequences that are too large or too small for the misbehavior are not as effective.

Work with the parent to determine an approach to consequences that is right for the family and child. One critical factor here is that *some discipline strategies can be traumatic reminders*. Consider these examples:

- A child who has experienced severe neglect is put into time-outs alone in her room by her foster family.

- A child who experienced hunger and malnutrition is told by her foster parents that the "logical consequence" of not eating her dinner is that she will not be offered any more food that night, no matter how hungry she gets.

- A child who was physically abused by his father is physically picked up and carried into his room for a time-out.

In each of these cases, given the particular trauma history of the child, a survival-in-the-moment state may be inadvertently triggered by the discipline strategy. If, in the course of a disciplinary episode, a child moves into a survival state, *nothing is learned*, and a great deal is lost.

> If, in the course of a disciplinary episode, a child moves into a survival state, *nothing is learned*, and a great deal is lost.

The final section of the HELPers Guide, on *planning for emergencies*, deals with what to do during a survival-in-the-moment state. Recall that as children transition through the four R's, what they need changes as well. In regulating states, the previously described parenting strategies can be highly effective. Some children can continue to respond to them in the revving state. But once a child enters the reexperiencing state—a survival-in-the-moment state—traditional parenting strategies no longer work. Not only can they be impossible to implement (try telling a child in a survival state to please go to his or her room for a 3-minute time-out), they also can function in the opposite manner to their intended outcome ("I notice that you're not breaking lamps even though you're angry! Oh—whoops, never mind!"). So a parent needs to learn when the child is in a survival state and what his or her best response options are at that time.

Work with parents to discuss how they can recognize their child's survival states, what they can do to minimize the triggers and stressors that cause these states, and how they can try to help their child—and themselves—during these moments. Over time, and as children move into the regulation-focused phase, this work will be greatly elaborated; but for now, helping parents to recognize those states and begin to try out strategies to minimize them is enough.

Planning for Emergencies

A good emergency plan can help to contain these crises. What does a good emergency plan do?

> HELPers Guide: Planning for emergencies

1. Helps parents determine a real emergency from a perceived emergency.
2. Helps parents determine the appropriate response for both real emergencies and perceived emergencies.
3. Gives parents a sense of control and order that contributes to more calmness in a state of emergency (or perceived emergency).

The HELPers Guide provides a structure for working with parents to come up with an emergency plan. The first goal is to help parents understand the difference between (1) a life-threatening emergency, (2) an emergency that warrants a call to the TST team or another crisis line, and (3) an upsetting event that is better off left until you meet again (and would, in fact, cause more disruption to the family if acted on as an emergency). Use concrete examples to talk through how and why you would categorize different events at different levels of urgency.

Once parents have a good understanding of what kind of event falls in which category, make sure they have a plan for what to do. For life-threatening emergencies the object here is not to teach cardiopulmonary resuscitation (CPR), but to just make sure the parent knows to call 911. For other emergencies—crises of child behavior, potential violence in the home, etc.—work with the parent to create a plan that involves both calling and doing. Whom should they call for what kind of problem? And what should they do? Of course, you will never exhaust the list of possible emergencies, but chances are good that for a family in the safety-focused phase you will have a very good sense of the types of emergencies this family is likely to face. Have a plan for these.

 Now rip the emergency plan off the packet. Hand it to the parent and ask where he or she will put it so as to know where to find it. We hope the parent never has to retrieve it.

Transitioning to the Next Phase

As families near the transition to the regulation-focused phase of treatment, their lives are likely a great deal more stable than they were when they started. It may have been quite a journey; therapists may have been through fire and back with families. This kind of work builds strong bonds, and families may come to feel that they couldn't do it without that team of therapists involved.

Depending on how TST is organized in any given agency, transitioning to regulation-focused work may mean terminating with a home-based team that has been intimately and intensively involved. It may mean shifting from three meetings a week to one. It may mean leaving a residential facility. Although there is much to feel good about as a family transitions out of the safety-focused phase, there may also be some loss, sadness, and even fear.

Finally, for providers who are anticipating terminating with a family (even if the family is transitioning to someone else on the TST team), take some time to focus on saying goodbye. Chapter 14 reviews the termination process in detail.

Closing Thoughts on the Safety-Focused Phase of Treatment

When a provider helps a family through the safety-focused phase of treatment, it is like jumping in the river to save the drowning child. No one said it would be easy. No one said there wouldn't be moments when you were scared, or thought things might not come out OK. But if a family has successfully moved beyond the safety-focused phase of treatment, something life-changing has occurred. The child is sitting on the banks of the river—perhaps dripping wet, cold, and scared, but out of danger. Take a moment to breathe. Take a moment to celebrate. The work is not over, but the most important part has been accomplished.

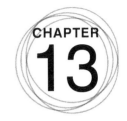

Regulation-Focused Treatment

*How to Help Children Regulate Survival States,
or How Therapists Can Be Construction Workers
on the Autobahn*

LEARNING OBJECTIVES

- To help children acquire emotion regulation skills
- To help children learn how to label and talk about feelings
- To help children learn coping skills for when they feel upset
- To help family members learn when, and how, they can help their child regulate survival states

---

ICONS USED IN THIS CHAPTER

Essential Point	Academic Point	Key Tool	Case Discussion

In regulation-focused treatment, we focus on building children's skills so that they don't switch to survival-in-the-moment reactions when a threat signal is perceived—or, if survival-in-the-moment begins, they are able to switch back. If a child starts TST in this phase, the environment is not deemed harmful (no "cats" can reach the child) or the child is not at risk of engaging in dangerous behavior if triggered by a perceived threat (cat hair). If a child started TST in the safety-focused phase, the environment is assessed to be no longer harmful and the child is no longer at risk to shift into dangerous survival states when triggered. The clinical picture of a child in regulation-focused treatment is such that he or she can be treated in a clinic or office and does not require (or no longer requires) community-based (or milieu-based) care.

What is regulation-focused treatment all about? It's about developing two capacities:

1. Developing *children's emotional regulation capacity*, so they can best navigate their world without switching to survival states.
2. Developing *caregivers' capacities to help and protect their children*, so their children can best navigate their world without switching into survival states.

Notice that these two capacities are exactly those noted in safety-focused treatment, but with the order reversed. These two capacities are also exactly what are required to address the trauma system. The emphasis in regulation-focused treatment is developing the *child's* capacity to regulate emotion, whereas the emphasis in safety-focused treatment is to develop the *caregiver's* capacity to help and protect. If a child started TST in the safety-focused phase, the work may have significantly reduced the amount of cat hair in the environment, but, within the bounds of reality, cat hair can never be fully eliminated (nor should it be fully eliminated). We want to raise strong children. Let's help them to manage the threats that will inevitably come their way. That is what regulation-focused treatment is all about.

The ultimate goal in regulation-focused treatment is to help the child succeed in getting through the day—and the next one, and the next one—without going into survival-in-the-moment states. This may seem like a fairly obvious goal—isn't that what treatment is all about? It is! Keeping a child out of survival-in-the-moment is important not only because it feels good to the child and to all involved, but also because the more regulated the child is, the more regulated he or she stays. Let us explain further.

TST was originally developed in Boston. An old city, Boston was originally developed by cows. Cows wandered the commons and made "cow paths." These cow paths became the easiest way to get from Place A to Place B, so people started riding their horses down these cow paths. Then they pulled their wagons down these paths, and pretty soon the paths became roads. Then the car came along, and down went gravel, and then pavement. Now we have highways where the cows once walked, because the paths most taken are the paths . . . most taken. So it is with the brain. If the "low road" of the amygdala is activated over and over again, it becomes the main highway in the brain. The poor, neglected cortical "high road" is gradually overgrown with weeds.

We need our kids to walk down the high road. Over and over again. Until it becomes the Autobahn. So that is what we are doing in the regulation-focused phase of treatment. We are pulling out all the stops to help kids stay off the amygdala road (and out of survival states) and get them thinking, talking, and implementing coping skills.

How Regulation-Focused Treatment Is Organized

One of the critical differences between the regulation-focused phase of treatment and the safety-focused phase of treatment is *level of risk*; children in this phase of treatment are at a much lower risk of being hurt than are those in safety-focused treatment.

We aim to build the child's skills to both prevent survival states and to facilitate the transition back to the regulating state once the switch to survival-in-the-moment occurs. We do this through a set of defined activities with the child and caregivers, under the following categories. We also continue the activities with caregivers, described in safety-focused treatment, to develop caregivers' capacities to help and protect children.

1. Building awareness
2. Applying awareness
3. Spreading awareness

1. **Building awareness**. How do we help the child understand the switch from his or her usual state to survival-in-the-moment? It is one thing for the TST team to understand exactly how this process works and have perfectly constructed priority problems to reflect this understanding. It is quite another thing for this understanding to be reflected in knowledge that the child can understand and then use. One of the three A's, awareness, is the only one that fully involves the higher-order brain systems necessary to regulate survival states. Helping children become more aware of how and why they are responding to the environment in the way they are responding, opens up an opportunity for them to respond differently. Survival-in-the-moment entails dramatically restricted choice. There is no freedom here. An environmental signal that connotes threat can only be responded to in one way: to survive in the face of it. Helping children become aware that the particular signal that leads to survival-in-the-moment states was not truly a threat to survival, opens up a new world of choices and the capacity to exercise their right to freedom. A lot can happen by building awareness.

2. **Applying awareness**. With the building of awareness, we introduce the capacity to choose in the face of a threat signal. This next component of regulation-focused treatment is about applying this choice. What can the child now do, in the face of a threat signal (remember: We're talking about

"cat hair," not "cat" at this point), other than his or her typical switch into survival states? How does the child use his or her awareness of how the switch occurs to make it less likely? It is one thing for the child to learn to be more aware of how this switch occurs; it is quite another thing to use this awareness to respond differently. A key function of the regulation-focused phase of treatment is to put this awareness into a format that the child will be able to *use* during treatment and after treatment ends. In this part of the process the child learns important emotion regulation skills.

> A key function of the regulation-focused phase of treatment is to put this awareness into a format that the child will be able to *use* during treatment and after treatment ends.

3. **Spreading awareness.** How do those around the child use their awareness of how the switch occurs in the child to make it less likely? Helping a child learn to use his or her awareness about how this switch into survival-in-the-moment states to achieve greater self-regulation is very important. It is equally important to help those around the child to support his or her regulation through *their* awareness about how the switch occurs, and work to (1) reduce the likelihood it will occur and (2) build their skills about how best to help if the child does enter a survival state. In regulation-focused treatment we also engage psychopharmacologists as needed, and continue to develop caregivers' capacities to help and protect children. This is how we help to spread awareness.

Treatment Structure

Whereas the bulk of the work in the safety-focused phase of treatment occurs in the community—in the home, schools, or residential facilities where children spend most of their time, day in and day out—regulation-focused treatment can be delivered in a more traditional clinic or office-based setting. Community-based work supporting the stability of the family may continue as a secondary focus of treatment, but the bulk of the work can now be office-based.

Regulation-focused treatment can be provided:

- In an office, school, residential, or home setting.
- By, or in close collaboration with, a mental health provider with a strong understanding of trauma and survival states.
- Directly to the child with active participation from the primary caregivers.

The Regulation-Focused Guide

 Just as we used the Safety-Focused Guide (SFG) to anchor safety-focused treatment, here we use the Regulation-Focused Guide (RFG) to anchor regulation-focused treatment (Appendix 9). The RFG is meant for providers and defines each component of this phase of treatment. If a provider is doing what is in the RFG, he or she is doing regulation-focused treatment under TST. The RFG is organized by the components of (1) building awareness, (2) applying awareness, and (3) spreading awareness. We also include additional components of psychopharmacology (when necessary) and continuing to care for caregivers. Throughout the chapter, the section of the RFG that corresponds to the section of the text is noted in a box in the left-hand margin.

 TOOL: Regulation-Focused Guide

> **What it is:** A treatment guide for the TST providers that describes concrete steps related to the regulation-focused treatment goals.
>
> **When to use it:** Throughout regulation-focused treatment, and occasionally in safety-focused treatment or beyond trauma.
>
> **Target goals:** To guide providers as they structure treatment around the primary components of regulation-focused treatment: building awareness, applying awareness, and spreading awareness.

Anchoring Regulation-Focused Treatment

Regulation-Focused Guide: anchoring regulation-focused treatment

There are two components to anchoring regulation-focused treatment. The first is similar to our anchoring process in safety-focused treatment. We want to adapt the overall treatment strategy for the purposes of the regulation-focused phase. The second is a bit different. It relies on agreements made in the treatment agreement letter for stabilizing the social environment. If the child starts in regulation-focused treatment, these agreements are important to make sure the environment will be stable enough to support the work. If the child started in safety-focused treatment, then you know how important these agreements are, within that phase, for stabilizing the environment so that the transition to regulation-focused treatment is possible. In this anchoring component of the regulation-focused phase, we want to make sure that we don't lose sight of the agreements that make the work of this phase possible. Let's now review each aspect of anchoring regulation-focused treatment.

The most important part of your preparation is to make sure you have a good-enough understanding of the child's TST priority problems.

The Adaptation of the Overall Treatment Strategy

As we described in safety-focused treatment and the sections on the SFG, we begin the phase by anchoring the TST Treatment Plan—particularly the overall treatment strategy—for the purposes of the specific phase of treatment. Your goal is to make everything you have already done as relevant as possible for the regulation-focused phase of treatment. You've already drafted an overall treatment strategy in Section 3.b of your TST Treatment Plan. If the child already started treatment in the safety-focused phase, then you've adapted the treatment strategy for that phase of treatment. Whether the child had started TST in safety-focused, or is starting in regulation-focused, the overall treatment strategy should be formulated for the purposes of regulation-focused treatment. Next you will see how we worded Emily's anchor for regulation-focused treatment, based on her overall treatment strategy statement (shown in Chapter 9). A version of this statement is also adapted for Items 5 and 6 of the treatment agreement letter. Throughout treatment in TST, that letter is referenced continually, including in the regulation-focused phase.

Here's Emily's regulation-focused anchor:

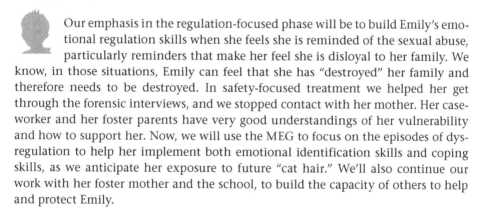

Our emphasis in the regulation-focused phase will be to build Emily's emotional regulation skills when she feels she is reminded of the sexual abuse, particularly reminders that make her feel she is disloyal to her family. We know, in those situations, Emily can feel that she has "destroyed" her family and therefore needs to be destroyed. In safety-focused treatment we helped her get through the forensic interviews, and we stopped contact with her mother. Her caseworker and her foster parents have very good understandings of her vulnerability and how to support her. Now, we will use the MEG to focus on the episodes of dysregulation to help her implement both emotional identification skills and coping skills, as we anticipate her exposure to future "cat hair." We'll also continue our work with her foster mother and the school, to build the capacity of others to help and protect Emily.

Continuing to Account for Agreements

If a child started in safety-focused treatment, true threats have been addressed and the child is now living in a safe-enough environment. There has also been a lot of work conducted to make sure the child's exposure to cat hair is under reasonable control. As detailed in the safety-focused chapter, our approach to these issues is largely predicated on the agreements we have struck with the relevant people to address these cat and cat hair issues. The establishing safety section of safety-focused treatment was all about making sure the agreements on these issues were kept and that they resulted in sufficient impact. For children who began in safety-focused treatment, regulation-focused treatment only makes sense if these agreements continue to be kept. In Point 2 of the anchoring section of the RFG, list the agreements about stabilizing the environment that must be in place for regulation-focused treatment to make sense. Also, here is where you write your plan for monitoring whether these agreements have actually been kept. You'll occasionally need to check in with the relevant caregivers or providers to make sure these agreements continue to be solidly maintained. Otherwise, things fall apart quickly. In such cases, you may need to send the child back to the safety-focused phase. Following is an excerpt from Appendix 9, filled in here for Emily.

What is the agreement, and with whom is it made?	Why is it necessary?	Plan to monitor agreements
Foster mother agreed to disallow phone calls and visits from Emily's mother during safety-focused treatment. This agreement needs to be continued during regulation-focused treatment.	Emily's mother has shown no willingness to modify her behavior related to communicating to Emily that she has harmed her family for reporting Jerry's abuse. It will be very difficult to build Emily's emotional regulation skills if she continues to receive this type of communication.	Check in with Emily and foster mother about this at least weekly.
Caseworker agreed to support foster mother in stopping phone calls and visits from Emily's mother. This needs to be continued during regulation-focused treatment.	As above.	Check in with caseworker about this at least every other week.

Implementing Regulation-Focused Treatment

Once you've completed the process of anchoring regulation-focused treatment by deciding how you will apply your overall treatment strategy for the purposes of this phase and deciding what agreements need to be monitored, treatment focuses on the three primary goals we described earlier:

- Building awareness, by making sure the child and family have knowledge (awareness) about how the child switches to survival-in-the-moment, at a level of detail that they can actually do something about it.
- Applying awareness, by helping the child and family take their knowledge (awareness) and actually do something about it.
- Spreading awareness, by making sure that anyone who interacts with the child, in settings where the child might switch to survival-in-the-moment, will know how to help.

In practice, regulation-focused sessions typically consist of the following activities and structure:

1. A brief check-in about the week to identify successful moments of regulation and, if they happened, incidences of survival states.
2. A Moment-by-Moment Assessment to understand any episodes of survival states that may have occurred, or revving states that were successfully managed and *did not* move into survival states.
3. A review and revision of the Managing Emotions Guide, or MEG.
4. A skill-building session that focuses on either of two types of skills:
   - Emotion identification skills (observing, naming, or expressing emotions)
   - Emotion coping skills (relaxation and affect management, or sometimes, cognitive skill building)

Many children and families in the regulation-focused phase of treatment have not yet developed a strong understanding of children's emotions and how they change. Without this understanding, a child's behavior will seem unpredictable. Unpredictable behavior gives you nothing to do differently next time. However, through careful observation of what happened leading up to the survival state and afterward, we can learn a great deal about a child's emotions and can usually identify a variety of things to do differently next time. Building awareness of a child's emotions, and how the child's three A's change as he or she moves through the four R's, is extremely valuable because:

- What triggers a child may be different in different states (e.g., the same joke that amuses someone in a regulated state may inflame him or her in a revving state).
- A child's coping capacity is different in different states.
- The way a caregiver can help a child is different in different states.

By knowing when children enter a revving state, caregivers can help them calm down while they still have access to their cortical high road, potentially preventing a survival moment. Children, for their part, can recognize that they are revving and need to implement coping skills or ask for help to stay calm. Equally important, by knowing when a child is in a reconstituting state (as opposed to regulating), caregivers can operate with an awareness of the likely vulnerable emotional state the child remains in and make judicious decisions about whether consequences might simply retrigger a survival state.

By knowing when children enter a revving state, caregivers can help them calm down while they still have access to their cortical high road, potentially preventing a survival moment.

A key tool for guiding this work is called the Managing Emotions Guide, or MEG (Appendix 10). This is a "working document" that is meant to be shared with, and used by, all the relevant TST team players. The MEG helps you create a detailed map of how a child's three A's change over the course of the four R's. Said less abstractly, the MEG tracks how a child moves through survival states, starting with identifying perceived threats and then charting how affect, awareness, and action change as the child moves toward and through a survival state. Along the way, the MEG identifies specific strategies a child can use to manage emotions, tailored to the capacities a child has (or doesn't have) as he or she moves through the various survival states. The MEG is a good friend in a time of need.

The MEG has two steps. The first step supports the *building awareness* work that defines this component of regulation-focused treatment. This work involves taking the team's understanding of the child's shift from his or her usual state to survival-in-the-moment states and building the child's awareness of this process in language tangible to him or her. In this process, we are integrating our understandings based on our Moment-by-Moment Assessments and communicating with the child in a way that he or she can understand. The second step of the MEG is the interventions part that inserts new skills or approaches to promote regulation in those difficult moments. That second step of the MEG also describes how people around the child can help him or her in those difficult moments. The component of regulation-focused treatment called *applying awareness* integrates the skill/strength interventions of the MEG, and the component called *spreading awareness* integrates the activities on MEG's second step related to how others can help the child.

TOOL: Managing Emotions Guide (MEG)

What it is: An individualized worksheet that identifies the way the child switches from his or her usual state to survival states and appropriate interventions for various stages of escalation and traumatic states.

When to use it: Throughout regulation-focused treatment, and occasionally in safety-focused treatment or beyond trauma.

Target goals: Child and caregiver will learn to identify triggers and patterns of escalation, and be able to intervene early in the cycle of survival states.

Building Awareness—Helping Children Understand Their Survival States

Step 1 of the MEG is not "square 1." We do not start at square 1 when we seek to build awareness in the regulation-focused phase of TST. We've already put a lot of time and effort into defining the TST priority problems. Of course, these are based on our work evaluating at least three episodes with Moment-by-Moment Assessments and then making decisions about the patterns that may link them. Our focus here in building awareness is to make sure all of this is most useful to the child and caregivers. Look at Tanisha's priority problem from her treatment plan shown in Appendix 5 on page 427:

That's a very well-constructed priority problem. Are you ready to use it? Maybe you are . . . but what about Tanisha? Does she understand how her switch gets flipped? What is her awareness of how her regulated emotional state shifts to survival states, and the types of threat signals that will repeatedly lead her into survival-in-the-moment reactions? You need to build a language with her, so that she may really understand how her priority problem works. You've already started building this language during ready–set–go, when you wrote your understanding of her priority problem in her treatment agreement letter. You wrote about this in a language she could understand, and it resulted in her signing off on the treatment agreement because, presumably, she understood it in a good-enough way.

Here's what you wrote in Section 3 of the treatment agreement letter about her priority problem. You discussed this with Tanisha and her mother, and this was part of the treatment agreement that ended ready–set–go.

> The main problem we see is that when Tanisha feels she is put in a position in which she has to choose between people she cares about, she gets very angry and then can do things to hurt other people. Sometimes, she doesn't even remember what she has done in such a situation. We've seen this happen most recently when her mother came to visit unannounced, when those family friends visited, and when that girl at school asked her to say who is her best friend.

The building awareness part of regulation-focused treatment starts with this understanding from ready–set–go and builds this understanding to a level of detail that Tanisha can really use. This level of understanding spans the full range of the switch (the four R's) and helps create a tangible, shared understanding with the child about the process: tangible enough that it can lead to ways the child will be able to use the understanding for new emotional regulation strategies.

The *building awareness* part of regulation-focused treatment helps create a tangible, shared understanding with the child about the process: tangible enough that it can lead to ways the child will be able to use the understanding for new emotional regulation strategies.

Building Awareness Activities

The MEG is one of several essential activities for helping to develop the level of understanding necessary to make meaningful change. Go to the Building Awareness Section of the RFG and we will walk you through the activities you need to complete for building awareness.

There are two main sets of skills related to emotion identification: *Observing and naming* skills focus on helping the child become aware of his or her emotions and to put words to the feeling. *Expression*, on the other hand, focuses on ways of not just labeling a feeling but allowing that feeling to be shared with another person, or even fully experienced by oneself. For children who experience numbing or avoidance of feelings, these skills may form the central portion of the regulation-focused work.

If the child you are working with has difficulty identifying the three A's across the four R's, select activities from the "Emotion Identification Toolbox" in Appendix 11 (or others that you know of) and implement them during the skill-building portion of the session.

Activity 1: Clarifying the Problem

Regulation-Focused Guide:
Building Awareness Activity 1:
clarifying the problem

This first activity is meant to double-check that you and the child are on the same page about the problem that you have decided to work on, recorded in Point 3 of the treatment agreement letter. Write your statement of the problem in this section of the RFG and talk with the child, and, if appropriate, the caregiver about it. You don't want to leave this activity feeling unsure that you and the child are on the same page. Obviously, this discussion has to be developmentally appropriate, given the age of the child. For younger children, caregivers will need to be more closely involved. We wrote the problem statement for Tanisha, in the previous section. We'll show you the problem statement for Emily and Briana next, to give you a bit more information about how these problems should be written.

For Emily:

> We've seen that when you hear something or talk to someone who makes you feel that you have done something bad to your family, you feel that you must hurt yourself or die.

For Briana:

> We've seen that when you see something about a boy or a man that reminds you of when your uncle removed his shirt before hurting you, that you feel terrified and then cut your arms and legs to feel better.

Show the child the statement. Read it to him or her. Talk with him or her about it. Do whatever you think is appropriate to make sure that you and the child share an understanding of the problem. Engage the caregivers as you see appropriate. Again, caregivers need to be more closely involved with younger children.

Activity 2: Exploring the Problem in Different Situations

In the first activity, you made sure you are on the same page with the child about the problem. In this next activity, you want to look at the problem—with the child (and caregivers)—in different situations. How do you do this? In a way, you've already done it

> Regulation-Focused Guide:
> Building Awareness Activity 2:
> exploring the problem in different
> situations

through your Moment-by-Moment Assessments, and then you developed your priority problem by seeing the patterns between them. Now you have your priority problem, and you can show the child how it works in different contexts. You should bring all your Moment-by-Moment Assessment sheets to this session (or sessions). You want to point out how the three A's work across the four R's for the child in different contexts. You want to point out the threat stimuli in each of the contexts and clarify that even though the threat may look differently in the different contexts, it is the same underlying threat. The purpose of this activity is to deepen the child's understanding about how his or her priority problem(s) works across contexts. This discussion is therapeutic in itself. A person who behaves extremely in many different situations inevitably feels out of control. When you help children see that their behavior and emotions in each of these contexts are very much the same, they may—for the first time—believe that there is some hope of their controlling their emotions and behavior. You are also building the language for the next activity, wherein you will be fleshing out, with the child, how the three A's shift across the four R's. You will be using the building awareness part of the MEG (Step 1).

Activity 3: Understanding How the Problem Happens (MEG—Step 1)

Activity 3 builds from the second activity. You have just helped the child understand how his or her problem of shifting into survival states works in different contexts. You have begun to build a language about the three A's and the four R's. Now you will use

> Regulation-Focused Guide:
> Building Awareness Activity 3:
> understanding how the problem
> happens

the MEG to build this awareness in a very tangible way. As you see from Step 1 of the MEG (Appendix 10), you and the child should consider each of the states: regulating, revving, reexperiencing, and reconstituting. Using the data from the Moment-by-Moment Assessments you've gathered, record your observations as well as the child's about how the environment tends to look in each of these four states. Record these observations about what the child feels, does, and thinks about in each of these states. Expanding the child's way of considering the way he or she shifts into survival-in-the-moment states will dramatically help you to intervene with their problems. An example of how that discussion might go for Tanisha follows:

THERAPIST: So we have our MEG in front of us and we have to fill out all these boxes based on what we just talked about with those Moment-by-Moment Assessments.

TANISHA: Where do we start?

THERAPIST: Exactly. It's a lot. Well, let's start with this first column over here that says *usual state*, or *regulating*. That's before all the trouble starts. We need to fill out how you were feeling, and what you were doing, and what you were aware of, before the trouble started. We have these three examples in front of us that we've just discussed. Anything come to mind?

TANISHA: Well, I was usually doing something I enjoy and my mind is really into it. Like reading. I love to read, and I don't want to be bothered when I read.

THERAPIST: And how are you feeling when you read?

TANISHA: Just so calm, and my mind is taken to places that are exciting. I'm not thinking of my troubles.

THERAPIST: So let's put all this information here in the MEG in that first column.

TANISHA: OK. (*Begins writing.*)

THERAPIST: (*after Tanisha has finished filling in the first column of the MEG*) I guess the trouble starts when someone or something pulls your attention from something you enjoy, especially reading.

TANISHA: Yeah. I hate being pulled away when I'm enjoying something. But it's not only that.

THERAPIST: What do you mean?

TANISHA: Well. We've gone over those three—what did you call them?—episodes. As we said last time, it's not only being pulled away from what I enjoy. It's when I feel pulled away and then torn between people. Like when Mom wants something that I know I can't do. Or when my grandma told me I had to play with that kid.

THERAPIST: And then I remember you said that you felt confused, frightened, and then angry.

TANISHA: Yeah. I don't know why, but I hate being pulled away from what I like to do and then being torn between what other people want. I get worried someone will get really mad at me.

THERAPIST: What you are saying is really important. Let's get it down in that revving column of the MEG.

This important process may take a session or two, but your goal is to use the information from the Moment-by-Moment Assessments and the child's understanding of the priority problem to guide the discussion for filling out this first step of building awareness on the MEG. This foundation sets up everything for what can be done to help when the child's new awareness is applied. An example of Tanisha's completed TST Moment-by-Moment Assessment Sheet is shown in Appendix 3.

WHAT DO YOU DO IF THE CHILD IS NO TANISHA?

A fair question. Tanisha, in this dialogue, shows great insight. She is able to make observations about her emotions ("I feel so calm, my mind is taken to exciting places"), name them ("I feel worried"), and express them ("I hate being pulled away!"). Not all children have these skills; building them is a fundamental part of the work of building awareness in order to learn to regulate emotions and behavior.

Activity 4: Identifying the Earliest Detectable Warning Signal

You may not be able to get this information, but if you do, it is golden. Often there will be a signal that the child might be able to detect that indicates the child has left the regulating state and is starting to rev into a survival-in-the-moment state. This signal,

Regulation-Focused Guide: Building Awareness Activity 4: identifying the earliest detectable warning signal

if detected early enough, offers an amazing opportunity to insert an emotional regulation skill at this point to quickly terminate survival-in-the-moment and shift back to regulating. The reason it is so important to detect this shift early is because a child's higher-order brain systems are still working well at this point. Survival-laden emotion is only beginning to creep in. Let's shut the door in the face of survival-laden emotion as quickly as we can (and lock it tightly!). What are these earliest detectable warning signals (EDWS)? They can be anything. Often the child simply pays no attention to them and never notices until you ask, "What is the first thing you notice or feel that indicates you are becoming upset?" It may be a feeling in the child's body or a specific perception that gets the whole painful process going. Whatever it is, it's so important to know about it. Some examples of an EDWS are:

- A 13-year-old girl noticed that her leg "twitches" before she becomes enraged and assaults others.
- An 8-year-old boy noticed that his vision becomes "blurry" before he gets panicked and needs to escape.
- A 17-year-old girl noticed that she hears "a lady laugh" before she loses time and cuts herself.
- A 10-year-old boy noticed that his "teeth grit" before he "becomes a tornado."

Now that you have helped the child have such awareness about survival states, it's time to help him or her to do something about it. Let's start applying this awareness.

Building Awareness Practice Tips

* Always frame a discussion about the four R's by starting with the child's *regulated* state and ending with the *reconstituted* state. Paying attention to the child's experiences of being in control is important both to help him or her recognize how these states differ from survival states, and also to bring attention to the positive moments.

* Successful regulation does not just mean being happy; times when the child felt upset, worried, sad, or angry but maintained control are extremely important examples of regulation and should be included as you fill out the MEG.

* Sometimes the sign of being in a revving state is feeling *less*, not more. Emotional numbing is a core symptom of PTSD, and for some children a traumatic reminder quickly leads to a shutdown of their whole emotional experience in a state of rigid control. They may control these feelings by avoiding situations that trigger any strong feelings, or avoiding thinking about things that stir strong feelings. Although in the short term these strategies may seem to help, in the long run they may prevent necessary and normal life experiences and emotions in the child. Have the child practice skill-building activities that help him or her experience emotions.

Applying Awareness—Helping Children Apply Awareness to Prevent Survival States

Successful emotional regulation does not mean experiencing just positive emotions.

If you've brought a child through the steps involved in building awareness, you've brought the child to the point where he or she has the possibility of feeling and acting differently the next time a threat signal is perceived. In applying awareness, we develop the child's repertoire of alternative response. This starts with identifying successful approaches the child is already employing to manage emotion, and helping the child apply these strategies to the survival moments. The information about these successful strategies comes from the child's strengths that you've already assessed. Applying awareness also employs new—tried and true—emotional regulation strategies that the child may never have used before. These are the regulation-focused exercises detailed in Appendix 11. Your role is to consider these many options and what you think will work with the child, and plan to insert them when the child is at risk to switch into survival-in-the-moment states. Like building awareness, the applying awareness section of the RFG provides a set of activities that should be followed. We detail each of these next. Use your RFG to follow along.

Activity I: Identifying the Tools to Use

In this section you take your knowledge of the child's priority problem at the level of detail you've derived through the building awareness activities and decide what tools you have to address the problem. Step 1

> Regulation-Focused Guide: Applying Awareness Activity 1: identifying tools to use

is really the process of laying the possible tools you may use in front of you and then deciding which you will use. This activity involves your preparation with your team and discussions with the child and family. There are two types of toolboxes you will use to select the tools you will actually use. The first comes from the child's strengths. In the treatment planning process, you identified ways in which the child had already employed personal strengths to manage his or her emotional states. These strengths are possible tools to use. Now that you know the child a little better, select those that you think might really help. We reach for these types of tools first, because we know they have worked before with the child. The second toolbox you use is from our list of regulation-focused exercises (in Appendix 11). This appendix provides a description of a great many emotional regulation skill-building approaches that have been shown to be helpful in the literature. Every child is different. Pick ones that you think will be helpful, because you will almost certainly need to reach for them. These regulation-focused exercises build either of two types of skills:

- Emotion identification skills (observing, naming, or expressing emotions)
- Emotion coping skills (relaxation and affect management, or sometimes cognitive skill building)

As is detailed in the next section, you will need to decide which tools to use—and when to use them—related to the four states of regulating, revving, reexperiencing, and reconstituting. Because the reexperiencing state can involve some danger, the safety plan developed in the safety-focused treatment phase will become a tool to use here. Ultimately, your decisions on the tools and approaches to use to apply awareness will be based on a discussion with the child and family.

Activity 2: Deciding When to Apply Each Tool (MEG—Step 2)

Activity 1 is conducted so you can best prepare to apply awareness. You've just surveyed the tools that you have at your disposal to help. Now you will work with the child and caregivers to plan which tools and

> Regulation-Focused Guide: Applying Awareness Activity 2: deciding when to apply each tool

approaches you will apply at various points in the dysregulation process. Your tool for planning all this is Step 2 of the MEG. Take out your MEG and examine this section. As you see, the MEG requires an approach that will promote regulation in each of the states of regulating, revving, reexperiencing, and reconstituting. MEG also distinguishes the activities that a child can do him or herself in each of these states, and those that require the help of an adult. You should consider the tools you have identified in Activity 1 of applying awareness, and think of where they would be most helpful in the respective *R* state. Broadly, the most important aspects of each of these states for promoting regulation are:

- *Regulating*: Activities and approaches that support a child's emotional regulation and sense of competence and autonomy, and that help to build positive relationships. Strategies to prevent threat exposure should be considered here as well.
- *Revving*: Activities and approaches that help to calm the child and keep events in perspective so that he or she can transition back to regulating.
- *Reexperiencing*: Activities and approaches for keeping the child safe, and to calm the child, so that he or she may safely transition to reconstituting.
- *Reconstituting*: Activities and approaches that help calm the child, to prevent a shift back to reexperiencing and facilitate a return to regulating.

Step 2 of the MEG provides a space for filling in possible activities and approaches for each of the four R's in two different categories: (1) things the child can do for him- or herself, and (2) things an adult or a friend can help the child do. In this section of the chapter, "Applying Awareness," we focus on skills the child can learn and implement. In the next section, "Spreading Awareness," we discuss what others can do.

Practice Tip:

- For some children, negative views of self or others may contribute to their entering survival states. In this case, introducing cognitive skill building is necessary to allow the child to overcome survival states. Although the bulk of cognitive skill building typically falls in the beyond trauma phase of treatment (detailed in the next chapter), if the triggers/stimuli identified in the priority problems point to cognitive perceptions as the source of the dysregulation, then introduce cognitive restructuring skills now.

Regulating State: Activities That Build a Sense of Competence, Autonomy, and Positive Relationships

The best way to set the stage for children to have lives and futures in which they are able to regulate emotion is to provide them with as many opportunities as possible to stay regulated. For many traumatized children, their shift into survival states begins to define them. They become the child who beats other children up, or the child who cuts herself, or the child who drinks and has unprotected sex. The tragic part of the way traumatized children are defined by others is how much this labeling begins to drive how they define themselves. When those around the child begin to define the child by his or her survival states, they miss the full picture of the child, including the many great things the child does and the skills and strengths that he or she possesses.

We promote children's capacity to stay in regulating states by giving them every opportunity to engage in activities that help them feel strong, effective, and regulated. The more we support a child to experience regulated states, and work with those around the child to make sure those happen, the more the child has the opportunity to redefine him- or herself. In the regulating column of the MEG, we take the child's strengths that we have identified and the activities that make the child feel good and in control and we list them here. In the spreading awareness part of regulation-focused treatment, we engage the relevant adults who may be able to help the child have more opportunities to engage in these activities to make sure the child has access to such regulating opportunities. Children who are struggling with powerful emotions and painful problems (*especially* these children!) need activities that make them feel good about them-selves, that allow them to practice independence, and that support the kinds of strong relationships that will carry them through life. You already have this information from the assessment form and treatment plan. Check out with the child and care-givers whether you've got it right. Adjust your ideas based on what they say, then write them down here; later we'll work on making them happen. We pro-vide an example of what a 15-year-old boy wrote in his MEG—Step 2 for the regulating state:

> Children who are struggling with powerful emotions and painful problems (*especially* these children!) need activities that make them feel good about themselves, that allow them to practice independence, and that support the kinds of strong relationships that will carry them through life.

Things you can do:

> Go running as often as I can after school.
>
> Try out for the track team.
>
> Get in the best shape I can.
>
> See if I can run a half marathon.

Things an adult or friend can help you with:

> My dad should encourage me more about track.
>
> I hope my mom will allow me to go to track after school and try out for the team.
>
> Don't punish me by saying I can't run. It's how I survive!

Revving State: Activities and Approaches That Help to Calm the Child and Keep Events in Perspective

In building awareness, you've developed the child's understanding of the impact of the threat signals and how they lead to the child's switch to survival states. In this part of applying awareness, you make the plan for what to do when the switch begins with the revving state. Importantly, you've also identified the EDWS of the child's switch to survival state. The EDWS gives you and the child the opportunity to elicit some calm before the emotion gets too far out of control. One of the examples given of an EDWS from the building awareness section was from a 13-year-old girl who noticed her leg twitching well before she got aggressive and assaulted people. That signal was used to initiate the emotional regulation tools she learned to use to shift back to regulating from revving.

In this section, form an agreement with the child on trying very hard to notice this identified EWDS and to apply an emotional regulation tool exactly at that time. It's important also to distinguish what a child can do on his or her own and what will require others. Obviously, activities that require others are harder to implement with the immediacy that may be needed to avert reexperiencing from revving, but there may well be strategies to identify with a helpful (and immediately available) adult. In the case of the 13-year-old girl, our approach was to have her raise her hand when she noticed her leg twitch and to ask her teacher to be excused from class, where she would then spend 10 minutes at the guidance counselor's office. Both her teacher and the guidance counselor agreed to this plan—and it worked! Work with the child and caregivers to identify and insert an emotional regulation tool as soon as the child notices the revving beginning. Such tools may be those that have worked for the child before (e.g., the child writing in a journal, listening to music, going to the gym to shoot baskets) or from an emotional regulation skill chosen from the list in Appendix 11. Work with the child to write this down in the second column of Step 2 of the MEG.

The list of activities chosen can grow and change over time. Some of the techniques that the child initially needs help implementing may, over time, become internalized so that he or she can to do them alone. Talking about what's bothering the child or getting a hug are strategies that clearly involve another person. Drawing pictures together, going on a walk, or doing relaxation exercises are all techniques that might eventually be employed by the child alone, but may initially need to be initiated and modeled by a parent.

The child may not have many things to put on this list when you start. That's where you come in. You've chosen one or more regulation-focused exercises (from Appendix 11) for specific activities that help a child regulate. What is most important is that the child develop these skills so that once he or she (or a caregiver) recognizes that a revving state is occurring, these skills can be used to transition back to the regulated state. We provide an example of what an 11-year-old girl wrote for MEG—Step 2, revving, below:

Things you can do:

> When I get that feeling in my stomach, do the favorite room exercise.
>
> If the favorite room does not work, do the imaginary school bus exercise.
>
> Use my journal in my desk at school to write.
>
> Listen to my iPod.

Things an adult or friend can help you with:

> Remind me to do favorite room or imaginary school bus exercise.
>
> Don't ignore me when I say my stomach feels that way.
>
> Don't tell me I can't use my journal or my iPod.
>
> DON'T YELL AT ME!

Reexperiencing State: Strategies for Keeping the Child Safe

If a child continues to escalate until reexperiencing happens, the whole playing field changes. Suddenly the same things that might have calmed a child earlier (e.g., joking around with him) may become a trigger. Interventions that might have worked 10 minutes ago (e.g., suggesting that she put on music) are irrelevant, and meanwhile the danger is escalating—the child is about to throw something or is curled up in a ball in a dissociated state. What now? In essence, this column in Step 2 of the MEG becomes a crisis management plan.

At this point, interventions are focused on maintaining safety and containing the child's behavior. Mutual regulation techniques often include reducing or eliminating the new set of traumatic reminders. For example, a child who cannot tolerate loud noise and high levels of stimulation when he or she is in a reexperiencing state could be taken to a quieter room, or other family members might be asked to leave the room. Consequences, which might be highly effective with a child during most times, may seem threatening and further escalate the behavior during these times. For instance, a time-out is not an appropriate strategy when a child is physically out of control. Instead, an intervention that focuses on calmly redirecting the behavior might be more helpful. This reexperiencing column of Step 2 of the MEG can also be used as an emergency crisis plan, as mentioned, so that parents have a list of numbers to call in an emergency.

Here's an example of what a 13-year-old girl wrote in the reexperiencing column of the MEG:

Things you can do:

> Try "walking and breathing" technique.
>
> Draw a really big picture on the butcher paper on the ground.
>
> Cheerlead self: "I can stay in control, I can stay in control, I can stay in control."

Things an adult or friend can help you with:

> Make sister leave the room.
>
> Don't yell, just talk normally.
>
> Put the big glass vase and your other breakable things where they can't be reached.
>
> If hitting head on wall, hold in big hug.
>
> Call TST team at 867-5309.
>
> If I can't calm down and I am worried about my own or someone else's safety, call 9-1-1.

Reconstituting State: Activities That Help a Child Transition Back to a Regulating State

As we described in Chapters 3 and 9, a reconstituting state is not to be confused with a regulating state, even though they may overtly look the same. The child is calmer than during a reexperiencing state, but can easily go back to reexperiencing if he or she doesn't feel safe enough. The best thing to do here is to make sure the perceived threat signal is removed (if possible). There also may be regulation-focused exercises (from Appendix 11) or other approaches that have worked in the past to facilitate the transition back to a regulating state. Talk with the child and family about what has been helpful in the past, in such a context, and insert these here. You may have selected an exercise from Appendix 11 that you think would be really helpful. Talk to the child and caregivers about whether they can do this exercise if they are in a reconstituting state and integrate that here. Here is an example of what a 10-year-old boy wrote in his MEG—Step 2, Reconstituting:

Things you can do:

> The deep breathing or the walking and breathing exercises can help.
>
> Closing my eyes and imagining I'm on a beach.

Things an adult or friend can help you with:

> I know if I'm like this, a hug can really help me.
>
> Reminding me to do deep breathing or walking and breathing.
>
> Tell me I'm not a bad boy.

Practice Point:

- Sometimes what the child did during a reexperiencing state has lasting effects or has caused other people to feel hurt or angry. Part of reconstitution can be coming up with a plan for what the child can do to repair some of the damage—literal or metaphorical. This is important not only to help diminish other people's feelings of anger, but also to help the child manage his or her own feelings of shame. Can a child put his or her allowance toward replacing a broken object? Can he or she write a letter of apology or help clean up the mess? These repair actions can be listed as part of the MEG—Step 2.

Activity 3: Getting Ready to Regulate

You've completed both Steps 1 and 2 of the MEG. These steps reflect the child and caregivers' full understanding of how survival states work for the child (Step 1: Building Awareness) and the plan for

Regulation-Focused Guide:
Applying Awareness Activity 3:
getting ready to regulate

inserting selected skills and approaches at each respective state of regulating, revving, reexperiencing, and reconstituting. Some of these skills and approaches are based on what has worked for the child in the past. Some are based on selected regulation-focused exercises. Now you will work with the child to anticipate exactly how the activities specified in the MEG—Step 2 will be applied in his or her world. Based on your Moment-by-Moment Assessments, you have knowledge of the types of situations that are trouble spots for the child and can rehearse with him or her how the child will handle the situation based on the decisions already made. This is also the time to practice in session. If you have selected a specific regulation-focused exercise, practice it in session until you, and the child, are confident the child will be able to implement it when the time comes. Give the child and caregivers homework to practice a given regulation-focused exercise or any other approach specified in the MEG—Step 2. The more a child prepares to regulate, and the more caregivers are prepared to help the child regulate, the more likely survival-in-the-moment states will be prevented.

Activity 4: Getting It Better

No matter how much a child and caregivers prepare and practice, there's nothing like a test in the real world to see if we've got it right. When Emily sees her mother standing on the sidewalk outside her

Regulation-Focused Guide:
Applying Awareness Activity 4:
getting it better

school, how will she respond? Will she stay in a regulated state, quickly return to regulating after starting to rev, or will she head right to reexperiencing? When Briana is at a friend's house and photos of the "hottest guys in school" are passed around, will she be able to follow the plan from her MEG and stay regulated?

In your sessions for Activity 4, you should ask about any situation in which the child was exposed to a threat stimulus and then assess his or her ability to implement the MEG plan and record the result. If the child can give you several examples of experiencing an exposure to cat hair and fully implementing the MEG, with well-regulated responses, you may be ready to transition to the final phase of TST, beyond trauma. If the child either was not able to implement MEG or the plan did not work, you need to understand what happened and refine the plan based on this information. The problem will usually fit within one of the following categories, each of which has a natural solution that you should implement, to refine the MEG:

- The skill or approach was right—*the child needed more practice.*
- The skill or approach was right—*the child needed someone's help to implement it.*
- The skill or approach was right—*the child missed the EDWS* (and then it was too late).
- The skill or approach was not right—*it was too complex to implement.*
- The skill or approach was not right—*it depended too much on others.*

Although these are the most common categories for the plan not to work, there are others. The important point is that you establish a process of testing whether the plan based on MEG—Step 2 works in a good-enough way and use this information to improve the plan. As you see, possible problems include the ability of other people to help the child. We've not discussed this much in this section, because it is the focus of the next section of regulation-focused treatment: spreading awareness.

Spreading Awareness—Helping Others Know How to Help

In applying awareness, a set of skills and approaches was selected according to the child's specific state of regulation or dysregulation. These were noted in the MEG—Step 2 under the categories of either "Things you can do" or "Things an adult or friend can help you with." The spreading awareness component of regulation-focused treatment is about "Things an adult or friend can help you with." If the plan depends on others, what *is* the plan to enable others to help? Spreading awareness is easiest (usually) to do with the child's primary caregivers; they (usually) accompany the child to treatment and therefore you can work to spread this awareness directly with them. If Tanisha needs her grandmother to help her write in her journal whenever she begins to rev (and to notice Tanisha's revving state), then this information needs to be communicated to Tanisha's grandmother in such a way that success is possible. What about others? The plan may depend on teachers, guidance counselors, foster parents, camp counselors, neighbors, or friends. We need a plan to engage them and enable them to help. Spreading awareness is about these activities. Use the RFG to help implement the three activities required for spreading awareness.

Activity 1: Listing Who Is Needed and Planning How to Engage Them

This activity is pretty straightforward. Start with what was written in MEG—Step 2 for "Things an adult or friend can help you with." Which adults? Which friends? Who are they and who should con-

> Regulation-Focused Guide: Spreading Awareness Activity 1: listing who is needed

tact them to communicate what we need from them? And what, exactly, do we need from them? To accomplish this activity, you should work with the child and caregivers to make such a list and decide on the approach for engagement. The plan could include a friend or neighbor coming to a session. It could include a school visit or a phone call to the relevant school provider. You will need to be closely involved in this communication. In this section, you should specify your plan to engage the people who are needed.

Activity 2: Engaging and Enabling Others Who Can Help

You've identified who needs to be involved and your plan to engage them. Now you need to engage them and help them understand what is needed of them. Sometimes the need here is very simple: perhaps a brief phone call from you to explain to a teacher how

> Regulation-Focused Guide: Spreading Awareness Activity 2: engaging and enabling others who can help

she can help a child implement a number counting regulation-focused exercise. Sometimes the need will be more extensive and will involve several sessions with someone to fully explain and practice their role in helping a child regulate. There are a great many possibilities here. The important point is that you bring onto the team the people whom you need to implement the plan specified in the MEG, and you communicate what is needed as effectively as you can. Here are some examples of spreading awareness:

- A meeting was held with the camp director and on-site medical staff before a child went to summer camp to provide the information contained in the child's MEG. The plan at camp was for the child to see the camp nurse three mornings per week to practice her regulation-focused exercises and for the camp counselor to be aware of her EDWS of nausea. The camp counselor is to help her listen to her iPod whenever such an EDWS is detected. The safety plan was also extensively discussed, and you agree to have a weekly check-in phone call with the camp counselor once camp begins.

- A child's babysitter comes to a session to learn about the safety plan and her role in helping with two regulation-focused exercises.

- A school meeting is held about a plan for a child to raise his hand when he notices his vision getting blurry (a reliable EDWS) and to be allowed to listen to his iPod, draw, or shut his eyes and imagine his "safe place" at that time. The recommended safety plan is also communicated at the meeting.

- A meeting is held between the residential care team, the child welfare caseworker, and the new foster mother who will care for the child after discharge from the residential program. The meeting is about communicating to the foster mother and the caseworker the information contained in the MEG and the specific role the foster mother can have in helping implement several regulation-focused exercises. The child's known threat signals and how they may be reduced within the foster home were also discussed.

Activity 3: Monitoring Whether It Worked

Regulation-Focused Guide:
Spreading Awareness Activity 3:
monitoring whether it worked

As always, we make decisions based on facts. The plans specified in MEG—Step 2, including the role of other people, may or may not work. We need to check it out. This monitoring is fully consistent with what was described for Activity 4 of applying awareness. Ask these questions the next few times the child is exposed to cat hair: Did the designated helpers help as planned? Was their help as helpful as planned? If not, refine the plan based on this information. Your assessment of the situation is consistent with what we described in Chapter 12 on advocating for needed interventions and services. Go through that same process here:

- Is the reason a misunderstanding? Then *communicate better.*
- Is the reason a practical barrier? Then *do your best to surmount the practical barrier.*
- Is the reason an unwillingness? Then *step it up.*

Reread pages 260–265 in Chapter 12 to refresh your memory about this process. Recall that when what we need is important enough, but we hit a wall with a person we need as part of this process, then we must advocate. In the examples given in the previous section, this may happen when the school declines to participate in its part of the plan, or if the child welfare caseworker does not think that what was communicated to the foster mother fits within her scope of work. We never advocate frivolously, but when we believe the participation is important enough and does fall within the person's scope of work, we advocate to make sure it happens.

Practice Point:

  * A revving child often pulls for strong emotions in a parent or caregiver.
    The "Things an adult or a friend can help you with" boxes may contain
    suggestions with asterisks next to them—these are ways a parent can
    engage *if he or she is regulated and entering the interaction with a constructive
    frame of mind.* Revisiting the section of the HELPers Guide that focuses
    on parental emotional regulation may be a critical part of helping some
    parents support their children's regulation.

Other Components of Regulation-Focused Treatment

Psychopharmacology

As detailed in previous chapters, some children will require psychopharmacology as part of their treatment plan. This is usually recommended within TST
to support, in the short term, the development of emotional regulation skills.
Dampening the survival circuits with psychotropic medication may help the
child to best take advantage of the skill building that is a core part of regulation-
focused treatment. The details of psychopharmacology within TST are provided
in Chapter 15. Most relevant to the regulation-focused phase of TST is this point:
You may find that a child who does not have a psychopharmacology intervention as part of his or her treatment plan may really need it (or an evaluation
for it, at least). This may be the case if you are finding that the child is not progressing in regulation-focused treatment as he or she should, because the child
becomes too overwhelmed. In such situations, consider a psychopharmacology
evaluation.

Continuing to Care for Caregivers

In safety-focused treatment we provided a strong focus on the needs of caregivers to be able to help and protect children. Although their needs may not be
quite as intense and immediate as in safety-focused phase, caregivers still need
to be cared for. You should continue to use the HELPers Guide in regulation-
focused treatment. You might occasionally select a session with a caregiver to
focus on specific elements of the guide that you see as relevant.

Closing Thoughts on the Regulation-Focused Phase of Treatment

Pause and consider for a moment what it means for children to accomplish the
aims of regulation-focused phase of treatment. It means that they no longer
enter survival states. It means that the people around them no longer walk on

eggshells or expect them to "blow." It means that the survival moments that used to define their lives, and the way people saw them, have disappeared and in their place is a string of moments of just being themselves: kids with ups and downs; kids who get along OK—just kids—kids who drive, all day, every day, on the proverbial Autobahn.

It doesn't mean life can't be improved . . . that children's hopes and beliefs about who they are and where they are heading couldn't be shined up a bit. Helping kids envision a brighter future, and themselves as a part of that future, is the focus of the next chapter and phase of treatment. Where *does* the Autobahn lead, anyway?

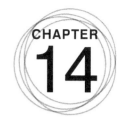

CHAPTER
14

Beyond Trauma Treatment

How to Help Traumatized Children
Move into a Better Future

with Liza Suarez

LEARNING OBJECTIVES

- To help children build their cognitive skills
- To help children tell their trauma story
- To help children leave their trauma in the past
- To help children leave their therapy in the past

ICONS USED IN THIS CHAPTER

Essential Point	Academic Point	Useful Tool	Case Discussion	Quotation

---

When a child no longer experiences survival states, a major threshold has been passed. Families breathe a sigh of relief as they begin to trust that their days will no longer be punctuated by moments of extreme emotion and behavior. By definition, a child who is in the beyond trauma phase of treatment lives in a

Lisa Suarez, PhD, is Assistant Professor of Clinical Psychology in the Department of Psychiatry at the University of Illinois at Chicago and co-director of the Urban Youth Trauma Center at the National Child Traumatic Stress Network.

environment that is not threatening; furthermore, the child is no longer vulnerable to entering survival states.* This is not to say, however, that everything is golden. The past experiences of trauma and associated survival states can leave some wear and tear. Children may be plagued by negative views of themselves, others, and their future, related to their experience of trauma and its consequences. Parents or other caregivers may harbor beliefs that the child is "difficult" or "damaged." The sometimes prolonged storm created by chronic emotional dysregulation may have obscured other real needs of the child. This final phase of treatment focuses on identifying and addressing these areas of concern; in short, the focus is on moving beyond the trauma so that a child's day-to-day life and sense of self are no longer defined by past events.

> This final phase of treatment focuses on identifying and addressing these areas of concern; in short, the focus is on moving beyond the trauma so that a child's day-to-day life and sense of self are no longer defined by past events.

How Beyond Trauma Treatment Is Organized

The primary goals of beyond trauma treatment are to help a child and family move beyond the trauma so that it does not define the child's sense of self and relationships, or how others view and treat the child. The beyond trauma phase also addresses how the child and family can derive lasting meaning from the experience of trauma and their efforts to overcome it. Finally, beyond trauma treatment is about saying goodbye to the TST team. The primary activities of beyond trauma treatment can be remembered via the mnemonic *STRONG:*

- **S**trengthening cognitive skills.
- **T**elling your story: the trauma narrative.
- **R**eevaluating needs.
- **O**rienting to the future.
- **N**urturing parent–child relationships.
- **G**oing forward.

Treatment Structure

As with regulation-focused treatment, the beyond trauma phase of treatment can be delivered in clinic or office-based settings. Typically, home-based work is less critical at this point since the social environment is no longer threatening;

---

*As noted in Chapter 13, some children become dysregulated due to their internal cognitions related to trauma (rather than external triggers); these children may need to process the trauma narrative in order to attain a fully regulated state.

however, in some cases ongoing work to continue to build the capacity of care-givers to be helpful and protective may be helpful.

Beyond trauma treatment can be provided:

- In an office, school, residential, or home setting.
- By a mental health provider with a strong understanding of trauma and trauma processing.
- Directly to the child with active participation from the primary caregivers.

 In practice, beyond trauma sessions typically consist of the following activities and structure:

1. A brief check-in about the week to identify any stressful events or situations.
2. A review of the Beyond Trauma Guide.
3. A review of therapeutic activities related to the Beyond Trauma Guide.
4. As needed: A brief regulation-focused exercise to help ground and transition the child.

The Beyond Trauma Guide

 As in all phases of TST, providers have a central tool that guides their work. In the beyond trauma phase, we provide the Beyond Trauma Guide (BTG), which can be found in Appendix 12. The BTG begins where all guides begin: Anchoring the treatment. Then, the BTG walks through the six primary goals of this phase of treatment, much like the RFG does for the regulation-focused phase of treatment. If a clinician is doing what is in the BTG, then he or she is doing beyond trauma treatment under TST.

TOOL: Beyond Trauma Guide

What it is: A treatment guide for the TST providers who implement concrete steps related to the primary beyond trauma treatment goals.

When to use it: Throughout beyond trauma treatment.

Target goals: To guide clinicians as they structure treatment around the primary treatment goals of beyond trauma treatment (STRONG): **S**trengthening cognitive skills, **T**elling your story, **R**eevaluating needs, **O**rienting to the future, **N**urturing parent–child relations, **G**oing forward

TST Priority Problems in the Beyond Trauma Phase

We've spent a lot of time talking about the importance of TST priority problems. We've got some good news for you. TST priority problems are not an important part of beyond trauma treatment. Don't fall off your chair. Stick with us a bit. What did you accomplish when "your" child graduated from regulation-focused treatment? He or she became regulated! What does that mean? Your child does not have shifts in the three A's across a very broad range of stressors. That does not mean the child never has uncomfortable feelings, or troubling thoughts, or engages in behavior that perhaps he or she shouldn't. It means that the three A's rarely shift together and there is much greater control over the process of shifting state. Accordingly, survival in the moment is in the child's past. And how did we define those TST priority problems?

Patterns of Links between Provocative Stimuli and Survival-in-the-Moment States

No survival-in-the-moment states. No TST priority problems. CONGRATULATIONS!

So . . . if there are no more survival-in-the-moment states and no more TST priority problems, what is left to do?

- Experiences of trauma and ongoing problems with shifts into survival-in-the-moment states can influence how others view the child and how the child views him- or herself. These problems take an ongoing toll on a child's developing personality. Accordingly, *strengthening cognitive skills* will help here.

- Experiences of trauma are laden with meaning of which the child may or may not be conscious. This meaning may have significant influence over the way the child regards him- or herself, the world, and the future. The child may feel completely alone with all of this if he or she has never shared his or her story with anyone. Accordingly, for these children *telling their story* will help here.

- The storm of trauma, cats, cat hair, and survival-in-the-moment episodes requires so much attention that other problems may have been missed. Sometimes once the storm clears, other problems are revealed that could not be seen from the eye of the storm. A problem such as ADHD, depression, or a developmental or learning disorder may now be apparent and should be addressed. Accordingly, *reevaluating needs* will help here.

> The storm of trauma, cats, cat hair, and survival-in-the-moment episodes requires so much attention that other problems may have been missed. Sometimes once the storm clears, other problems are revealed that could not be seen from the eye of the storm.

- Trauma keeps people stuck in the past and defines them as victims of past events. Beyond trauma treatment is the time to put the past, and its trauma, away. It's time to look to the future from what may have been learned from the trauma, its aftermath, and efforts to overcome it in treatment, to create a healthier and happier future. Accordingly, activities in *orienting to the future* will help here.

- Let's not forget parents and families. They have gone through a lot too. The trauma and its aftermath usually have important meanings personally and for their relationship with their child. Over the course of TST, we've been building parent–child relationships; our HELPers Guide focuses on this critical goal. In beyond trauma treatment, we continue to *nurture the parent–child relationship* and anticipate how it could continue to be nurtured after treatment ends.

- Finally, it's time to say goodbye. A lot of great work has been accomplished. The therapeutic relationship has deepened. The child, family, and providers will not be working together again. Our *going forward* component focuses on saying goodbye and anticipating life without TST (and its providers).

Anchoring Beyond Trauma Treatment

As with earlier phases of treatment, Beyond Trauma begins with anchoring the treatment. This means we adapt the overall treatment strategy and Treatment Agreement Letter to be consistent with the goals of

> Beyond Trauma Guide:
> Anchoring Beyond Trauma
> Treatment

Beyond Trauma treatment. For children moving into Beyond Trauma treatment, the emphasis will shift to ways of thinking that are unhelpful and perpetuate negative emotions. We identified these problematic trauma-related cognitions in the assessment and treatment planning process. Beyond Trauma is the phase to address them.

1. **The adaptation of the overall treatment strategy.** Building on the information learned through assessment and treatment planning, and through earlier treatment phases if applicable, you now develop a treatment strategy focused on the goals of Beyond Trauma. Here is how we wrote Emily's anchor for Beyond Trauma:

   > Our emphasis in the Beyond Trauma phase of treatment will be to help identify certain ways of thinking that Emily has that are unhelpful to her, and cause her to feel sad and to withdraw. We know that Emily still worries she has "destroyed" her family and has been disloyal to them. While these worries no longer lead to survival states, she continues to feel very sad and sometimes withdraws from activities when she feels this way. We will work with Emily to help her learn to notice when she has thoughts that are

unhelpful or inaccurate, and help her develop alternative ways of thinking that are both more true and more helpful. We also will work with her to figure out why she continues to have a particularly difficult time with free-reading period at school, and to see if there are things that could help with that. Finally, we will continue to work with her foster mother around how best to help Emily when she feels sad and begins to withdraw.

2. **Continuing to account for treatment agreements.** As with earlier phases of treatment, treatment agreements continue to be important. While the social environment in Beyond Trauma is by definition not threatening, there may continue to be important ways that it could be more helpful to and protective of the child. Especially as trauma processing progresses, unnecessary "cat hair" may make it more difficult for the child to manage feelings and he or she may experience a resurgence of survival states. Agreements that have been made about protecting the child from such cat hair should be revisited.

3. **Identification of tried and true emotion regulation strategies.** During regulation-focused treatment, specific regulation strategies were identified that likely became the child's "go-to" strategies for managing emotion. During the course of Beyond Trauma, trauma processing may lead them to temporarily encounter more difficulties with emotion regulation, and more sensitivity to perceived threats in the environment. Regulation strategies that were particularly effective in the past should be revisited, and kept close by during Beyond Trauma.

Implementing Beyond Trauma Treatment

Strengthening Cognitive Skills

Thoughts float in and out of our heads all day long. Some thoughts are helpful and contribute to a sense of well-being, give us motivation, and help us feel good about ourselves and our work. For instance, try this one on:

> "If I read this chapter, I will really build my knowledge around TST. I may not understand it all at once, but I know I'm understanding some of it, and I will be better able to help kids. Over time I know the TST team will help me really consolidate this learning, too."

At other times, however, thoughts are unhelpful. They bog us down, make us feel like things won't work, and make it harder to persevere with our task at hand. For instance . . .

> "I never get this trauma stuff, and these authors have totally failed at explaining things well so far. I'm sure they will make this chapter obtuse and unreadable too. Even if I did do what they say, it probably wouldn't make a difference in my work. Mental health treatments never work."

Feel like reading on? OK, you get our point. Of course, if we really have written an obtuse and unreadable chapter, then no amount of positive thinking will change that. On the other hand, what if we wrote a good chapter? What if, should you persevere and read on, you would find it helpful? The unhelpful thought above might prevent you from even trying, and in a self-fulfilling prophecy, your sense that treatments don't work would be reinforced.

By the way, for the remainder of this chapter please *DON'T* think about the words *obtuse* and *unreadable*.

Traumatized children sometimes have a preponderance of unhelpful and inaccurate thoughts, and part of our job is to help them notice those thoughts and replace them with more helpful and accurate thoughts. These form the foundation of cognitive skills.

> Traumatized children sometimes have a preponderance of unhelpful and inaccurate thoughts, and part of our job is to help them notice those thoughts and replace them with more helpful and accurate thoughts.

Wait—didn't we just say, "Don't think about the words *obtuse* and *unreadable?"* Did you just think them? It turns out that simply telling someone to stop thinking about something (like the words *obtuse* and *unreadable*) have the opposite effect; the unwanted thoughts intrude and appear just as you are trying to make them go away. So another key cognitive skill is thought stopping, or gaining a set of skills to manage intrusive thoughts. Within the beyond trauma phase four main sets of cognitive skills are built:

1. Cognitive awareness
2. Thought stopping
3. Positive thinking
4. Catching, calling, and changing unhelpful thoughts

For children who are transitioning from the regulation-focused phase of treatment, cognitive awareness skills will build on their past work. Whereas in regulation-focused treatment a great deal of attention was paid to noticing one's *emotions*, cognitive awareness skills brings that same kind of attention to one's *thoughts*. Sometimes basic cognitive skills have already been introduced through the MEG (Appendix 10); this work continues and is deepened in this component of strengthening cognitive skills. Recall how the MEG helps kids notice how their three A's (affect, awareness, action) change over the four R's (regulating, revving, reexperiencing, reconstituting)? Whereas the focus of the MEG is to think about the change across states in the three A's, a first step in strengthening cognitive skills is to help children understand how within each of the four R phases the *three A's are connected!* Let's take the example from Chapter 5 of Lucy, the girl who is skipping rope when a boy rushes past (chasing a ball) and bumps her. Here is a brief look at Lucy's MEG:

Regulating	Revving	Reexperiencing	Reconstituting
Affect: *Happy.*	**Affect:** *Fearful and mad.*	**Affect:** *Enraged, panicked.*	**Affect:** *Tired, feels lonely, ashamed.*
Awareness: *Aware of being in school, at recess, trying to remember the jump-rope jingle.*	**Awareness:** *Remembers when the boy came after her brother with a knife. Thinking "he hates me and he could hurt me too."*	**Awareness:** *Feels like it is happening again. He's out to get me.*	**Awareness:** *Aware of being in the principal's office. Sense of self: "No one likes me—I'm always causing problems."*
Action: *Skipping rope, playing*	**Action:** *Freezes, stops playing.*	**Action:** *Jumps on the boy and starts hitting him.*	**Action:** *Sitting quietly.*

Now, let's take a closer look at the three A's in the revving column. We could begin to map out their connection like this:

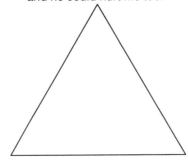

Awareness: Intrusive thoughts about brother being killed, thinks "that boy ran into me because he hates me, and he could hurt me too."

Action: Freezes and stops playing.

Affect: Fearful and mad

In this situation Lucy's *thoughts* (a central component of awareness) influence her affect and action. Some people describe this interrelationship as a *triad* of thoughts, feelings, and behavior.

Helping Lucy understand the way that thoughts, feelings, and behavior go together builds her *cognitive awareness skills.* What can Lucy do to manage her feelings in this situation? One of the most helpful strategies for her may be *thought stopping.* Thought-stopping strategies are concrete, immediate ways of distracting oneself from an intrusive, upsetting thought that is interfering with one's ability to function. In collaboration with her provider, Lucy might decide that one of the interventions listed on the MEG is to try imagining she is "changing the channel" by clicking a TV remote control whenever she begins to see the scene of her brother's murder.

Sometimes a child's thoughts may not be obviously related to past trauma but nonetheless are negatively biased. Recall from Chapter 5 the way *safety signals* can shape a child's expectation of the world around him or her. Sometimes signals of danger or carelessness have suffused a child's world and shaped his or her way of thinking. Although the TST treatment team will have worked like crazy to bring down the signals of danger and bring up the signals of care, sometimes a child's *way of thinking* needs to be addressed as well.

Strengthening cognitive skills helps a child notice how thoughts relate to feelings and actions, and to build concrete skills for stopping unwanted thoughts and challenging and changing unhelpful thoughts.

> Sometimes signals of danger or carelessness have suffused a child's world and shaped his or her way of thinking.

Once the child understands how thoughts can shape feelings and behavior, he or she can begin to explore the usefulness of *positive thinking*. Positive self-talk, a concept described by Cohen, Mannarino, and Deblinger (2006), refers to focusing on positive and optimistic thoughts about oneself or the task of coping with the trauma. Positive self-talk is a good companion skill to use in conjunction with both thought stopping and cognitive awareness. The therapist should initially have the child attempt to generate alternative thoughts on his or her own, and if the child has difficulty, the therapist can help. It is a good idea to have the child take the list of alternative thoughts home to revisit whenever necessary.

Make sure that the alternative thoughts you help the child generate are real—that is, don't encourage a child to think "I won't be mugged again in my neighborhood" if it might, in fact, happen. If the social environment is still distressed and the child is accurately perceiving the lack of safety, focus on things the child *can* control. For instance, "I know I can knock on a neighbor's door or call for help if I'm feeling scared in the neighborhood" acknowledges the potential threat while giving the child a greater sense of control.

Understanding how our thoughts affect our feelings and behavior, and being able to put a quick stop to unwanted thoughts and focus on positive self-talk, are a good start. But to really, fundamentally change one's view of oneself, the world, and others—and to really be ready to process a past trauma—more skills are needed. Children need to learn how to identify unhelpful or inaccurate thoughts, to challenge these thoughts, and to replace them with more helpful thoughts. This final set of skills—catching it, calling it, changing it—can be extremely powerful for children to learn.

How do you help children change their thoughts? First, it is important to make sure children understand that they are not "thinking wrong" or should just "look on the bright side" when, in fact, there is a huge dark cloud in the sky. Rather, the goal is to help identify when they are having particularly *unhelpful* and *inaccurate* thoughts. These *unhelpful* and *inaccurate* thoughts are considered "thinking traps" (Albano & DiBartolo, 2007). These thinking traps include the following:

- **Probability overestimation:** Believing bad things are way more likely to happen than they really are. For example:

  "If I stay home for my sister's stupid birthday party instead of hanging out with my friends tonight, they are all going to be mad at me and think that I don't like them."

- **Catastrophizing:** Expecting that the very worst thing possible will happen, and that you won't be able to deal with it if it does. For example:

  "On the bus ride to the away game, I will probably get motion sick and throw up all over. I would be so embarrassed I would never be able to face people again!"

- **All-or-nothing (or black-and-white) thinking:** Viewing a situation as only being one way or another without considering other possibilities in between. For example:

  "Everyone hates me."

- **Fortune telling:** Predicting something bad is going to happen in the future. For example:

  "Ballet class is going to be terrible and boring."

- **Discounting the positive:** Ignoring the good aspects or telling yourself they don't really matter. For example:

  "It doesn't matter that I got a good score on my math test, I still won't get an A this semester."

- **Focusing on the negative:** Paying attention to the bad parts of something without seeing the whole picture. For example:

  "The fair is going to be so crowded, it probably will take forever to get on the rides—what's the point in even going?"

- **Emotional reasoning:** Thinking something must be true because you *feel* like it is, while ignoring evidence to the contrary. For example:

  "When Daddy spilled my lemonade, he must have done it on purpose because I feel like he was being mean. When he says it was by accident, he must just be lying."

- **The "shoulds":** Having a set ideal of how you or others *should* behave and believing it would be very bad to act any other way. For example:

  "I should have known better, I shouldn't have let this happen to me. I guess that makes me a bad person."

The first step in *changing* an unhelpful thought is to *catch* it.

The first step in *changing* an unhelpful thought is to *catch* it. Although most children will not memorize the above types of thinking traps, they can often readily begin to think about "helpful versus unhelpful thoughts," "accurate versus inaccurate thoughts," and "worry versus calming thoughts."

Once children begin to be able to identify unhelpful thoughts, they can then learn to *challenge* them, or "call them." The goal here is not to suggest that these thoughts are just "in your head" or that problems aren't real and will just vanish "if you just think about it differently." Rather, you want to help the child sort out what the facts are; what these facts suggest about themselves, their world, and the future; and whether there are alternative ways of thinking about a situation that may be more accurate and ultimately more helpful. In essence, you want to encourage children to become detectives. When a child falls into one of the above thinking traps, help him or her review the situation by asking the following "detective questions":

- "What, exactly, happened in the situation? 'Just the facts, ma'am.'"
- "Have you ever been through a similar situation? What happened?"
- "Have you ever had a similar thought? What happened?"
- "Now consider the thought you had about this situation. What is the evidence for it being true? What is the evidence for it being different?"
- "What is an alternative, more calming thought that could be true about this situation?"

If the evidence points to the fact that the child may have fallen into a thinking trap, then a different, more helpful and accurate thought can be identified. If, however, the evidence points to the fact that this negative thought might, in fact, be somewhat accurate, then help the child to review which aspects of the situation he or she may have control over, or help the child think about ways in which his or her strengths and abilities could help him or her handle the adversity. Consider Ethan:

 Ethan is a 10-year-old boy who told his therapist that he believed his mother didn't love him. The therapist, rather than blithely saying "But of course she does!", instead probed a little more to ask what had led Ethan to believe this. Ethan then told his therapist that just the other morning his mother had made that statement to him. On further probing, it appeared they had had a big fight, and his mother had yelled that she didn't love him in the midst of great emotion. The therapist worked to help Ethan see that although it is true that his mother had said she didn't love him, there were other times when she expressed her love and showed him tremendous positive regard. Although there was some evidence for his negative thought ("She doesn't love me"), there was also some evidence to the contrary, so Ethan was able to come up with an alternative thought: "Sometimes Mom gets really upset with what I do, but she gets over it and still loves me." The therapist also worked with Ethan's mother to help her see the damage that can be done by saying things in the heat of the moment and used the HELPers Guide to provide her with some concrete emotion regulation strategies.

The four cognitive skills (cognitive awareness, thought stopping, positive thinking, and catch it–call it–change it) do not necessarily proceed in any given order. Sometimes cognitive awareness skills (structured by the Cognitive Awareness Log, introduced below) can be introduced first, and then thought stopping or positive thinking can be used as shortcuts to rapidly cut off unhelpful thoughts that have been identified through the log. Other times thought stopping can be taught quickly to help manage intrusive, disruptive thoughts and then later the more detailed work of the log can be introduced. Depending on the child's needs and skills, a therapist can move back and forth between these various tools to help a child best manage his or her unhelpful thoughts.

Step 1: Strengthening Cognitive Skills: Using the Cognitive Awareness Log

Beyond Trauma Guide:
Implementing Beyond Trauma
Step 1: Strengthening Cognitive
Skills

The Cognitive Awareness Log (CAL; Appendix 13) will help both the child and family structure their learning around cognitive skill building. Remember our friend, the MEG, from regulation-focused treatment? Now let us introduce you to CAL. At the outset of beyond trauma treatment CAL will consume a great deal of time in the session, and the associated cognitive skill building will directly inform the child's work on CAL.

🔧 TOOL: Cognitive Awareness Log (CAL)

What it is: An individualized worksheet that identifies thoughts, feelings, and behaviors associated with negative emotions as well as adaptive, alternative thoughts.

When to use it: In the early stages of beyond trauma treatment and in later stages in response to particular stressful incidents; sometimes during regulation-focused treatment.

Target goals: Child and caregiver will learn to identify links between the child's thoughts, feelings, and behaviors as well as adaptive ways of countering automatic thoughts.

The CAL is the primary tool for strengthening cognitive skills. Just as the MEG helps children observe and learn about their emotions, the CAL helps children observe their thoughts and the way those thoughts relate to how they feel and act. For children who have been using the MEG, you can first introduce this idea by beginning to connect how their *awareness* (their thoughts) relates to their *affect* and *action*. The CAL can then be introduced as a way of delving deeper into observing thoughts and practicing cognitive restructuring techniques.

The CAL helps children observe their thoughts and the way those thoughts relate to how they feel and act.

When first introducing the idea of how thoughts, feelings, and behaviors go together, it is often helpful to provide the child with a hypothetical situation. The therapist might say something like the following:

> "Let's say you are walking down the street during the middle of the day, and you hear someone running behind you. You glance behind you and see a boy from your class running toward you, and it looks like he is holding something. He's yelling at you to stop. You think to yourself 'That guy from my class is chasing me, and it looks like he might try to hurt me.' You then feel panicked and you start to run as fast as you can. You later realize that you must have dropped your wallet earlier when you were walking down the street. You feel disappointed because you have no idea where it is at this point.

> "Now let's change the scenario a little bit. You are walking down the street and you hear someone running behind you. You glance behind you and see a boy from your class running toward you, and it looks like he's holding something. You think to yourself 'That guy from my class is trying to get my attention. I wonder what he wants.' You feel calm and comfortable and walk toward him. Sure enough, you had dropped your wallet, and he is trying to give it back to you. You feel relieved and happy. Do you see how your thoughts affected the way you felt and behaved in each scenario? That's why it's so important to pay attention to your thoughts and attempt to change them if they are making you feel bad or making you act in ways that are not helpful."

Once the child can easily see the connection between the thoughts, feelings, and behavior described in this example, and can understand how alternative thoughts might have led to different (and better) outcomes, you can then apply the same idea to the child's own experiences. The CAL structures this discussion. As with the MEG, the CAL is best used in relation to a real-life situation that has come up recently for the child. Begin by asking about any particularly challenging or upsetting situations that occurred over the week, or if the child is worried about something coming up. Review what happened or the upcoming challenge, what the child was/is thinking, how the child felt/feels, and what the child did next/could do next.

A Moment-by-Moment Assessment is critical to help identify the specific thoughts and feelings a child has, which form the foundation of the CAL worksheets. In this phase the Moment-by-Moment Assessment emphasizes *thoughts, from the Awareness component of this assessment:* "What were you thinking? What went through your head?" You may need to prompt children with additional questions to help them articulate their thoughts. For example:

- "What were you thinking about yourself and your ability to handle it?"
- "What did you think others were thinking about you?"

- "What did you think might happen next?"
- "What did you think were the possible outcomes?"

Working together, and using the information gleaned from the Moment-by-Moment Assessment, fill out the icons on the first page of the CAL. Then, still working together, review the CAL detective questions. Focus on the facts and help the child think through the answers. Once this is done and the child seems able to separate fact from feeling, move to one of the two next sections: either "CAL to the Rescue" (for children who are ready to build cognitive restructuring skills) or "Thought Stopping with CAL."

For children who identify unwanted, intrusive thoughts that seem to immediately derail them, flip to the "Thought Stopping" section of the CAL. Work with the child to select a concrete thought-stopping technique for him or her to plan on using the very next time (and every time) that unwanted thought happens. Verbal (saying "Stop"), and/or visual ("Picture a big STOP sign in your head") techniques can be used to interrupt an intrusive thought.

The following case example illustrates the use of thought stopping:

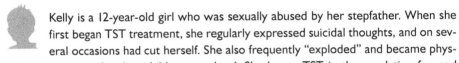 Kelly is a 12-year-old girl who was sexually abused by her stepfather. When she first began TST treatment, she regularly expressed suicidal thoughts, and on several occasions had cut herself. She also frequently "exploded" and became physically aggressive with other children at school. She began TST in the regulation-focused phase, and it was discovered that these explosive and physically aggressive episodes repeatedly followed affectionate signals from peers, which sometimes involved physical contact (e.g., hair stroking, shoulder massage). These types of signals triggered survival-in-the-moment states because, it was determined, the sexual abuse was frequently preceded by that type of physical contact from her stepfather. Kelly developed strong emotion regulation skills and was determined to be ready for the beyond trauma phase. There were, however, other problems that emerged. Kelly seemed somewhat quiet and morose at home. Her mother reported that she spends a great deal of time in her room tidying it up to the point of perfection, and that her school grades are slipping. Recently she was supposed to complete a book report and the night before it was due had not even started it. "Who cares," she said when her mother asked about it, "I can't write a good report, so why even bother!"

Kelly's therapist met with her and learned that every time Kelly starts reading her book, she has recurring, intrusive thoughts about her perpetrator. She states, "I just can't get his words out of my head. He told me that if I told anyone what he did to me, then I would never see my mom again. When I think about it, I feel sick to my stomach."

Although a critical step in Kelly's treatment will later involve in-depth processing of these intrusive thoughts and images, the initial goal in the beyond trauma treatment phase is to help her put a stop to thoughts that are distracting and upsetting. The therapist might help Kelly combat these intrusive thoughts by saying something like the following:

> "As soon as you realize that you are hearing his voice in your head, I want you to picture a large stop sign, and I want you to yell to yourself, 'Stop!' You can even yell 'Stop!' out loud if you are by yourself."

It is important for the therapist to be able to help the child see the difference between *controlling* intrusive thoughts when necessary versus *avoiding* all thoughts of the trauma all of the time. Teaching thought-stopping skills is not meant to discourage children from having any thoughts about the trauma whatsoever. This skill should be used to help children stop thoughts that are limiting their ability to function (e.g., Kelly getting that book read for her book report) and distract themselves from those thoughts so that they are better able to handle the tasks of daily life.

After the therapist has helped Kelly learn thought-stopping techniques, the therapist can also help her generate a list of alternative thoughts on which to focus instead of the threats that her abusive stepfather made. These more adaptive thoughts might include:

> "It's over now."
>
> "I know my mom is safe."
>
> "He can't hurt any of us any more."
>
> "There are lots of people protecting me."

For children who are ready for cognitive restructuring skills, the "CAL to the Rescue" section can be completed. Help the child identify a more accurate, helpful thought that could have been the response to the same situation. What might the child have felt then? What might the child have done? When the CAL identifies a negative thought that recurs for a child, rather than completing a new CAL every time he or she has that thought, the therapist can encourage the child to jump to thought stopping by saying something like the following:

> "So Ethan, now we know that when the thought 'Mom doesn't love me' pops into your head, you feel really awful and sometimes that awful feeling also leads to you doing things that aren't all that helpful. We also talked about how a more accurate thought might be 'Mom gets really upset when I do certain things, but she still loves me.' How about the next time you notice that unhelpful thought pop into your head, you picture a big STOP sign in your head, and imagine someone calling out loudly 'STOP!'"

Similar to the MEG, the CAL is a tool that should be used collaboratively among the caregiver, child, and provider. The worksheet can be used to anticipate a difficult upcoming situation and after the child has faced an upsetting or challenging situation, whether at home or at school. For younger children, the caregiver and child are asked to fill out the worksheet together at home. Adolescents may prefer to fill it out on their own. The child then brings the completed CAL to the next treatment session for review. The child is asked to complete one CAL per week, *at a minimum*, and preferably three or more.

Telling Your Story

The second, and possibly most important, treatment domain within the beyond trauma treatment phase entails developing and processing the trauma narrative.

This form of treatment has also been referred to as "gradual exposure" therapy (e.g., Cohen et al., 2006, 2012; Deblinger & Heflin, 1996; March, Amaya-Jackson, Murray, & Schulte, 1998; Pynoos & Nader, 1988), which is a cornerstone of most treatments for traumatized children.

Sometimes there can be great reticence on the part of the child, caregiver, or even a provider to talk about what happened to the child. It may seem that talking about it will just make things worse, and that it is best just "left behind." However, for a child who is consistently plagued by thoughts of the trauma or in other ways lives his or her daily life with a painful awareness of the past, just "ignoring it" or wishing it away is anything but helpful. Helping the child develop a narrative around what happened, reconsider the ways in which he or she can think about certain aspects of the narrative, and sharing the narrative with caregivers can be extremely powerful and healing.

In order to help children and caregivers understand why talking about the traumatic event is helpful, Cohen and colleagues (2006, 2012) provide a very effective metaphor (cleaning a physical wound) for therapists to use in treating traumatized children and their caregivers. The therapist might say something like the following:

"Let's pretend that a little girl your age is riding her bike along a bumpy road, falls off of the bike, and scrapes her knee. In order to make sure that the girl's knee does not become infected, it will be important to clean out the wound, right? So even though cleaning the cut may hurt at first, it helps the wound to heal much faster and it will stop hurting over time. If the girl were to leave the cut and not wash it out, it would end up hurting more and more over time because it is likely to get infected. It's kind of the same thing when we begin to talk about the trauma because at first, it hurts. But the more we talk about it, the less it hurts, and the less likely it is to hurt over time."

Trauma processing occurs in two (sometimes overlapping) components: building a trauma narrative and cognitive restructuring. The first component is to help the child develop the narrative about what happened. The method of narrative development that the therapist chooses to use should match the skills and interests of the child. For example, if a child enjoys singing or writing rap music, the trauma can be processed using song lyrics or raps. Other examples include making collages; drawings; or writing poetry, play scripts, or books. Whatever the medium, the key is to help the child put together a story about what he or she experienced, including facts, feelings, and a sense of time that separates past, present, and future.

As the narrative develops, negative thoughts will likely be uncovered; ongoing work with the CAL will help to continue to build the child's cognitive skills, now in relation to emotionally laden material. In fact, bringing to light the negative thoughts is a very important part of building the trauma narrative; the therapist can encourage this part by asking questions throughout the narrative, such as:

- "How did that make you feel?"
- "Did this change the way you think about yourself and others?"
- "Did you start doing things differently as a result of this?"

Understanding how trauma may have shaped the way children feel, think, and do things can also help them separate who they are from what happened to them. Cognitive restructuring skills can then be brought to bear on any negative imprints left by the trauma.

> Understanding how trauma may have shaped the way children feel, think, and do things can also help them separate who they are from what happened to them.

Much of the purpose of doing a trauma narrative is accomplished simply in the act of putting the story together. However, most children need encouragement and coaching to elaborate the story. The following paragraph is taken from Kelly's initial trauma narrative, which she wrote as part of making a book, and exemplifies the level of detail that can be expected after a child's first pass at a trauma narrative:

"As usual, my stepfather came into my room when I was at my desk doing homework. Mom always works her shift at that time, so he knew it was safe for him. He opened my bedroom door. I didn't look up. He came behind me, rubbed my shoulders, said I was tense and I must have had a bad day. Then he had sex with me. When he did it, I was crying. He told me to take my clothes off. I almost ran out of the room, but then he locked the door. When my mother came home, I finally told her what was happening. She said to him, 'Why did you do that?' and he said, 'What did I do?'"

The next narrative illustrates the ways in which the therapist was able to help Kelly expand on her previous narrative and incorporate more detail, including her own feelings, observations of others' emotions and reactions, additional traumatic aspects, as well as "rescripting." *Rescripting* refers to the child's attempts to, literally, rewrite the ending of his or her own trauma experience. It is a useful means of helping the child gain a sense of mastery or identifying potential unhelpful thoughts that may need to be addressed.

> Kelly wrote:
>
> My stepfather was mean. He had sex with me. When he did it I was crying, but he is not in my family now, so he can't hurt anyone in my family. I was mad when he did it to me. He came to my room and started rubbing my shoulders. It made me feel all hot and prickly. He kept whispering things in my ear, saying "You must be stressed, you must be tense" and it was hot and yucky, I felt sick to my stomach. Then he told me to take my clothes off. I almost ran out of the room, but he locked the door. I felt mad when he asked me to take my clothes off. I also felt like I must have done something wrong, like he was punishing me for something. He pulled my clothes off and threw them on the floor, and he whispered in my ear, "You messy girl, you." Then he pushed me down on the bed. The worst part was when I was trying to get up and he pinned me down and covered my mouth. When my mother came home from work I told her what happened . . . that he had sex with me, even though he told me not to tell anyone or he'd kill my mom. First I told my mom, "Dad had sex with me." My mom got mad. Her face looked really angry. When he came home from work, my mother said, "Why did you do that?" and he said, "What did I do?" I felt mad when I heard them arguing. I felt like I shouldn't have said anything because then they wouldn't be fighting. I was scared that he would hurt my mom. This is what I wish would have happened: I would get my brothers and sisters ready at the front door and when my stepfather came to my room, I would run past him, run to the front door, and run to my aunt's house with all of my brothers and sisters.

There is obviously a great deal of material to work with in the previous trauma narrative. As an example, Kelly's narrative contains elements of self-blame, such as "I felt like I must have done something wrong, like he was punishing me for something" and "I felt like I shouldn't have said anything because then they wouldn't be fighting." Cohen and colleagues (2006) describe the use of *progressive logical questioning* to address inaccurate or unhelpful thoughts. The following example demonstrates how a therapist might use this technique with Kelly to address her statements of self-blame:

THERAPIST: Can you help me find a sentence in this chapter that may be unhelpful or untrue?

KELLY: Maybe the sentence about how I must have done something wrong?

THERAPIST: When you say that you felt like you had done something wrong, that's really a thought. Can you tell me what the feeling is?

KELLY: Guilty. Like it was my fault that it was happening because he was trying to punish me for something.

THERAPIST: So when you think to yourself that you must have done something wrong, that makes you feel guilty. You also said that it felt like he was punishing you. What do you think he was punishing you for?

KELLY: Well . . . I did forget to clean my room that day.

THERAPIST: Now let's think about that for a minute. We may never know why your stepfather hurt you in the way that he did. But it sounds like he has a lot of problems and that his reasons for hurting you have absolutely nothing to do with anything that you did. But what if what you're saying is true? Everyone makes mistakes sometimes, right? What if you had forgotten to clean your room? Do you think that means that your stepfather has a right to punish you in that way . . . to rape you?

KELLY: No. I don't deserve that just because I didn't clean my room.

THERAPIST: That's right. Can you think of *anything* that you could have done that would have made it OK for your stepfather to rape you?

KELLY: No. It wasn't fair. I don't deserve to be treated like that, even if I do something wrong.

THERAPIST: You're absolutely right. Raping someone is a terrible thing to do and should *never* be used as a form of punishment. It is also illegal, and that is why your stepfather is going to jail. So instead of thinking to yourself, "I felt like I must have done something wrong, like he was punishing me for something," what could you think to yourself that might be more helpful and accurate?

KELLY: I know that I didn't do anything wrong, and even if I made a mistake, he should never have raped me. I didn't deserve that. No one deserves that.

If left unaddressed, cognitive distortions can become extremely damaging in that they can develop into permanent, global statements related to the child's self-concept. Consequently, helping a child identify and change unhelpful and/or inaccurate thoughts about the traumatic event is a critical step in ensuring his or her future psychological health. Because these thoughts can be so powerful, it may take several sessions to fully process their meaning and help the child generate more adaptive thoughts. These negative thoughts may also have affected the way the child views self and relationships more generally; understanding these broader effects of trauma, and helping the child to see and address them as well, is very important. The following dialogue provides another example of how to address an unhelpful thought:

THERAPIST: Can you find another sentence in there that may be unhelpful?

KELLY: I guess it's not helpful to think that I shouldn't have said anything because it made them fight.

THERAPIST: What makes this thought unhelpful? What does it make you feel when you think about it?

KELLY: It's unhelpful because I feel guilty again. Like it's my fault that they were fighting.

THERAPIST: What do you think would have happened if you hadn't said anything?

KELLY: They wouldn't have been fighting. He wouldn't have tried to hurt my mom.

THERAPIST: That might be true. But can you think of anything bad that might have happened if you hadn't said anything?

KELLY: He probably would have done it again . . . I mean, raped me. And maybe not just me . . . maybe my sister too.

THERAPIST: So by telling your mom, you were protecting yourself and also your sister. Those are two very important reasons for telling your mom, don't you think?

KELLY: Yeah. I guess if I hadn't told her, he could still be living with us . . . and still abusing me.

THERAPIST: It sounds like you made a very smart and also very brave decision to tell your mom what he did. And your sister is very lucky to have you looking out for her. So let's go back to the unhelpful sentence that we started with: "I felt like I shouldn't have said anything because then they wouldn't be fighting." What would be a more helpful thought to have?

KELLY: If I never said anything, my stepdad could still be abusing me and my sister. It was important to tell my mom so she could help protect us.

It is important to note that the therapist should not begin to address cognitive distortions in the child's narrative until the child has written the entire narrative. If the therapist were to address unhelpful thoughts too early, it may make the child inhibited and reluctant to write about thoughts or feelings that may be considered inaccurate or unhelpful.

The creation of a book is an ideal way of helping the child process the trauma; there is evidence that the act of writing about the trauma can be healing in itself (Donnelly & Murray, 1991; Esterling, L'Abate, & Murray, 1999). However, it is critical that the child write about thoughts and feelings associated with the trauma because research suggests that the integration of thoughts and feelings within the trauma narrative is essential for improving psychological health (Pennebaker & Francis, 1996). As suggested by Cohen and colleagues (2006), the therapist should start by having the child begin with neutral information such as name, birthdate, grade in school, etc., in order to help him or her begin to feel comfortable with the process. Next, the therapist should help the child move toward gathering "facts" about the trauma, such as what happened, where did the trauma take place, who was there, etc. Finally, the therapist should help the child process thoughts and feelings associated with the traumatic incident(s) described and address cognitive distortions that are likely to arise during the writing of the trauma narrative. This part is described in more detail later in the chapter.

Step 2: Telling Your Story: Using the BTG

The first step in developing the trauma narrative is to make sure that the child is ready for trauma processing. Are the child's cognitive skills sufficiently mastered so that he or she can apply them in day-to-day situations? Moving to the trauma narrative

Beyond Trauma Guide:
Implementing Beyond Trauma
Treatment Step 2: Telling Your
Story

before the child has developed the necessary cognitive skills can be counterproductive, so if the child is not ready, then return to the "Strengthening Cognitive Skills" section, Step 1 of the treatment, in the early part of this chapter.

Next, the clinician must think through whether the narrative will be about a single event or series of related events, or instead is the story of chronic upheaval and trauma. Consider these two children:

 Lou is a 14-year-old boy who lives with his parents and younger brother. When Lou was 12, he attended a sleep-away camp where a male counselor repeatedly abused him sexually. Lou continues to experience intrusive thoughts about the abuse and avoids sleeping over at friends' houses. Later in the year his class is planning on taking a 3-day trip to Washington, DC. Lou has become increasingly anxious about this event and begun to avoid going to school.

Jerry is an 8-year-old boy who was severely neglected as an infant. His mother used heroin regularly when he was a small child, and when he was 3 years old Jerry was placed in foster care. During his first foster home stay an older foster sibling became extremely aggressive with him, and he was moved to a new home when bruises were discovered up and down his back. Jerry then went through a period of about 4 years during which he bounced from foster home to foster home due to his "wild, erratic, and aggressive behavior." For the past year he has been stable in a therapeutic foster home and no longer demonstrates physical aggression. He continues to struggle with poor self-esteem and seems distrustful of those around him, often making statements such as "I probably won't be part of this family for long—no one really wants me as their kid." His current case manager, who has been with him for 3 years, has known him longer than anyone else in his life.

Lou and Jerry could both benefit from trauma processing; however, the approach to building a narrative with each of them will need to be quite different. Lou's "story" is one of substantial stability and love, punctuated by a defined period of terrible abuse. Jerry, on the other hand, looks back on a blur of a life. His memory of his passage from one home to the next is fragmented. No one in his life can tell the complete story of how he moved from place to place; case notes, "his file," and his current case manager hold bits and pieces of his story. For Jerry, building a narrative is as much about bringing coherence and order to his history as it is about processing specific events. We call Lou's story a *specific-event trauma narrative*. We call Jerry's story a *chronic trauma narrative*. A guide for each of these two narratives is included in the BTG (pp. 479–490).

At times, a combination of approaches may be helpful; for instance, in the course of developing his story, Jerry may dwell on the aggressive foster sibling, and the specific period of his history may be worth exploring in more detail (as in the first narrative approach).

Once the general narrative approach has been identified, the child's particular strengths in communication should be considered. Is the child an artist? A singer? A storyteller? A writer? Although telling or writing will be a necessary part of the story, the process can be made more engaging by building on the child's inherent strengths and interests. For a very young or cognitively limited child, replaying the story through pretend play can be used. Some examples of ways of approaching the narrative include:

- **Collages or drawings**. Provide three large pieces of paper labeled *Past*, *Present*, and *Future*. Ask the child to complete collages for each of these time periods and then interview the child. During the interview include questions about the facts of each time period, as well as the emotions the child experienced.
- **Poetry**. Use existing poems to provide inspiration or a starting structure for the child. For example, Wallace Stevens' "Thirteen Ways of Looking at a Blackbird" could be read, and then the theme of "Thirteen Ways of Looking at My Life" could be used. Another good poem is Robert Frost's "The Road Not Taken": Read the poem, then have the child or adolescent write one poem about "The Road behind Me," one poem about "The Road I'm on," and one poem about "The Road I'm Going to Take." After the child is done writing, interview him or her about the poetry to help the child elaborate on the facts, feelings, and chronology of his or her life.
- **Pretend play**. Provide the child with relevant props (e.g., dollhouse, dolls, car, if a car accident is involved) and ask him or her to show you what happened. As the play progresses, you can ask questions about how the doll is feeling, what the doll is thinking, etc.
- **Writing a story**. Starting with a title page and Chapter 1, help the child outline and write a story. Children who are less comfortable writing can dictate. Using a computer allows for easy revisions and adding in elaborations.

- **Cartoons**. Cartoon scripts easily lend themselves to adding thought bubbles.

Next, the trauma narrative is begun.

Every trauma narrative will look different, and the guidance and prompts used with each child will need to be tailored by the therapist. For instance, children who experienced trauma at a very young age may not even have verbal memories of what happened—

> Every trauma narrative will look different, and the guidance and prompts used with each child will need to be tailored by the therapist.

although the experience may have deeply affected them, telling the story about it may be different than for a child who remembers and can describe the traumatic event. The BTG provides outlines for the two types of trauma narratives we have been discussing. These outlines, which can be adapted and changed to reflect the developmental stage of the child and his or her specific experiences, are used as tools to help therapists think about the type of questions that would be helpful in getting a narrative started. As the child progresses through the narrative, the therapist should make notes in the "Notes" section about potential areas to revisit during the trauma processing section. Unhelpful or inaccurate thoughts can be flagged and talked through later, after the narrative has been fully developed.

Finally, the work of trauma processing should be in done in tandem with Step 5 in the BTG, "Nurturing Parent–Child Relationships." A critical part of narrative development and processing is sharing the story with the child's parents or other caregivers; a critical part of making sure the sharing is productive is first working with the parents to make sure they can receive the story in a way that helps the child. This point is described in more detail later in the chapter.

Reevaluating Needs

As described previously, trauma and its aftermath comprise a storm that requires so much attention that other problems may be missed. Once the storm clears, sometimes other problems are revealed that could not be seen from the eye of the storm. For children who have experienced survival states on a regular basis until recently, other needs may have been overlooked. Now that the storm is clearing, we need to look anew and ask ourselves: "Is trauma the only story here? Or does this child have other, real needs that have been obscured by the trauma responses until now?"

Let's think about Kelly for a minute. Her clinician identified negative thoughts as a target of treatment and initiated cognitive skill building in response. However, the clinician was an astute observer and noted that whereas Kelly had a great number of negative thoughts about her abilities in relation to reading, this pattern did not seem to be present in other academic areas. In fact, Kelly felt quite sure about her abilities in math. Kelly's mother reported that the reading assignments did not seem overly hard and that most children in the classroom seemed to be handling them relatively well. Kelly's teacher noted that reading seemed to be a particularly difficult time of the day for Kelly and that she was not keeping pace with her peers. Might there be another problem at play here?

In consultation with Kelly's clinician, Kelly's mother decided to request a reading evaluation. Indeed, the results showed that Kelly was struggling with mild dyslexia, which was contributing to her frustration and negative self-view. Additional support around reading was implemented at school, and Kelly's frustration diminished.

It is easy to see how, for a child who just a couple of months ago was exploding on a regular basis in response to relatively mild provocations at school, her frustration and negative mood around reading could be overlooked. Those reading-related reactions might even have been understood, inadvertently, as a trauma response. But no amount of emotion regulation skill building would remove the central problem of a reading disability. Now that the smoke has cleared, the TST team must look with fresh eyes at the child and her difficulties to determine if other problems are at play and if other interventions are needed.

Step 3: Reevaluating Needs: Using the BTG

Beyond Trauma Guide: Implementing Beyond Trauma Treatment Step 3: Reevaluating Needs

The BTG provides a list of common problems that may require additional intervention. At the outset of the beyond trauma treatment phase the clinician conducts a reevaluation of the child in terms of his or her functioning and any potential problems. Areas that require further assessment are flagged, as are areas that clearly need further intervention. Once these other needs have been identified, a plan can be put in place for either:

1. Providing the intervention through the ongoing therapeutic relationship, or
2. Referring out for additional evaluation and/or intervention.

Whether or not the TST team can provide the additional interventions needed depends on both the specific needs of the child and the specific skill sets of the TST providers. Empirically based approaches to addressing most problems are readily available, and if the TST team is not trained in these models, then a referral should be made to an outside provider.

Step 4: Orienting to the Future

> We must never forget that we may also find meaning in life even when confronted with a hopeless situation, when facing a fate that cannot be changed. For what then matters is to bear witness to the uniquely human potential at its best, which is to transform a personal tragedy into triumph, to turn one's predicament into a human achievement. (Frankl, 1962, p. 135)

In his book *Man's Search for Meaning*, Viktor Frankl (1962) describes his tragic experiences in a concentration camp during World War II and his resulting creation of "logotherapy," a meaning-centered form of psychotherapy that focuses on "the meaning of human existence as well as on man's search for such a meaning" (p. 121).

For a child and family who have experienced suffering or borne witness to that suffering, it is essential to try to understand the meaning in what has come before—and what lies ahead. Current treatments for traumatized children often overlook the necessity of helping children make meaning out of their traumatic events. It is likely that the acquisition of meaning-making skills following a traumatic event can serve as a protective mechanism and buffer children from future symptom relapse. Meaning-making skills can provide children with hope for the future and allow them to focus on the positive aspects of their lives as opposed to dwelling on the tragedies that they were forced to endure. In essence, the activity of creating meaning out of a traumatic experience allows children and families to put the event(s) in context so that they are no longer consumed by the past but can move into their future.

> Meaning-making skills can provide children with hope for the future and allow them to focus on the positive aspects of their lives as opposed to dwelling on the tragedies that they were forced to endure.

According to Frankl (1962), two of the central experiences that contribute to finding meaning in life are creating or doing something, and experiencing another human being in all of his or her uniqueness. In this step of *orienting to the future*, we encourage children to move toward these experiences through helping them (1) see themselves as worthy of healthy, intimate relationship; and (2) identify and work toward life goals.

The Self as Worthy of Healthy, Intimate Relationships

After a traumatic event, children's identities sometimes change for the worse. After being abandoned by a parent, a child may see himself as "unwanted" or "lost." After being raped by her stepfather, a child may see herself as "damaged" or "worthless." These maladaptive identities may be even more difficult to change if the trauma has been chronic. Even after a child has processed his or her thoughts and feelings about the abuse, negative self-images may persist indefinitely unless they are directly addressed, challenged, and modified.

The cognitive skills already practiced in this phase of treatment will have begun to address negative self-images. For children whose falsely negative self-images persist, additional emphasis on examining and challenging these self-views is needed. This can be done through eliciting the child's self-perception and having the child compare it to his or her "real" self.

Especially for adolescents, who are at a time developmentally when they reflect on their identities and place in the world, this natural exploration and confirmation of self may be fostered through dialogue or other creative outlets. Below is a story of how one child's image of herself transformed over treatment:

> Victoria is a 16-year-old Sudanese girl with an extensive and complicated trauma history. While in the Sudan as a child, she was raped by militia and threatened with female genital cutting (FGC). In order to escape undergoing FGC, she ran away from her village and ultimately to the United States. When she arrived in the United States at age 16, she was experiencing major depression and PTSD. She had attempted suicide twice.
>
> Victoria was an exceptionally talented artist. At the start of treatment, she drew several pictures that resonated with themes of emptiness, loss, and powerlessness. Her self-portrait showed a girl with a blank expression, and she explained that the girl did not have hope.
>
> As treatment continued, Victoria's therapist encouraged her to explore new themes with her art. She painted a series of paintings about the process of FGC rituals, showing young girls being prepared for this procedure. She explained that she wanted the world to understand what was happening back in Africa. Toward the end of her treatment, she shifted her topic yet again and did a series of portraits of self and others. Each of these was of a young woman, beautiful and physically powerful looking. One she described as "finding love." Another she described as a self-portrait of herself crossing a bridge, leaving the horrors of the past behind her.

For some children, focusing on ways in which their survival of the trauma helped them to learn something important about themselves or life can be an important way to emphasize their self-worth. In the course of the trauma narrative the child may already have been asked to consider what he or she learned in the process. Generally, children are able to identify more and more "lessons" as time goes by. These lessons that children may have learned from their traumatic experiences may take on many different forms. For some children, the lessons can pertain to things that they learned about themselves, things they learned about others, or things that they learned about life in general.

Finally, the CAL will continue to be an important tool. Use the CAL to help children identify their thinking traps around self-image and identify more helpful ways of thinking about who they are and the ways in which the trauma has, or has not, changed them.

Working toward Life Goals

The true meaning of life is to be discovered in the world rather than within man or his own psyche, as though it were a closed system . . . being human always points, and is directed, to something or someone other than oneself—be it a meaning to fulfill or another human to encounter. (Frankl, 1962, p. 133)

In the preceding quotation, Dr. Frankl talks about the importance of being a part of the world, not just in the closed system of one's own psyche. And, with TST, the ultimate goal is to transition away from the *trauma system* and into the world. Looking beyond oneself and, in some way, to "point" toward others can happen in small, immediate ways and also by mapping a course toward larger, longer-term goals.

Your work leading up to the beyond trauma phase can facilitate this type of discussion about the meaning of goals. The assessment process includes the identification of goals as a central part of treatment engagement. In beyond trauma we take these goals and explore their meaning to the children as they imagine themselves contributing to the benefit of other people. Why does Tanisha want to become a teacher? Why did this goal have such a hold on her that she was able to use it to get through the difficult work of recovering from trauma? In this phase of treatment, your conversation with Tanisha might reveal the following:

- "I want to be a teacher because I want to help kids."
- "I'm good with kids, and I want to give back and help kids who don't have what I have."
- "With what I went through with my mom, I know how it can be. I can help others from my experience."
- "My grandma is my hero. She protected me. I know how hard it was for her to say no to my mom. But she did, to protect me. I want to be brave for kids the way my grandma was brave for me."

Your work exploring and reinforcing these thoughts will mark Tanisha's present and future. Think about how meaningful it would be for Ms. Williams to be part of this conversation. Trauma assaults the deepest parts of human beings. But humans are remarkably strong. They make meaning of their experiences. They can transform their experiences into things that are amazing. Your job is to be the midwife of that miraculous process.

Here is another story of transforming a traumatic experience during beyond trauma:

Michael is a 17-year-old boy who was in a serious car accident one year before treatment began. He had several broken bones but was able to heal rapidly.

Unfortunately, his girlfriend of 1 year had been in the passenger seat and experienced severe injuries to her head and her neck. She is now completely paralyzed from the neck down.

When Michael began therapy, he was extremely guilt-ridden over his girlfriend's situation and was experiencing major depressive symptoms, including suicidal ideation. He also had symptoms of traumatic stress, such as frequent nightmares, flashbacks of the accident, and avoidance of the site of the car crash.

Once his emotion regulation skills were strong enough, Michael began to spend a great deal of time with his girlfriend, offering her emotional support and providing her with information about new technologies that may be able to assist in her recovery. Providing her with hope was healing for Michael as well. He also began fundraising efforts at his high school to raise money for his girlfriend so she may be able to afford the newest advances in medicine. At his high school homecoming dance, Michael was able to raise money through ticket sales; $5 of each ticket was given to his girlfriend's fund.

> By the end of this phase, children should not only be able to think about the future but to see themselves as effective creators of a meaningful future.

By the end of this phase, children should not only be able to think about the future but to see themselves as effective creators of a meaningful future. If children are able to shift their views in this way, they have initiated a brand new journey with a different destination in mind, one that has the potential for reparative experiences and new ways of looking at the world.

Orienting to the Future: Using the BTG

> Beyond Trauma Guide: Implementing Beyond Trauma Treatment Step 4B

By this time in treatment a provider may have a clear sense of how the child sees him- or herself. Sometimes, however, it is less clear. As a provider begins working to help a child focus on the future, it is important to first understand how the child sees him- or herself. Sometimes this can be done through a simple conversation, but other times structured activities may help the child articulate implicit evaluations of his or her own self-worth. Consider using the following activities to guide the conversation:

- "Draw yourself as a cartoon character. Talk about how cartoonists take elements of a person and exaggerate them. What would your cartoon character be? What would it look like? How would it act? Now think about how this cartoon character is the same or different from the actual *you* that you perceive."

- "Make yourself a superhero. What superpowers would you have? All superheroes have an 'Achilles heel.' What is your superhero's vulnerability or weakness? Now think about how this superhero is the same or different from the actual *you* that you see."

- "If someone wrote a short story in which you were the main character, what would they say about you?"
- "Describe the kind of person you aspire to be. Now think about how you are alike or different from what you aspire to be."

Once a self-image has been articulated, help the child complete a CAL related to any unhelpful and inaccurate thoughts. If you structured the conversation using some of the preceding ideas, revisit the

> Beyond Trauma Guide:
> Implementing Beyond Trauma
> Treatment Step 4C

character or superhero and help the child consider other ways of thinking about strengths/weaknesses that are more realistic and helpful.

It will be important to use what Carol Dweck (2006) calls "growth language" in these conversations. Specifically, focus on how a child's actions and efforts determine who he or she is—rather than having an

> Beyond Trauma Guide:
> Implementing Beyond Trauma
> Treatment Step 4D

innate identity that is fixed and can't be changed. For instance, if a child wins a game, praise his or her actions ("Wow, you really focused on this game—you must have been paying very careful attention to the cards I played!") rather than praising some innate characteristic ("Wow, you are *so* smart!"). The first kind of praise identifies behaviors a child can consciously do again—that is, focusing and paying attention. The second kind of praise suggests that if the child loses next time, he or she might not be so smart, after all. Applying this kind of "growth mindset" to self-image can help children feel that they are not just simply "who they are," but rather can become who they *want to be* through working toward a vision. In the words of Victor Frankl (1962):

 Man does not simply exist, but always decides what his existence will be, what he will become in the next moment. By the same token, every human being has the freedom to change at any instant. (p. 154)

Step 5: Nurturing Parent–Child Relations

Throughout earlier intervention modules, TST structures activities to strengthen parents' relationships with their children. Now the strength of those relationships will be critical as children develop a trauma narrative and share it with their caregivers.

One of the deepest desires of childhood—or perhaps life—is to be truly seen and understood by another. When a child skins his or her knee on the playground, gets up, runs across the playground to Mother and *then* begins to cry, it is not "faking it"; rather, it is an expression of the universal need to communicate pain to, and be understood by, those with whom we are most intimate. When a parent "kisses the boo-boo" as a way to make it better, he or she is communicating to the child "I see you, I understand you got hurt, and I care about you."

When we are talking about a traumatic experience, rather than a skinned knee, the magnitude has changed—but the rest remains the same. Part of the healing process is being able to share with others, in a safe and secure setting, the pain of the trauma and to have a parent demonstrate "I see you, I understand you got hurt, and I care about you." But unlike a skinned knee, traumas are often fraught with powerful emotions for caregivers, as well as children. Feelings of guilt, shame, anger, remorse, or disbelief can prevent a parent from responding in a helpful way. Part of nurturing parent–child relationships in TST is preparing a parent for the critical job of seeing, understanding, and expressing care as the child shares. Sometimes caregivers believe that their children will "only feel worse" after talking about the event, and so they avoid any discussion of the trauma in an effort to prevent their children from getting upset. For this reason, many caregivers will benefit from psychoeducation regarding the benefits of openly discussing their children's thoughts and feelings surrounding the traumatic event. In addition, some caregivers have difficulty hearing about their children's experiences due to their own (the caregivers') unresolved traumatic reactions or feelings of guilt that they did not protect their children. It may become necessary to refer caregivers to individual therapists during this phase of treatment in order to address their own symptoms.

Nurturing Parent–Child Relations: Using the BTG

Beyond Trauma Guide: Implementing Beyond Trauma Treatment Step 5: Nurturing Parent–Child Relationships

Before encouraging a child to share a trauma story with a parent, it is important to carefully assess the caregiver's own progress with regard to processing the trauma. Because the key element of building the parent–child relationship in the beyond trauma phase of treatment is the joint sharing and open discussion of the trauma, it is essential that the caregiver is able to offer support to the child during the joint sessions.

The BTG lists several indicators that a parent is *not* ready to talk about the trauma with the child:

- Parent blames child.
- Parent becomes overwhelmed talking about trauma.
- Parent disbelieves child.
- Parent fails to see the value of talking about trauma.
- Parent demonstrates unhelpful or inaccurate thoughts about trauma.

Some of these concerns may be easily overcome through a few individual meetings with a parent. Other times a referral for a parent to manage his or her own feelings and thoughts around the trauma is necessary. Finally, sometimes a parent may not be "ready" for the child to share the trauma. In these instances, the clinician may decide to help the child either share the trauma with someone else with whom the child is close or let the child know that the therapist sees, understands, and cares about the child.

Once the child and parent are both ready to discuss the trauma, joint sessions (or parts of session) are held. Save a few minutes at the end to check in individually with both the parent and child to see how the experience felt to each of them.

If using the child's book as a guide, the therapist should plan to review approximately three chapters per session with the caregiver and the child. It is useful for the child to read the chapters to the caregiver and then to have the caregiver offer his or her own thoughts and feelings after the child is done reading. The caregiver should also be able to offer praise to the child. Teach the parent about *growth mindset* praise; for example, saying "You've really worked hard to learn how to manage your feelings around this" communicates that the child has an active role in overcoming the trauma.

The therapist may wish to help prepare the caregiver ahead of time as to what kind of statements may be helpful or unhelpful in this situation. For example, after Kelly read her narrative to her mother, her mother stated: "I'm so sorry that happened to you. It makes me very sad to hear how upset you were, but I'm so proud of you for being able to talk about it." When Kelly's mother met with the therapist alone, she stated, "I completely blame myself for what happened. I should have kicked him out of the house way before that. I guess this just confirms that I'm a horrible mother."

Clearly, this latter statement would not have been helpful for Kelly to hear, and thankfully, Kelly's mother was insightful enough to suppress these statements while in session with Kelly and discuss them later during her individual time with the therapist. If necessary, the therapist may find it useful to conduct a role play with the caregiver (e.g., parent pretends to be the child, and the therapist pretends to be the parent) if he or she appears to be having some difficulty providing support to the child during the joint session. In the case of Tanisha and Ms. Williams, such preparation work will be essential, given Ms. Williams's feelings of guilt about how she raised her daughter. The sharing of the trauma narrative, as described previously, has the potential to be transformative for Ms. Williams as well as for Tanisha.

It is important for the child and the caregiver to discuss the "hardest parts" of the narrative to think about and/or talk about. Without this important component, it is likely that the child and/or caregiver will be at greater risk of future avoidance and possibly the resurgence of trauma symptoms.

Step 6: <u>G</u>oing Forward

A child's journey through treatment can be long, full of joy and pain, at times uncertain, and ultimately life-changing. A therapist is witness and partner in all of this. Treatment must end eventually. The child, parent(s), and therapist, must say goodbye, and doing so can be difficult for everyone involved. Saying goodbye also has critical therapeutic value regarding everything this chapter is about: leading a meaningful life beyond the trauma of the past.

Before talking about how we like to bring therapy to a close in TST, we need to acknowledge that you may not ever get here. Although in a perfect therapy world treatment ends when everyone involved is ready for it to end, that doesn't always happen. An intern finishes her rotation and has to transfer a family midstream, a child's symptoms improve and Mom doesn't see a need to bring him to therapy anymore, or sometimes a family just stops coming and you don't ever learn why. These can be difficult endings, because so much is left unfinished or unsaid. Although maybe we don't see the child again, we can guess that it is hard for him or her.

And it's hard for the therapist, too! Unplanned endings can leave a therapist wondering what he or she did wrong, or that the treatment offered wasn't enough. Maybe the child is still having a lot of trouble, and the therapist feels like a failure. It's hard for everyone not to have closure.

But it's also important not to despair just because you didn't make it all the way through beyond trauma. Truthfully, healing rarely happens in a straight line. Maybe family members have done all they can do for now—but you've given them a gift of opening the door to treatment, and they will come back when they are ready for the next step. Maybe you've expressed that one compliment that the child is going to hold in his or her heart during the hard times ahead. Maybe you'll never know that, but you can rest assured that there's meaning in the therapist–client relationship that is impossible to see on the surface.

Special Vulnerabilities of the Traumatized Child at the End of Treatment

Traumatized children often have long and painful histories of loss and abandonment. The notion of the ending of treatment may provoke memories and emotions related to these experiences. Sometimes these experiences occurred at a very young age, before the child was able to really store declarative memories of them. In these cases, the child may still respond to stimuli related to the end of treatment with emotions around loss and abandonment, but not know why he or she is responding in such ways.

The therapist should expect some exacerbation of symptoms around the time of the end of treatment. In a way, this is a good test of the child's new emotional regulation and cognitive processing skills. The essence of the treatment approach during this increase in symptoms is to help the child use new skills to manage emotion related to the end of treatment and to help the child and family see that they can use these new skills to manage stressors after treatment ends.

In rare cases, the child may experience a significant decompensation during the end of treatment. In this case the therapist should review the events leading to the decompensation with the treatment team in order to determine whether the decision to end treatment was premature. The team should also be vigilant about whether there is any missing information that may have precipitated the decompensation, such as undisclosed environmental stressors or undisclosed episodes of emotional/behavioral dysregulation.

Three Steps to Helping the Child and Family Go Forward (without You)

Saying goodbye is a topic that is bigger than this book. We offer here, however, a few thoughts on how to bring TST to a meaningful end—both for the family and the therapist. These thoughts are organized according to three basic steps:

> Beyond Trauma Guide:
> Implementing Beyond Trauma
> Treatment Step 6: Going Forward

1. Anticipate the goodbye early.
2. Acknowledge the meaning of the work.
3. Acknowledge the meaning of the relationship.

Saying goodbye is a highly personal and individualized process. There are a great many variations to this process depending on the people involved and their shared memory of the therapy. The ultimate aim of saying goodbye is to create a sustaining and meaningful memory of the therapy and the therapeutic relationship.

When considering each of the three steps, it is important to consider the child's memory of the trauma and how it has affected him or her, in relation to the memory the child will have of the therapy and the therapeutic relationship and how it will sustain him or her. In many ways, the process of saying goodbye brings to the forefront exactly why therapy works: *It creates meaningful and sustaining memories that are exactly counter to the memories of trauma.*

I. ANTICIPATE THE GOODBYE EARLY

Trauma Memory. Loss for the traumatized child is usually precipitous. Suddenly the person on whom the child depends is gone. In cases where such a loss could be anticipated, no one took the time to prepare the child or to help him or her with feelings related to loss. Over time the child learns that no one is dependable or trustworthy. The child expects that no one will treat his or her feelings with care.

TST Memory. The TST clinician is vigilant about the child's feelings related to loss and abandonment and is fully accountable for his or her role in caring for these feelings (TST Principle 5: Insist on accountability, particularly your own). This accountability begins with the initial treatment agreement, whereby the child and family should know how long treatment is likely to last and the boundaries and limits of the clinician's role for helping them. Nothing sets up a child who is vulnerable to abandonment more potently than false promises. As treatment progresses, the clinician should have a good understanding of the child's and family's vulnerabilities to loss and abandonment. These should be proactively referenced during the course of treatment to anticipate and manage feelings related to the end of treatment.

2. ACKNOWLEDGE THE MEANING OF THE WORK

Trauma Memory. Many traumatized children learn that their efforts don't matter. This can begin at the time of the trauma when all efforts to escape are ineffective and all words indicating *stop* are not attended. It may continue when the child's work at school or at home does not seem to matter to the adults in his or her life. Healthy development requires that the child have a basic sense of pride in his or her efforts to do good things. If this sense of pride is not acknowledged and mirrored by adults, it shrivels and dies. The repeated experience of unacknowledged pride creates memories and expectations within traumatized children that they are ineffective and that nothing they do matters.

TST Memory. The TST clinician is vigilant about acknowledging the child's efforts and good work. This acknowledgment is expressed throughout the treatment. The period leading to the end of treatment should be used to reflect on and review the child's effort and work. The child should be encouraged to feel proud of what he or she has accomplished. This sense of pride should be acknowledged, supported, and mirrored back to the child by the clinician. All of these interactions between child and clinician create powerful, meaningful, and sustaining memories that go exactly counter to many of the memories related to the trauma, as detailed above.

3. ACKNOWLEDGE THE MEANING OF THE RELATIONSHIP

Trauma Memory. Children who have experienced interpersonal trauma have memories of relationships riddled with conflict, strife, betrayal, violence, loss, and abandonment. There are a great many consequences to these memories. Perhaps at a most basic level these memories indicate to children that they are unloved and unlovable, uncared for and unworthy of care. The consequences of these memories and expectations, among other things, lead to lifelong difficulties with relationships and sense of self.

TST Memory. As described in Chapter 5, the TST clinician takes great care to acknowledge the meaning of the relationship. The work of TST is a highly interpersonal process and is built on the foundation of a safe, trustworthy, and accountable therapeutic relationship. The TST clinician acknowledges the meaning of the therapeutic relationship frequently in the course of treatment. As treatment moves toward a close, the meaning of the relationship is acknowledged and discussed explicitly. This may be the child's first experience of an adult who expresses care, concern, and empathy.

Here is a story of an 8-year-old boy who was ending treatment:

 Gregoire had been attending treatment for almost a year, and his therapist and mother joyfully noted that his depression was gone, and he was succeeding well in school. The therapist decided it was time to begin the process of ending therapy. The first day she brought it up, Gregoire wanted to play "doctor." He was the doctor, and he made the patient (therapist) wait for a long period of time in the waiting room. He finally was able to see the patient and examined her heart. He stated that her heart was very ill, and that she would need to come back. This same theme was replayed for several weeks. Finally, on one of the last days of treatment, Gregoire examined the patient's (therapist's) heart one last time. He then picked up a plastic chainsaw from the shelf and proceeded to "operate" on the patient's heart.

"There," he said, "I've fixed your heart. Now you are all better, and you can't come to see me anymore."

Gregoire's play with his therapist very eloquently shows the sad tradeoff of the therapeutic relationship. The "doctor" (therapist) had made Gregoire share his heart and helped him to feel better, but the cost of getting better is that Gregoire could no longer see his therapist. Gregoire poignantly expresses his readiness for therapy to end during this play sequence, but he is immeasurably helped in this process by a clinician who has consistently acknowledged the meanings of the work and the relationship.

Bridging to the World Beyond

Recall the treatment Principle 10, *Leave a better system*? Until now you have been a part of that system, helping to build a system, being a strong and supportive part of that system. Now, time to leave. But what else is in place? What else needs to be in place? How can you make sure that when your meetings with the child end, the rest of the world picks up?

If you are working with a child in a higher level of care, such as residential treatment, then you likely are used to considering "step down" or referrals to less intensive treatment as a child transitions out of your care. But there are many other parts to the system that, regardless of what level of care a child needs, should be part of the supportive system for a child. Think about the child's life goals and what the child needs to get there. Some of those needs may be related to continued support around the specific work you've begun: continuing additional supports through the child's IEP at school, ongoing psychopharmacological treatment, or ongoing supportive counseling. Some of the needs, however, may relate more to life goals and helping the child bridge to the broader world of hopes and aspirations. If the child wants to be a jazz musician, she needs a trumpet and some lessons. If a child continues to struggle with shyness, he needs structured after-school social activities. You know by now what the child needs; part of *going forward* is working with parents and other advocates to find ways to put these things in place so that next week, when Tuesday at 4:00 P.M. rolls around, instead of heading to your office the child is walking into the music room, trumpet in hand.

What about You (Yes, YOU)?!

Helping a child to reach the point of treatment's conclusion is no small task. In fact, you should feel considerably proud for having impacted a child's development and future in such an important way. It should be a time of celebration between you and the child/family and between you and your team. The end of a treatment should be marked, noted, celebrated, and remembered. It is not only the child who needs to have these types of memories to keep going. Remember, you have left a child with a better system.

Going Forward: Using the BTG

Although termination is a very individualized process, the BTG will help you make sure that the three basic steps are accomplished. We repeat:

1. Anticipate the goodbye early.
2. Acknowledge the meaning of the work.
3. Acknowledge the meaning of the relationship.

Here is a simple truth: Goodbyes are hard. Sometimes avoiding them is easier. Even the best among us may find ways to put off the conversation.

"Gee, she looks so sad today about what happened at school, probably not a good day to bring up termination . . . "

"Gosh, I really want to cover this material, and she seems really engaged—best not to derail things and lose time by bringing up termination . . . "

"Hmm, I really enjoy meeting with him and don't want to disappoint him. . . . He probably needs me. . . . He probably would fall apart if I terminated . . . maybe summer is a better time to transition anyway. . . . Plus, we still have a few weeks—I mean, days—I mean, oh gosh, we're out of time. Bye!"

Don't let it happen. Schedule it in. Start the conversation. Start the conversation yesterday.

Depending on the age of the child, helping him or her to visualize the length of time left in treatment can help. Marking the time on a calendar, including other events of importance (both before *and* after the termination date), can help. Younger children may want to make a paper chain with a loop for each remaining meeting. Perhaps each day when they take the loop off, you can write a message together on it about what you enjoyed doing together. Whatever you do, just make sure that termination doesn't take anyone by surprise.

As you lead up to the goodbye, focus the child and his or her family on the world beyond. Review any needs you identified during the "reevaluating needs" component of the treatment model and make sure systems are in place to address these. Then think beyond those areas to the life goals and what needs to be in place to support the child in reaching them. On the next page is an example of how one clinician made an after-treatment plan for an 8-year-old girl, Ella, who has a love for animals:

People and places that support child in life goals	Already in place?	Barriers to keeping or putting in place?	Plan to overcome barriers
Animal shelter (volunteering)	N	Need to work out transportation to/from	Another child from the school goes there every Tuesday; Mom to look into carpooling
Dr. Frank, ongoing medication	Y	Mom not sure medication still helpful	Tell Dr. Frank to reevaluate and discuss with Mom; suggest ongoing monitoring if meds discontinued
Elderly neighbor who has a dog often has been kind to Ella: suggest Ella walk her dog daily and visit	N	Ella shy about offering	Mom to visit with Ella and neighbor and suggest arrangement
Primary care physician: Ongoing nutrition support around addressing obesity	Y	No	

As you can see, Ella may still need some mental health supports (Dr. Frank), but other parts of her life—fostering her love of animals in a way that also encourages her self-esteem, making sure a health need is addressed—are just as important. Devoting attention to these other needs as you draw to a close communicates this importance.

Closing Thoughts on Beyond Trauma

Working with a traumatized child is a journey. For a brief (in the scheme of life) period of time you have walked a road with a child. Think back to where you started. Maybe she was that child who was drowning in the river. Maybe he was that child whose life was defined by moments of entering survival states. Maybe she was that child who thought she'd been damaged in irreparable ways. And now? It's not to say there won't be challenges again. Every life worth living has challenges to overcome. But you have worked to give these children an invaluable gift. You've given them the skills to meet those challenges, you've worked to knit together a world around them that can support them through those challenges, and you've given them the confidence that they are someone, worthy of love and capable of doing, that can overcome those challenges. Congratulations. Job well done.

CHAPTER

15

Psychopharmacology

How Psychopharmacology Is Integrated within TST

There is no magic pill. TST is about focused services integration. Psychopharmacology can be a very useful service, but it must be integrated into care thoughtfully and clearly. Although we review various medications that can be useful for traumatized children, our main focus is about how the *principles and practice* of psychopharmacology fit within TST.

> There is no magic pill.

This chapter also describes the psychiatric consultant's role within TST and should be read carefully by all members of the TST treatment team. Psychiatric consultants should read the chapter to understand how their practice can and should be altered to fit within TST. Other providers should read this chapter to understand how to best use these services.

The first principle of TST is "Fix a broken system." This means that interventions are devoted to the trauma system, defined as:

- A traumatized child who is not able to regulate survival-in-the-moment states.
- A social environment and/or service system that is not able to sufficiently help the child to regulate these survival-in-the-moment states.

Psychopharmacology, like all TST interventions, works toward this goal of fixing the trauma system and is closely integrated with other TST interventions. The advantage of considering psychopharmacology within the framework of TST is that the wider context of interventions are *built-in*. In other types of psychopharmacology practice, the psychopharmacologist is often practicing in isolation and either has to weave other interventions together around the psychopharmacology interventions or must spend a great deal of time communicating with other providers in order to understand what services are being provided and how these services fit together with the psychopharmacological interventions. Psychopharmacology within TST can be much more efficient than in other types of practice because this type of communication is, again, built-in.

The Role of the Psychiatric Consultant

There are a number of specific functions on a TST team for a psychiatric consultant. These include:

1. Direct psychopharmacological intervention.
2. Consultation on when a child needs a medical or neurological evaluation.
3. Consultation on diagnoses and differential diagnoses.
4. Oversight of the team's management of psychiatric emergencies.
5. Communications with other medical providers and with psychiatric inpatient units.

In practice, a number of different medical professionals have the training to offer direct psychopharmacological services. These include psychiatrists, neurologists, behavioral and developmental pediatricians, and clinical nurse specialists. Whoever fills this role should have the breadth and depth of expertise necessary to perform the specific functions listed above. If it is not possible to have a psychopharmacologist with the knowledge base to provide such expertise, pairing a practitioner with a psychiatric consultant for additional consultation or supervision can work.

Psychopharmacology and the Survival Circuits

As we reviewed in Chapter 2, psychopharmacology and psychotherapy work together on specific brain pathways to diminish the amygdala's "hostile takeover of consciousness by emotion" (LeDoux, 2002, p. 226). These pathways, which we call the *survival circuits*, have evolved to help individuals survive in the face of threat and are central to the psychopathology of traumatic stress. In particular, when an individual with traumatic stress is presented with a stimulus that reminds him or her of the trauma, the response is immediate and extreme. As detailed in Chapter 3 we call these responses *survival-in-the-moment states* and define them as:

> *an individual's experience of the present environment as threatening to his or her survival, with corresponding thoughts, emotions, behaviors, and neurochemical and neurophysiological responses.*

During these emotional states the child is, to some degree, responding to the traumatic event in the present. When signals in the environment suggest threat to the child, the child shifts from his or her usual state to a survival-in-the-moment state. These shifts are ultimately maladaptive as, in reality, survival is not at stake—now. The child's brain is unable to discern that he or she is no longer under immediate life threat. Sometimes these environmental signals of threat are very subtle (e.g., a type of glance, a tone of voice), and the child's extreme response appears "out of the blue" or, at least, grossly disproportionate to the situation. Unless these signals are assessed and the child's vulnerability to them is recognized by understanding his or her trauma history, the child may be treated erroneously for problems other than traumatic stress.

The aforementioned understanding of the nature of traumatic stress is fully embedded within the TST assessment process, detailed in Chapter 9. In particular, all providers and their teams are trained to conduct Moment-by-Moment Assessments of each episode of dysregulation to determine the patterns of survival-in-the-moment. These patterns serve to define the clinical problems that are addressed in TST. These clinical problems are defined in one (and only one) way: by what we call a TST priority problem, which involves:

> *patterns of links between provocative stimuli and survival-in-the-moment states.*

A great deal of attention is dedicated to obtaining high-quality information that would determine a small number of TST priority problems. The psychiatric consultant's assessment should contribute data to arriving at the understanding of these problems. Once the TST priority problems are determined, all clinical intervention is aimed at remediating them, and psychotropic agents will occasionally be part of that integrated approach to intervention. Within TST, interventions are meant to work in the following way:

1. Social-environmental interventions work to diminish threatening stimuli.
2. Psychotherapeutic interventions provide skills to regulate emotional states.
3. Psychopharmacological agents work with skill-based interventions to contribute to emotional regulation, when clinically indicated.

> The psychiatric consultant stands arm in arm with the rest of the treatment team members to work toward diminishing the stimulation and to give the child increasing emotion regulation skills.

The psychiatric consultant, accordingly, stands arm in arm with the rest of the treatment team members to work toward diminishing the stimulation and to give the child increasing emotion regulation skills. In TST, all interventions fit together to "fix a broken system" (Principle 1).

A number of specific psychopharmacological agents are known to diminish the reaction of this emergency response system or survival circuit—in essence, medications that diminish the reactivity of the amygdala so that survival-in-the-moment states are diminished. Medications known to inhibit the amygdala, either directly or indirectly, include benzodiazepines, selective serotonin reuptake inhibitors (SSRIs), tricyclic antidepressants, mood stabilizers, and antipsychotics. This range covers an awful lot of medications. In fact, the amygdala has been implicated in a wide range of psychiatric disorders.

What about PTSD?

We reviewed PTSD in Chapter 3. We believe the disparate groupings of PTSD symptoms are a good start but are only the surface markers (symptoms) of the reactivity of the survival circuit. As described, the main target of psychopharmacological intervention is to reduce survival-in-the-moment states.

This definition of treatment target covers a wider range of symptoms than PTSD but more narrowly constrains the focus of intervention to one process (i.e., *how specific stimuli lead to specific responses*). Again: These processes are mediated by the dysfunction of the survival circuits.

"Think Things and Not Words" (Differential Diagnosis)

It is not entirely clear that words used to describe different clinical problems truly describe different processes in nature or are, in fact, different words for the same thing. Justice Oliver Wendell Holmes's (1899) famous admonition to "think things and not words" is very relevant here. Is it PTSD or ADHD? Is it PTSD or depression? Is it PTSD or rapid-cycling juvenile bipolar disorder? Is it both? Is it all?! Is differential diagnosis different than comorbidity? Is there a more useful way of thinking about all this? Again: "Think things and not words"!

> It is not entirely clear that words used to describe different clinical problems truly describe different processes in nature or are, in fact, different words for the same thing.

⭐ The brain can unravel only in certain ways, depending on the systems that are affected. The brain is comprised of systems (e.g., attentional system, social communication system, motivational system, or fear/threat appraisal system). If traumatic events influence these systems, then the types of problems expressed by the traumatized child would look similar to other conditions that are called by other names but influence the same systems. Our ways of arguing about whether these children *really* have ADHD or a bipolar or psychotic or depressed condition may leave us thinking about words, not things. If the brain processes underlying other conditions are the same or similar to brain processes related to the effects of traumatic events, it would be expected that medications helpful to other conditions would also be helpful for traumatic stress. Consider how traumatic stress likely shares processes important for other conditions.

Traumatic Stress and ADHD

The traumatized child may be processing internal information (e.g., traumatic memories, anxiety) at the expense of processing of external information (e.g., school lessons). Furthermore, there may be impulsive behavior and increased motor activity when the child is confronted with a reminder.

Traumatic Stress and Bipolar Disorder

In situations of high threat or stress the child may shift rapidly among different, intense affective states. These rapidly changing states may be accompanied by impulsive behavior.

Traumatic Stress and Depression

Traumatized children can experience a dramatic shutting down of emotional responses, such that they appear and feel numb and have difficulty feeling pleasure. In addition, there may be difficulty with and alterations in attention, sleep, and appetite.

Traumatic Stress and Psychosis

The appraisal systems of traumatized children can misperceive sensations and reality. The sexually abused child, for example, sometimes hears the voice of the perpetrator. The Vietnam veteran sometimes hears the blades of the helicopters coming. Are these hallucinations, illusions, or perceptual distortions of some sort? If a hallucination is an internally driven perception of external stimulation that does not correspond to the external reality of that perception, then it is hard to argue that these two examples are not hallucinations. Similarly, the abused child who scans the environment for signs that others might hurt her and misinterprets benign signals as threatening may be called delusional. If a delusion is a fixed, false idea, it is hard to argue that this problem is not a delusion.

Our overall approach to psychopharmacology is to make a clinical decision about whether a given target symptom is related to survival-in-the-moment or not. If this target symptom is consistent with survival-in-the-moment, then we start with a medication to diminish amygdala responding.

Adaptation

Before we get specific about different medications, we must consider the crucial concept of *adaptation*. Our discussion of the survival circuits depends on the understanding that the life threat is in the past and the traumatized child is not fully able to discern that he or she is in a safer context. In the safety-focused phase of treatment, however, there are true threats of harm. Therefore the traumatized child's symptoms may be important adaptations to help with *real* threats to survival. Consider the following examples:

> The traumatized child's symptoms may be important adaptations to help with *real* threats to survival.

- The child who does not want to go to sleep because he or she is afraid of being abused in the night hours.
- The child who lives in a neighborhood where there is a gang war and who spends a lot of time scanning the environment for sources of threat.
- The child who avoids going to school because someone has threatened to kill her.
- The adolescent who is aggressive with his mother's boyfriend to protect her from getting beaten up.

These examples may seem obvious but in busy psychopharmacological practice, particularly when it is disconnected from other therapeutic interventions, the adaptive nature of a child's response can easily be missed and treated like a symptom. From our point of view this is a significant clinical and ethical problem. Treatment efforts in this situation must be aimed at *decreasing the real threat in the environment*.

What to Choose?

 The TST psychiatric consultant must choose a medication or medications to help. Which ones?

Here is a secret that is simply true:

Psychopharmacology involves witchcraft.

To clarify (because we do not want to get thrown out of the psychopharmacologist's coven!):

Psychopharmacology does not only involve witchcraft. It is constrained by a scientific literature and scientific teaching.

Nevertheless, psychopharmacology does involve the mixing of "potions" that are often chosen without a great deal of existing scientific evidence. What are our potions?

We do not believe our approach is the only approach. As we noted, many different medications can work to diminish amygdala reactivity. Based on our understanding of safety, side effects, and effectiveness, we recommend a first-line approach to help stabilize the survival circuits and then other approaches for special cases.

First-Line Approach

Our practice is to start with an SSRI such as fluoxetine, sertraline, or paroxetine. The SSRIs have been shown to help with anxiety, arousal, intrusions, impulsivity, depression, and numbing. In some cases of severe anxiety/arousal that is significantly affecting functioning and psychotherapy engagement, a benzodiazepine (e.g., clonazepam) can be helpful in the shorter term, as the initial response to an SSRI often requires a number of weeks. Once this level of anxiety and arousal is diminishing, the benzodiazepine can be tapered and the SSRI continued.

Second Line

Other medications tried next include:

- Benzodiazepines alone
- Tricyclic antidepressants, such as imipramine or desipramine
- Atypical antipsychotic medications, such as risperidone or olanzapine. (These medications should be reserved for severe anxiety that does not

respond to other medications, particularly when the anxiety/arousal leads to disorganized thinking.)

Special Cases

The following variations to our usual first-line practice occur when a given specific problem is prominent:

Insomnia

- Make sure the child is not consuming products that are known to interfere with sleep (e.g., cigarettes, coffee, soda, illicit drugs).
- Sedating antidepressants such as trazodone and doxepine
- Benzodiazepines (not short-acting)
- Alpha$_2$-adrenergic inhibitors such as clonidine or guanfacine

Impulsivity

We discuss behavioral dysregulation in Chapter 3. Survival states sometimes become expressed in aggressive, risky, or self-destructive behaviors. As these types of behaviors are often expressions of the survival circuits (behaviors used to survive, even though survival is not currently at stake), the usual first-line interventions should be tried first. There are two cautions with this recommendation, however:

- There is currently controversy about whether the SSRIs lead to increased impulsive and risky behavior. In our experience, these medications are more likely to help than hurt. However, as increases in risky behavior are possible with SSRIs, the child should be monitored closely, particularly in the weeks after this medication is initiated.
- Benzodiazepines can lead to disinhibition. It is our experience that, similar to the SSRIs, a judicious use of benzodiazepines is more likely to help than hurt. Nevertheless, as disinhibition is well documented following benzodiazepine treatment, these medications should be chosen as third- or fourth-line treatments for impulsivity and monitored carefully.

Medications that can also be helpful for impulsivity and should be considered following a trial with an SSRI (and sometimes in addition to it, depending on the clinical circumstances) are:

- Mood stabilizers such as lithium, valproic acid, and carbamazepine
- Alpha$_2$-adrenergic inhibitors such as clonidine or guanfacine
- Atypical antipsychotics such as risperidone or olanzapine

Beware that impulsive behavior can sometimes be a first sign of alcohol or drug abuse. It is important, therefore, to keep a high index of suspicion about drug abuse in an impulsive adolescent or preadolescent.

Depression and Numbing

Traumatized children can experience a dramatic shutting down of emotional responses that can significantly interfere with their functioning and responsiveness to skill-building interventions. Sometimes traumatized children get depressed.

Medications that can help with this shutting down of emotional responses, including major depression, are:

- SSRIs
- Tricyclic antidepressants
- Other antidepressants such as bupropion and venlafaxine

Disorganized/Idiosyncratic Thinking/Perceptual Distortions

- Start with the first-line approach, as problems related to the appraisal of reality may be driven by survival-laden affect.
- As a second line, or occasionally as adjunct to this first line, use an atypical antipsychotic agent such as risperidone or olanzapine.
- Occasionally, if high levels of anxiety, disorganized and distorted perceptions and thinking, *and* risky behavior are present, we recommend starting with an atypical antipsychotic agent.

Inattention

- Start with the first-line approach, as problems related to inattention may be related to survival-laden affect.
- As an adjunct to this first line, use a stimulant.
- If the above approach does not work, consider bupropion or a tricyclic antidepressant.

The Practice of Psychopharmacology in TST

 The psychiatric consultant should be familiar with the 10 treatment principles described in Chapter 6 for TST interventions. These principles guide all TST interventions, including psychopharmacology, and should be considered an overarching guide to psychopharmacology practice. We list these 10 principles again here. Details about their use are given in Chapter 6.

1. Fix a broken system.
2. Put safety first.
3. Create clear, focused plans that are based on facts.
4. Don't "go" before you are "ready."
5. Put scarce resources where they'll work.
6. Insist on accountability, particularly your own.
7. Align with reality.
8. Take care of yourself and your team.
9. Build from strength.
10. Leave a better system.

Psychopharmacology fits closely with other treatment modalities in TST. In the first phase of TST—safety-focused treatment—the main use of psychopharmacology is to avert crisis. During these phases, when the social environment is unstable and the child is at high risk to engage in dangerous behavior, psychopharmacology can be used to help to prevent psychiatric emergencies, psychiatric hospitalizations, and out-of-home placements. Once the child transitions to the more advanced phases of treatment, the main goal of psychopharmacology is to enhance emotion regulation skill building.

An important part of TST is helping the child acquire the skills to (1) manage emotion, (2) process the trauma(s), and (3) create meaning out of the experience(s). This idea assumes that it is the building of these skills that will be most instrumental in helping the child function better over the course of his or her life. Accordingly, the primary goal of psychopharmacology within TST, when crisis is not such a salient part of the clinical picture, is to support these skill-building interventions. This goal is accomplished within TST via the very high degree of communication that is "built-in" for all providers, the full integration of psychopharmacology within the larger TST treatment plan, and the phase-dependent clinical decisions that are integral to psychopharmacology within TST.

> The primary goal of psychopharmacology within TST, when crisis is not such a salient part of the clinical picture, is to support skill-building interventions.

Psychopharmacology is, in this way, explicitly an adjunct or supportive intervention within TST. When the survival circuit is triggered, the child is often too aroused or disorganized to engage in skill-building interventions. Psychopharmacology is used to diminish the reactivity of the survival circuit so that skill-building interventions can occur.

Whenever psychopharmacology is used within TST, it is done with a high degree of integration with other interventions and providers. Psychopharmacology decisions are influenced by information from the team, are supported by the team, and effect decisions by other team members. TST psychopharmacology is best characterized as a *team intervention*.

Day-to-Day Psychopharmacology Practice

Referral to psychopharmacology intervention works like referral to any of the interventions. It fits within the overall TST Treatment Plan. The psychiatric consultant is a part of the TST team meetings and can offer valued input to team discussion. All decisions about an intervention modality are team decisions and are based on the defined treatment plan. In this way, the psychiatric consultant is never confused about the "referral question."

The Initial Meeting

When the psychiatric consultant has his or her first meeting with the family, he or she should have a copy of the draft TST Treatment Plan (Chapter 10) that fully outlines the results of the assessment and preliminary plans for treatment. At this meeting the psychiatric consultant should:

- **Confirm the child's and family's understanding of why they were referred and how psychopharmacology can fit within the rest of the family's care.** It is extremely important at this initial meeting that the child and family understand that the psychiatric consultant is part of the team, works very closely with the rest of the team, and that medications, if they are recommended, are only a part of the overall treatment plan.

- **Understand family concerns about psychopharmacological interventions as early as possible and dispel any misunderstandings.** Families frequently have negative reactions to the possible use of medications and addressing these concerns up front can go a long way to building the alliance.

- **Reassess the initial evaluation of emotional and behavioral dysregulation and psychiatric diagnoses.** The psychiatric consultant has particular expertise in these assessments and should confirm this initial assessment.

- **Assess the usual domains covered in a psychopharmacological evaluation** (e.g., prior treatment history, medical history).

Ongoing psychopharmacological practice within TST shares many elements with usual psychopharmacological practice. Follow-up meetings are usually scheduled every 1–2 weeks until an effective dose of medication is found. Once the child is more stable, follow-up appointments are usually every month. The psychiatric consultant's confidence in the treatment is enhanced by the much higher degree of communication and treatment integration than is usual. Treatment will also vary somewhat depending on the phase of TST. The following section describes how psychopharmacology is used in the different phases of treatment.

Psychopharmacology across the Phases of Treatment

TST occurs in three treatment phases that are defined by different levels of dysregulation in the child and different levels of instability in the child's social environment. These phases are reviewed in detail in Chapter 10, on treatment planning. The three phases are safety-focused (Chapter 12), regulation-focused (Chapter 13), and beyond trauma (Chapter 14). Details about interventions provided in each phase are offered in each respective chapter.

SAFETY-FOCUSED PHASE

During the safety-focused phase of TST, the child may be exhibiting dangerous behaviors during survival states; in addition, the social environment may be harmful or insufficiently helpful and protective. Accordingly, the team is often in communication with child welfare, the police, psychiatric inpatient units, and hospital emergency rooms. The referral for psychopharmacology, in this context, is relatively urgent in order to help regulate the child so that a psychiatric hospitalization is prevented. The social environment may, however, be so unstable that the psychiatric consultant is not confident that parents or guardians can consent or will use the medications appropriately. In this case it may be difficult to avoid psychiatric hospitalization. Social services agencies are frequently involved and can at times either facilitate this consent or give consent themselves. During the safety-focused phase, the psychiatric consultant's expertise in risk assessment can be invaluable to the team. The psychiatric consultant should give his or her opinion on the level of risk and, if the team is still unsure, assess risk directly with the child and family. The psychiatric consultant can also be helpful to the team via communication with medical/psychiatric staff on inpatient units and in emergency rooms.

 The psychiatric consultant must assess whether the presentation of a given symptom is really an "adaptation," as described above. In the safety-focused phase of treatment there are true threats of harm to the child. Such behaviors as aggression, vigilance, lack of sleep, and avoidance may be ways of *staying alive*, and, if so, should never be medicated.

The psychiatric consultant must assess whether the presentation of a given symptom is really an "adaptation."

During this phase, the TST team is conducting interventions in the child's home to diminish the triggering stimuli that repeatedly lead to dysregulation. Receiving the information about what is occurring in the home is critical for psychopharmacology practice. The psychiatric consultant may have initiated a medication, for example, to help with the child's ability to regulate emotion. The child may initially not improve or even get worse. In this context, the psychiatric consultant is often inclined to increase the dose or to change medications. However, if the TST team provides information that there are increased stressors in the home, this information will be very important for the psychiatric consultant to consider so that symptoms are not erroneously "chased" with medication. Home-based care during this phase can also be very helpful for the team to assess the family's compliance with medications and any barriers to compliance. This information can similarly be integrated into the psychopharmacological treatment plan.

REGULATION-FOCUSED PHASE

In the regulation-focused phase, the environment is more stable than in the safety-focused phase. The child is usually not engaging in dangerous behavior during survival-in-the-moment states. The regulation-focused phase is largely defined by office-based emotion regulation skill training. In this phase, TST most resembles "typical" psychopharmacological practice. The therapist is trying to help the child regulate emotion. The child may need medication to make the best use of this psychotherapeutic intervention. As described, when a child is having significant difficulty regulating emotional states, he or she may need medication to diminish arousal so that emotional skill training is optimized.

The main psychopharmacological decisions in the regulation-focused phase concern whether medications are necessary to help the child acquire emotion regulation skills. Accordingly, the psychopharmacologist's communication with the child's therapist will be very important for him or her to learn about the child's progress in emotion regulation skill training and if emotional states are interfering with this treatment. Children with mood disorders, ADHD, or disorganized thinking will need medication if these problems interfere with psychotherapy.

BEYOND TRAUMA PHASE

During the beyond trauma phase of treatment, the environment is more stable and the child has sufficient emotion regulation skills to cognitively process the trauma through a trauma narrative. Many children will not need medication during trauma processing, and some children will be tapered off their medications. As in the regulation-focused phase, psychopharmacological decisions will concern how to help the child best take advantage of the psychotherapeutic interventions that define the phase. Learning occurs with an optimum level of arousal. Cognitive processing of the trauma is meant to increase arousal so that there can be some extinction of the trauma response. It is important, therefore, to avoid medicating this increased arousal *unless* it interferes with the child's functioning. Close consultation with the child's therapist will be important so that the psychiatric consultant will know:

1. When to expect this increase of arousal related to trauma processing.
2. Whether this increase in arousal is interfering with functioning.

The therapist can be very helpful in providing information about whether the level of arousal was expected and should be treated with medication.

One component of the beyond trauma phase is to *reevaluate needs.* Occasionally, other existing psychiatric problems will emerge once the "storm" of traumatic stress abates. During the initial phases of treatment, while the focus is on stabilizing environments and preventing survival-in-the-moment states, it is hard to see other problems. Once these more immediate problems are handled, it may become clear that the child has an ongoing mood, attentional, learning, or developmental disorder. The psychiatric consultant may therefore be called to reevaluate the child during the beyond trauma phase of treatment.

Closing Thoughts on Psychopharmacology

Psychopharmacology can be a very useful intervention for children with traumatic stress. Used within TST, psychopharmacology must be highly integrated with other TST interventions. Broadly speaking, the goal is to avert crisis in the earlier phases of treatment and to enhance skill-building interventions in the later phase of treatment. The psychiatric consultant is a full member of the team and should always conduct care consistent with the principles of TST.

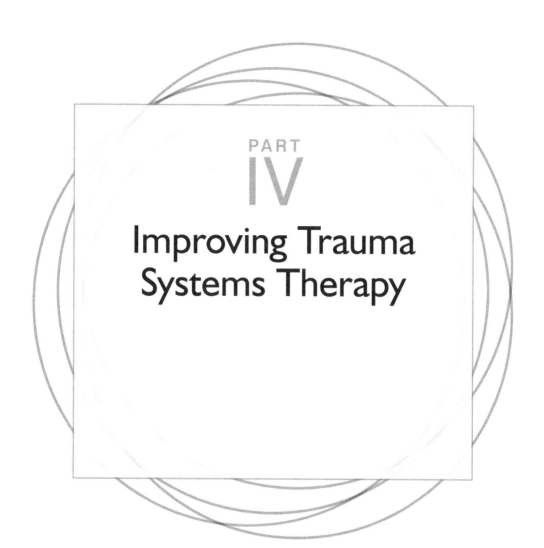

Improving Trauma Systems Therapy

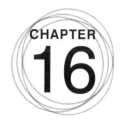

CHAPTER

16

Democratizing Trauma Systems Therapy

How a Community of TST Users Has Created a Process of Continually Improving TST and Adapting It to an Ever-Widening Variety of Settings

---

LEARNING OBJECTIVES

- To describe the process of lead-user innovation for TST

- To describe how lead-user innovation has resulted in many improvements in the TST model

- To detail the adaptations to TST so it can be used for a variety of settings and populations

---

ICONS USED IN THIS CHAPTER

Essential Point	Academic Point	Danger

When the iPod was released on October 23, 2001, it completely changed the game for how people listened to music. Announcing its release, Steve Jobs described it as a Mac-compatible music player with a 5-GB hard drive that could put "1,000 songs in your pocket." Wow! Hard to release a product with more impact than that. Here's a question for you iPod users: Why does the iPod you now listen to hardly resemble the amazing product that Apple released on October 23, 2001? For some of you, your iPod is embedded in an iPhone with

363

integrated cellular, web, and Wi-Fi connection; *and* corresponding photography and video capacity at astonishing resolution; *and* integrated with a zillion possible apps that enhance your music listening experience and your experience with everything else connected to that thing you hold in your hand. And it's in color! For some of you, your iPod is embedded in your iPad. For others, you have an iPod alone that, itself, hardly resembles that ancient contraption from October 23, 2001. Still others are using the MP3 players, cell phones, etc., from other companies built from ideas related to that first iPod.

OK. What's the point of this diversion into modern digital technology? Technologies are never-ending stories based on the experience of people who use them. Apple, like all good businesses, works very hard to understand the experience of the people who use their products (e.g., the iPod) to continually improve them over time. The experience and ideas of users are continually integrated into the improvement of useful technologies. And what is a psychotherapy model? A technology! It is a specified and standardized set of processes that must be followed in a close-enough way to achieve a set of results related to human needs. A psychotherapy model specifies and standardizes the processes that must be followed—by mental health providers—in order to achieve a set of results related to mental health problems. And that brings us to TST.

We see TST as a technology that specifies and standardizes the processes to provide integrated trauma-informed care across the child services system. We have embraced a form of innovation within TST to enable our technology to continually improve and not get fixed in time (like the iPod in October 2001). Innovation can be fostered by a business organization (like Apple) that licenses and protects their intellectual property for their product (like the iPod), but continually works to understand the needs of users and integrate that understanding into improvements to the product. Innovation can also be fostered within a community of users who work to improve a product by sharing their ideas and innovations, where no intellectual property is claimed. That is the route we chose for TST. It has led to a great many benefits for the quality of the model itself, for the needs of the great many practitioners who use it, and of course for the children and families who benefit from its use. Broadly, the improvements in TST have occurred in two categories:

> Innovation can be fostered within a community of users who work to improve a product by sharing their ideas and innovations, where no intellectual property is claimed.

1. Improvements to the model itself, implemented in all settings that use TST.

2. Improvements in the capacity to adapt TST to a wide variety of settings, with specifications for how the model can be adapted to each of these settings.

This chapter describes how we work with a community of TST users to continually improve TST in these two ways. We begin with a description of how innovation works within TST and then describe how this has led to a model with a much higher level of utility than when we started. We then detail the way that this innovation process has led to adaptations in a wide variety of settings and provide detail on those adaptations. Since many readers have interests in settings other than where TST was originally developed (outpatient mental health in an urban clinic), we provide a lot of detail about these adaptations so that you can see how TST can be implemented in a setting you care about.

Democratizing TST

As we described in Chapter 1, the initial development of TST began around 1999. The first version of the manual was completed in late 2001 and after a great deal of refinement based on its use, it was published in book form by Guilford Press (Saxe, Ellis, & Kaplow, 2006). The version you now hold in your hands was released 9 years later. The ideas contained within TST come from an ever-widening community of users who have, over the years, agreed to work together to implement new ideas to help traumatized children and families, evaluate their utility, and then decide whether they should be integrated into the model. We began with a handful of clinicians who worked together on a clinical team in one clinical setting. We spent about 3 or 4 years tinkering with the model by slowly integrating and evaluating different approaches until we felt we had a model that we thought had a chance of achieving meaningful results. As we wrote this new book, it became clear to us how different it was from our previous book because we were able to integrate so many new ideas and innovations that had been developed and found to be useful by so many people over these years.

> The ideas contained within TST come from an ever widening community of users who have, over the years, agreed to work together to implement new ideas to help traumatized children and families, evaluate their utility, and then decide whether they should be integrated into the model.

TST has become a never-ending story based on a community of users. If we had stopped when we completed our manual in 2001, or when our first outcome study was published in 2005, or when our first book was released in 2006, it would have been like stopping the development of the iPod after its release in October 23, 2001 (we are not claiming that TST is as groundbreaking as the iPod—that's up to you to determine). We believe this tendency to stop improving a model has become a big problem in the field of psychotherapy development. A psychotherapy model gets developed and evaluated, a clinical trial gets published about the model's efficacy, and the development of the model then largely stops—because any change to the model becomes a fidelity violation and means that an implementation of the model, with this change, cannot be supported by the *evidence base* of the clinical trial. We are creating a field of 2001 iPods!

Early in the development of TST, one of us (G. N. S.) stumbled upon a book called *Democratizing Innovation*, by Eric von Hippel, the director of the Innovation programs at the Massachusetts Institute of Technology's Sloan School of Management. Von Hippel was interested in the phenomenon of *lead-user innovation*: innovative ideas that come from the lead users who are expert practitioners in their fields and need improved technologies to improve their performance. These lead-user practitioners form communities to innovate the technology they want to improve and commit to freely reveal their innovations and results to help each other improve the technology. In *Democratizing Innovation*, von Hippel describes the experience of communities of computer programmers collaborating as they tinkered with open-source software to improve the utility of the software, communities of mountain bike aficionados collaborating to improve the performance of their bicycles, and communities of surgeons collaborating to improve the performance of their surgical equipment.

What about a psychotherapy model? What about TST? Could we *democratize* psychotherapy development? Could we democratize TST? We sought von Hippel's technical support as we planned to do this. The first step, he said, was not to claim intellectual property for TST but to freely reveal it so that many people would have license to innovate. This was a controversial move. Wouldn't this give people the license to steal and claim the ideas we had worked so hard to develop, as their own? Wouldn't this take control away from the developers so that anything could be called *TST*? Wouldn't this throw fidelity out the window and make evaluation impossible? Maybe. But wouldn't following the usual recipe of psychotherapy model development, evaluation, and publication simply be launching a 2001 iPod locked, more or less, forever in time? Certainly. And we did not want to do this. So what did we do?

- We did not (and do not) claim intellectual property. TST is public property.

- We embraced the notion of minimal fidelity, a fidelity standard that we believe should be practiced wherever TST is implemented. This standard becomes the platform on top of which all innovation occurs.

- We created processes for individuals and agencies that use TST to communicate with each other and share their innovations. This network of users became what we now call the *TST Innovation Community*: agencies around the nation that implement TST and work with us, and with each other, to continually improve TST.

- We provided technical assistance to TST lead users to standardize and evaluate innovations.

- We created processes for users to try out new innovations to decide whether we should integrate them within the overall TST model. These processes included using our Innovation Community to get invaluable feedback on what should be included in the revised treatment model that forms the core of this book.

Following these processes to democratize TST has led to a great many benefits for the model, as described above. Many innovations that emerged within our community of users have now been integrated within the overall model. People have also adapted the model to settings and clinical problems that we never imagined when we set out to design TST. Why is this process so powerful? There are many answers for this question, but the one we find most compelling is this: Democratizing innovation respects the informational limitations of the "expert" and leverages the full range of expertise required to improve a technology. Stated more practically: The authors of this book, collectively, have many areas of expertise: the impact of trauma on children, psychotherapy and pharmacotherapy for traumatized children, intervention development and evaluation, organizational management, child advocacy. The authors of this book also, collectively, have a great many limitations to their expertise that are critical for their treatment model to work in reality. These limitations include:

> Democratizing innovation respects the informational limitations of the "expert" and leverages the full range of expertise required to improve a technology.

- How foster care and mental health systems operate in the state of Kansas, such that a model meant to be adapted to these systems for their integration can take root in the settings it will be implemented.
- How residential care in rural Texas works, such that a model can take root in the residential programs where it will be implemented.
- How a middle school in inner-city Boston operates, such that a model can take root in that school.

None of us (G. N. S., B. H. E., A. D. B.) knows very much about any of these areas. But we know the people who *do* know a lot about such matters. They are the people who bring us in to help them. *Democratizing TST* then brings *them* in as full partners in the innovation process. Next we detail how democratizing TST has led to considerable improvements in our model and flexibility in its adaptation.

Improving TST Based on Integrating Innovations from a Community of Users

If you compare the book you hold in your hand to the book we published on TST in 2006, you will notice a great many differences. As described, these differences did not just bubble up in our minds as we were writing this book. They emerged within a community of TST users and developers, implementing TST in a wide variety of settings over the last 9 years. Some ideas were abandoned because they did not generate sufficient utility. Other ideas gelled within the community and spread across it, based on utility. Over time it became clear which ideas/innovations should be kept within TST, and which should be abandoned. Importantly, this process also told us which ideas from our model published in 2006 should also be abandoned. At the time of its publication, TST was being used with a much smaller community of users over a shorter period of time. To save you the trouble of comparing the two books, we list some of the innovations added to, and subtracted from, the TST model based on the collective experience of a community of users.

- We simplified the number of phases from five (surviving, stabilizing, enduring, understanding, and transcending) to three (safety-focused, regulation-focused, and beyond trauma).
- We created much more specificity about what should be done in each phase, with guides for providers and families that anchor the work in each phase.
- We eliminated treatment modules and integrated the activities that would define each module (e.g., advocacy, psychopharmacology) within the respective chapters that cover the three phases of treatment.
- We "tightened" the process of implementing TST by operationalizing this process in steps, from assessment to treatment planning to treatment engagement to treatment implementation. We created worksheets and guides for each step.
- We revised our (minimal) fidelity approach based on how providers are performing each of these steps.
- We are much clearer on the type of information that needs to be gathered in the assessment process and how this information needs to be used to guide decisions in the treatment planning process.
- We created a more powerful process for treatment engagement by starting the assessment with knowledge about the child's and family's most important goals and priorities and requiring the treatment team to consider how addressing any problem in treatment needs to address the child and family priorities.
- We created a treatment plan document designed to communicate what is most important, in a language that is much more tangible to the family.
- We integrated an organizational planning process to help agencies that implement TST support their programs.
- We expanded ways to address secondary traumatization in several sections.
- We created more specific approaches for addressing the needs of parents.

- We made our Foundations chapters (Part I) more practical and better connected to the rest of the book.
- We integrated processes for innovating in TST (in the chapter you are now reading).

Adapting TST to a Wide Variety of Settings Based on Integrating Innovations from a Community of Users

We initially created TST as a trauma-informed outpatient mental health treatment model to address the needs of children and families in urban settings. We had not really considered how these ideas might be applied to other settings. Fortunately, many people emerged from those other settings to help us. TST has now been adapted in a great many settings based on adaptations created within our community of users. Newer members of our community have picked up some of these adaptations. In this section we detail some of the more developed adaptations that are more commonly implemented. We have two purposes for this description. First: to illustrate how the process of democratizing TST has led to such adaptations in such a variety of settings. Second: to give you details about these adaptations so that you can consider whether any of these might fit for the setting in which you work, or for the children for whom you care.

Space precludes a full description of each adaptation. We simply describe why TST was thought to be a good fit for the intended setting or population and provide an outline of the ways it was adapted to make it a better fit.

TST in Residential Care Settings

Fit for Setting

As described, TST was initially developed as an outpatient mental health treatment for children with traumatic stress who lived in the inner city of Boston. How could such a treatment benefit children, and providers, in residential care settings? Providers and administrators in residential settings first became interested in TST because of the way it could address the social environment of the residential milieu. The residential milieu is a place where behavioral disruptions were increasingly recognized as trauma-related. How could the milieu form an essential part of the social environment such that it could be addressed in TST? Moreover, residential programs were interested in a trauma-informed model of care that could create a common language for all providers, including the non-professional direct-care staff.

TST has now been used in several residential care programs across four states. It was first adapted for residential care at Children's Village in Westchester County, New York, approximately 8 years ago. Shortly thereafter, it was used in residential programs operated by KVC Health Systems in Kansas. KVC now has the most extensive experience using TST for residential care, in several large residential programs.

Adaptations to Improve Fit

• The therapeutic milieu is considered an essential part of the social environment. Since children live in this setting, it provides an important opportunity to understand survival-in-the-moment states and thereby derive high-quality information about the nature of each child's clinical problems.

• Direct-care and clinical staff members are trained together about all aspects of TST. They are particularly encouraged to collaborate to conduct Moment-by-Moment Assessments. Since direct-care staff members spend far more time with children than clinical staff, their observations are pivotal for identifying TST priority problems.

• The TST team is expected to include both direct-care and clinical staff. The logistics of enabling direct-care staff to join the TST team is a very important part of organizational planning in residential programs.

• The TST organizational plan is expected to address all services that interact with the child (e.g., psychology, social work, psychiatry, school, direct care, recreation). Representation from these "divisions" of the residential program are expected to be part of the leadership team for the development of an integrated approach to using TST in the residential care setting.

• Residential care settings are usually affiliated with schools located on the site of the residential program. The school should be integrated into the functioning of the TST team so that information from the school can inform the TST treatment plan, and decisions made for the plan can be implemented in the school.

• The social environment of the child's home should be integrated into the work of the team. Children sometimes arrive at the residential program because there are knowable problems at home that must be addressed in treatment. If the TST priority problem relates to the home environment, this information must be explicitly integrated into the TST Treatment Plan. Every effort must be made to integrate families into the treatment, if the work in the residential program is to generalize beyond the walls of this program.

• If the social environment of the home is thought to be insufficiently helpful and protective or even harmful, this information must be fully integrated into the treatment plan. If discharge is planned to an insufficiently helpful and protective or a harmful social environment, without providing due diligence to address the problems, then the residential program becomes an insufficiently helpful and protective or a harmful environment, itself. Children know what is going on at home. If the residential program is ignoring these realities, the program becomes full partners in perpetuating the problem. Children cannot be expected to trust providers in the residential program if they do not perceive any effort to address the obvious (to them) realities of distress and threat at home.

> Children know what is going on at home. If the residential program is ignoring these realities, the program becomes full partners in perpetuating the problem.

- Legal advocacy is vigorously applied when a child welfare service plan is in place that does not account for the aforementioned realities.

- A great deal of caution is used before physical restraint is applied. Although it may, in certain moments, be necessary to preserve safety, it also provides evidence to all children who observe the restraint that the residential setting is a place where large people overpower small people, and even tie them up. Cat hair is now all over the milieu. Witnesses will have their own survival-in-the-moment states related to that reality. Accordingly, restraint can paradoxically create more danger than it prevents.

TST in Foster Care Settings

Fit for Setting

Children in foster care have been removed from their families because the child welfare authorities have determined sufficient maltreatment has occurred to mandate such removal and placement. Clearly, traumatic stress reactions are common among children in foster care. The ongoing maltreatment, the removal from family, and the placement with a family that is usually unknown to the child set the stage for ongoing traumatic stress and survival-in-the-moment reactions. Agencies seeking TST for their foster care programs have typically wanted a trauma-informed program that can prevent foster care placement disruptions and facilitate reunification with families, when appropriate. TST was first applied in foster care by the Jewish Board of Family and Child Services (JBFCS) and partnering agencies in New York City. It has now been used in many foster care programs in several states. KVC Health Systems in Kansas has used TST for foster care and spread it to several states in the Midwest. The child welfare system in the District of Columbia has embraced TST across its foster care system and forms the largest dissemination and adaptation of TST for foster care. Our New York University team is working with the foster care authorities in New York City and State for large disseminations of TST for children in the Bronx and Ulster County, New York.

Adaptations to Improve Fit

- Teams are created that include mental health clinical providers and foster care caseworkers. Caseworkers and foster care staff provide the home-based component of TST intervention during the safety-focused phase.

- Knowledge about the child's TST priority problems is pivotal for enabling a child to maintain foster care placement and to transition back to his or her family, if such transition is appropriate. Information for Moment-by-Moment Assessments comes from the child, the caseworker, foster parent, birth parent, or any other observer so that high-quality information can be generated for why a child switches to survival-in-the-moment in specific, definable moments.

> Knowledge about the child's TST priority problems is pivotal for enabling a child to maintain foster care placement and to transition back to his or her family, if such transition is appropriate.

- Foster care placement disruptions are often driven by the child's repetitive shifts to survival in the moment. Foster families can be frustrated (and frightened) by the seemingly "out-of-the-blue" nature of the child's survival-in-the-moment states. Accordingly, information about these states, as defined by the child's TST priority problems, can be very helpful for foster families. A foster parent with a child who, for example, shifts to survival-in-the-moment with specific struggles around food and mealtimes, could be helped to understand how these struggles could be minimized and survival-in-the-moment reactions prevented.

- Placement decisions are informed by an understanding of a child's vulnerabilities, defined by their propensity to shift into survival-in-the-moment states (TST priority problems). Some foster parents may have a greater capacity to address a child's priority problems than others. In preparation for the placement of any foster child, the foster family should understand the child's specific vulnerabilities, as described, and receive support from the foster care agency to manage them.

- Reunification decisions are informed by an understanding of the child's vulnerabilities, defined by his or her propensity to shift into survival-in-the-moment states (TST priority problems). Before reunification is considered, the role of specific family members' contributions to the child's priority problem is examined with a view to whether there has been sufficient improvement. If a child's survival-in-the-moment states typically involve suicidal or violent behavior, and these states have repeatedly been driven by specific interactions with family members, it is not surprising that they would recur upon reunification, if there has been no effective intervention with those family members.

- The environment to which the child might return, like all environments considered within TST, is assessed for whether it is sufficiently helpful and protective or harmful. Reunification decisions are based on this determination. The

TST principle to *align with reality* is the operative principle when reunification is considered. If there is uncertainty about this reality, the four questions for "when the reality is hard to see," described in Chapter 9 (pp. 177–178), are applied.

• If a legally binding plan (from a judge or child welfare authority) clearly deviates from reality, as defined above, such that there are clear and present dangers, the team has an obligation to strenuously advocate. This is an occasion when a child is clearly drowning in the river, as described in Chapter 1. Never be a bystander in this context.

TST with Refugee Populations

Fit for Population

Refugee populations have a high prevalence of traumatic stress related to war and political violence in their nation of origin and the experience of displacement and resettlement. The cultural stressors related to resettlement create particular difficulties within the family context. Agencies seeking TST for refugee populations typically are looking for trauma-informed programs that address the social environment, integrate the cultural context, and connect to the wider services system. The program leading the adaptation and dissemination of TST for refugees is the Center for Refugee Trauma and Resilience at Boston Children's Hospital who have worked with refugee agencies in Massachusetts, Maine, Minnesota, and Kentucky.

Adaptations to Improve Fit

• The refugee child's home environment is shaped not only by the particular family members but also by the larger culture of origin that influences the family's goals, behavior, and way of relating to the world beyond. Mental health clinicians typically cannot understand and appreciate the cultural nuances of cultures they are not a part of; cultural brokers (members from the refugee community who have a deep understanding of their own culture) and representatives from the resettlement culture and mental health service systems culture are integral members of the team. Cultural brokers can help with language translation and, perhaps more importantly, the translation of cultural meanings that relate to such areas as trauma, emotional disorders, and mental health intervention. The identified cultural broker is an integral member of the TST team.

> The refugee child's home environment is shaped not only by the particular family members but also by the larger culture of origin that influences the family's goals, behavior, and way of relating to the world beyond.

• Broader community outreach provides a foundation from which the specific TST program can operate. Refugee communities can have great wariness toward those in authority, and mental health providers are seen as authority figures. The engagement of the community and a process of co-learning about both the community's primary concerns and the way trauma may be related help community members to develop strategies to overcome stigma and support their children to receive the services they need.

- The inclusion of cultural and religious practices that children and family members find comforting and helpful can be very important. These practices are identified, assessed, and integrated as strengths during the treatment planning and engagement process and included in the emotion regulation interventions. Partnering with religious leaders can be very helpful here.

- The stigma of mental health problems and intervention can present large barriers to engagement with some refugee communities. Accordingly, it can be helpful to base TST refugee programs in less stigmatized settings, such as within primary care or schools. The Boston Children's Hospital team has achieved great success in refugee programs for Somali families there by basing these programs in schools. In addition, nonstigmatized skill-building groups offered in a school setting allow families and children to begin engagement with TST ideas and team members in a way that doesn't single out their children as in need of services, but instead acknowledges the ubiquity of cultural stressors and supports all refugee children's adjustment to a new cultural setting.

TST with Substance-Abusing Adolescents

Fit for Population

The rates of trauma and victimization histories are high among adolescents presenting for substance abuse treatment. Childhood trauma exposure increases risk for later substance use, criminal activity, anxiety disorders, etc. Youth that exhibit comorbid substance abuse and posttraumatic stress problems show greater clinical severity, increased functional impairment, and greater involvement with multiple service systems when compared to youth with only one of these conditions. Agencies seeking TST for substance-abusing populations typically are looking for a treatment approach that can address how substance abuse may be related to traumatic stress reactions, and integrate the way the youth's social environment may contribute to these problems, across multiple services systems. The organization that has most directly adapted TST for treating substance-abusing adolescents is the Urban Youth Trauma Center of the University of Illinois at Chicago's Institute for Juvenile Research, under the guidance of Liza Suarez. The center's staff has engaged agencies in several states, including Illinois, California, and Texas, in adapting TST for adolescents with substance abuse.

Adaptations to Improve Fit

- Substance-abusing behavior is considered dangerous related to a shift to survival-in-the-moment states. Moment-by-moment analyses gather information about the patterns of these shifting states so that the contributors to the adolescent's substance abuse can best be understood.

- Interventions for substance abuse integrate the aforementioned understandings about survival-in-the-moment states. During safety-focused treatment, the environmental contributors to the behavior are prioritized. During regulation-focused treatment, the child's emotional regulation skills are prioritized.

- As the youth's substance abuse deepens, stimuli related to trauma (cat hair) diminish in importance due to the process of chemical dependency. Environmental cues related to substance abuse grow in importance. Trauma-related stimuli may continue to be contributors throughout, but their relative importance diminishes. Accordingly, TST may be more effective earlier in the chemical dependency process than later.

  > TST may be more effective earlier in the chemical dependency process than later.

- The treatment engagement process—ready–set–go—is supplemented by motivational interviewing because there is a strong literature supporting its effectiveness with this population.

- Psychoeducation about substance abuse and its interaction with symptoms of traumatic stress are integrated in ready–set–go.

- ⚠ The psychiatric consultant has a particularly important role in TST for substance abuse due to the well-known medical consequences of intoxication and dependency. The use of psychotropic medications is considered with particular caution in this population.

- Behavioral management techniques are particularly emphasized with substance-abusing adolescents. These techniques are used in the HELPers Guide introduced in safety-focused treatment and continued throughout the three phases of TST. Such behavior management strategies include increased substance abuse monitoring and appropriate limit setting, particularly around drug use and high-risk behaviors.

- Substance abuse treatment strategies such as teaching parent–teen communication skills, recognizing and planning for substance abuse cues or trigger situations, recognizing and planning for substance abuse cravings, and teaching cognitive and interpersonal problem-solving techniques and other relapse prevention techniques.

TST in Schools

Fit for Setting

Children with traumatic stress can have particular problems in schools, and schools located in communities with high rates of trauma can have difficulties with a host of problems related to traumatic stress. Children who experience survival-in-the-moment reactions in schools can be highly disruptive in the classroom; they may then get suspended and become quite avoidant of school, leading to high rates of absenteeism. Children with traumatic stress may also be quietly dissociative in class and not learn at their intellectual capacity. Children with survival-in-the-moment responses frequently are seen as unmotivated disciplinary problems or as angry and overreactive. This common but inaccurate view of survival-in-the-moment states by teachers often leads them to respond in ways that are not helpful and may even exacerbate the problem. A child who has been suspended for disruptive behavior, or who has a poor school attendance history, or who does not pay attention in class is a child at high risk of school failure and/or dropping out. Schools seeking TST typically are looking for an integrated treatment approach that can help them work with the children they are most worried about (for reasons described above). They seek a program that can fully engage the social environment of the school and the teachers and other staff members to better understand the school-related problems of traumatized children. The program with the most experience adapting TST for school-based settings is Connecting With Care (CWC), a school-based counseling program run by Lisa Baron and Bob Kilkenny of the Alliance for Inclusion and Prevention in Boston. CWC partners with local provider agencies to place mental health professionals into Boston public schools on a full-time basis.

Adaptations to Improve Fit

> The TST program in the school setting integrates within the school culture and performs a vital consultative role helping teachers and other school staff members recognize how traumatic stress can influence learning at school.

- The TST program in the school setting integrates within the school culture and performs a vital consultative role helping teachers and other school staff members recognize how traumatic stress can influence learning at school. Trainings should be offered by the TST team and direct classroom observations conducted to provide consultation to classroom teachers with particular difficulty.

- The organization plan within the school should be drafted with a leadership team that integrates representation from all specialties that will be involved in the care of children. These included special education, physical education, security, and regular classroom teachers, as well as representation from the principal's office.

- There should be an evaluation plan that directly addresses the concern of the school (particularly the principal's office). Such a plan should track key educational indicators such as absenteeism, classroom disruptions, critical incidents, and school performance.

- The assessment of children should include classroom observation, particularly if there is concern about behavior in the classroom. This should be integrated into the Moment-by-Moment Assessments.

- Most schools do not have dedicated teams of mental health providers (although many have a small capacity for learning and behavioral consultation). Schools will typically refer to local mental health agencies for the children who cause concern, but that work then is usually quite disconnected from the school and does not address the social environment. Successful programs have formed partnerships with local mental health agencies so that clinicians from those agencies join the TST team and conduct the mental health intervention integrated with the work of the team and with fidelity to TST. Such providers, obviously, add to the mental health capacity of the TST program in the school. The interagency agreement between the school and the mental health clinic allows the mental health clinicians to bill for services, as usual, under the mental health clinic's license. This can be financially advantageous to the mental health clinic because providing intervention at the child's school reduces "no-show" rates.

- The child's family is integrated into the care. A child who needs safety-focused treatment suggests the presence of a very clear problem, even danger, at home that needs to be addressed. Mental health agencies that provide home-based care for children and families with acute need should be integrated into the program and engaged through interagency agreements, as described above. These children may also be highly disruptive in class. In such a situation, things will not improve without the integrated home-based services that are part of safety-focused treatment. These are the children who are usually thought to be too difficult to handle in school. They typically get psychiatrically hospitalized and then lose their school placement.

- The TST team evaluates the child's IEP for its suitability related to the impact of traumatic stress on the child's learning at school. TST providers attend the IEP meetings of the children with whom they work. There should be an agreement, reflected in the program's organizational plan, about how the situation will be handled if the TST team and the school's educational program disagree about IEPs.

Closing Thoughts on Democratizing TST

We started with a sort-of iPod from October 2001 and gave it to an ever-broadening community of users and innovators. Then we watched the magic happen as these people began to adapt it to their needs. In the process, the treatment model called *TST* became considerably, and increasingly, more useful than it was when it was first launched, and is now available to any organization that wants to use it. And it has been specifically adapted to a wide range of settings and for a diverse range of populations of traumatized children. We cannot wait to see where this will go next. As the years continue, we are less and less able to predict where people will take TST. And that is very exciting for us. We hope you will join this ride.

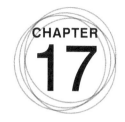

Extending Trauma Systems Therapy Beyond Trauma

Using the TST Approach to Help Children with Non-Trauma-Related Problems

---

LEARNING OBJECTIVES

- To describe how the TST approach can be used for mental health and developmental disorders other than traumatic stress.
- To describe how the different components of TST may be applied in this pursuit.

ICONS USED IN THIS CHAPTER

Essential Point

Case Discussion

As you have read, TST is about addressing two core problems that define the trauma system. These core problems—as you are no doubt very familiar with—involve the traumatized child's transition from his or her usual state to an extreme emotional state related to survival in specific, definable moments, and to the incapacity of those around the child to help prevent this transition and to support regulation when it occurs. Let's take trauma out of the mix for now. Let's not talk about survival-in-the-moment, for just a moment (but we might bring it back). Let's consider four children who do not have traumatic stress:

- A 17-year-old girl with depression feels like she wants to die because of a breakup with a boyfriend.
- An 8-year-old boy with autism assaults a classmate who "gets too close."
- A 12-year-old boy with ADHD assaults his mother when she puts pressure on him to clean his room as he is trying to do his homework.
- A 16-year-old girl comes home intoxicated from a party, upset because another girl said her dress was "trashy."

These children, of course, have very different problems from each other, but what do they have in common? Each of the problems, at some level, involves the child's transition from a usual state to an extreme emotional state, in a definable moment. The problems of these children also involve the incapacity of those around them to help prevent the transition and to support their regulation when it occurs. Sound familiar? A great many mental health and developmental problems involve the dysregulation of emotional states in certain contexts. Can the TST approach be adapted to help children and families with these disorders?

> A great many mental health and developmental problems involve the dysregulation of emotional states in certain contexts.

State Dysregulation as a Core Problem for Many Disorders

In order to explore this possibility, it is necessary to consider the role of state dysregulation for specific disorders. If the symptoms/emotions/behaviors that define a given disorder do not fluctuate together in certain moments, or if fluctuations occur but are not context dependent, then the TST approach may not be useful. On the other hand, our experience tells us that the problems that need to be addressed in many of disorders involve fluctuations in emotional states in specific, definable moments and contexts. Some may say that the episodes of state dysregulation for other disorders are not context dependent and do not involve environmental triggers. Maybe. But has a Moment-by-Moment Assessment determined this, or is it just assumed? As we discussed repeatedly through this book, it is very common for the episodes of dysregulation in children with traumatic stress to be considered context independent, or "out of the blue." But when Moment-by-Moment Assessments are conducted for each episode, patterns begin to emerge that could not be seen until the facts were gathered.

Obviously, much further research needs to be dedicated to clarifying the state transitions involved in a variety of psychiatric and developmental disorders. Even for disorders that do not appear to have significant emotional state transitions and/or the transitions are largely context independent, there may be key periods where context is important, and this should not be missed. The value of recognizing context-related dysregulation is that it points to important strategies of intervention. Although we don't mean to overgeneralize, in our experience, and with some burgeoning support from the empirical literature, the following generalities may be true:

1. Individuals with depression are vulnerable to signals of loss and have patterns of emotional state transition characterized by sadness, hopelessness, anhedonia, and self-destruction when faced with signals of loss.

> The value of recognizing context-related dysregulation is that it points to important strategies of intervention.

2. Individuals with autism spectrum disorders are vulnerable to signals suggesting social demands and/or discrimination and can become agitated and aggressive when faced with these social signals.

3. Individuals with attention-deficit disorders are vulnerable to signals that either pull their attention from activities that draw their interest, or place unrealistic demands on their ability to attend to multiple tasks at once.

4. Individuals with a host of disorders involving repetitive behaviors/habits (e.g., eating disorders, substance abuse disorders, impulse control disorders) are vulnerable to signals that make them feel bad about themselves. The problematic, repetitive behaviors occur within emotional states precipitated by these types of signals. The specific signals are determined by the individual's history.

If you are an attentive reader, you will notice that these four examples violate a rule described in Chapter 10 on treatment planning: We understand that problems need to be addressed based on facts and not on theory. The four examples may be true, but they are based on our theories about how a problematic behavior or emotion *might have occurred*. This will only get us so far.

 If you are assessing a patient with the following problems, how will you get to the relevant facts to ascertain what you need to do?

1. A 17-year-old girl has episodes of sadness, hopelessness, anhedonia, and self-destruction four times in the last year.
2. An 8-year-old boy has assaulted classmates four times in the last year.
3. A 12-year-old boy assaulted his mother four times in the last year.
4. A 16-year-old girl came home intoxicated four times in the last year.

Notice we did not describe anything about the child's history or diagnosis. What would you do to assess each child? What facts would you gather about each child's four problematic episodes? Would you jump to a theory or would you gather the facts about the context, emotions, and behaviors in each episode so that you might see a pattern? And what if you did see a pattern? Wouldn't it be helpful to know what to do?

Here's what we think: The three A's, the four R's, and the two E's detailed in Chapter 3 are more relevant than we might guess for a wide variety of problems and disorders. And therefore . . . the Moment-by-Moment Assessment process and identification of priority problems will be very helpful and relevant for a much wider variety of disorders than traumatic stress.

How the TST Approach Can Apply to Disorders Other Than Traumatic Stress

If you are still with us about this possibility, then consider the following ideas for how the TST approach could be applied to a much broader array of problems and disorders than traumatic stress. We're very interested in your thoughts about these ideas:

- Within TST, the trauma system is central to the problem of child traumatic stress. The trauma system construct is a version of the old *goodness-of-fit* notion of child development and psychopathology that Chess and Thomas (1991) proposed many years ago. Our version places the developmental problem of emotional state dysregulation as central, but goodness of fit has been applied, and can be applied, to a great many psychiatric and developmental disorders.

- A core part of the trauma system is the shift to survival-in-the-moment states mediated by brain circuits sculpted over the course of evolution to promote survival (i.e., survival circuit). This concept was detailed in Chapter 2. Although we are not sure about the following, we think it's worth considering: When a person transitions to *any* extreme emotional state, might the survival circuit be at the bottom of it?

When a person transitions to *any* extreme emotional state, might the survival circuit be at the bottom of it?

- Survival-in-the-moment reactions are based on what we described as the *building blocks* of emotional dysregulation. These building blocks are defined by the two E's, three A's, and four R's that we detailed in Chapter 3. These building blocks are relevant to any disorder that includes shifting states as a part of its psychopathology.

- The way states shift, or not, is greatly influenced by the social context embedded in a social environment. As we described in Chapters 4 and 5, the social environment is comprised of human relationships and human communication that can involve signals of threat and/or safety. These ideas are critical for both family relationships and the therapeutic relationship and have implications well beyond traumatic stress.

- In order to prepare to implement treatment, TST includes a formalized assessment, treatment planning, and treatment engagement process. In essence, this process results in the delivery of a set of integrated interventions, defined within three sequential treatment phases. The phases are determined within a two-dimensional grid that graphs the stability of the social environment and the child's degree of dysregulation. This grid is fully applicable to any disorder involving state dysregulation and, accordingly, the resulting three intervention phases are also highly applicable. This application is clear by examining the primary goals of each respective phase: If the child has a disorder *and* his or her social environment is unsafe, the first priority is to make the environment safe (safety-focused treatment). If the child's disorder involves repetitively shifting emotional states, the next priority is to help him or her regulate these states (regulation-focused treatment). Once the storm of environmental threat and distress abates and the child is more regulated, the next question is "What else is needed?" (beyond *something* treatment). Similarly, the focus of all intervention within TST is toward a very small number of priority problems, each defined in the same way: as *patterns of links between provocative stimuli and dysregulated emotional responses.* These problems are determined by a Moment-by-Moment Assessment of each episode and a formalized process to facilitate the identification of the patterns between episodes. As described, this process is also widely applicable.

- Shifting from the applicability of our clinical approach to our organizational approach: The organizational processes we detailed in Chapter 8 all concern how an agency organizes its services to provide integrated, effective care within a program that is sustainable and meets organizational goals. There's little here exclusive to trauma. Similarly, our dissemination approach described in Chapter 16, on democratizing TST, is based on a lead-user innovation approach used in many fields. Although we were the first to apply this powerful approach to mental health interventions, we believe that it can be useful for any mental health intervention.

Closing Thoughts on Extending TST Beyond Trauma

We built a treatment model to help traumatized children and families and have been glad and gratified to see it benefit so many children and families. Over the years, on many occasions, we have received comments such as "What you are describing is just good care—it doesn't need to apply only to traumatic stress." Our usual response has been to say something like, "We designed this treatment specifically for the problem of child traumatic stress, and we don't want to make any claims beyond what we feel confident to make." In the process of writing this book, we revisited this issue several times, and as we considered it, we began to think about how the ideas of TST could be extended beyond trauma. And as we thought about it, we were surprised by how easy it was to see how this could work (as sketched above). We still don't want to make claims that go beyond our level of confidence. We have never tried to extend TST beyond trauma before. But, as we have described repeatedly, TST is a never-ending story based on the experience of a community of users. We write this chapter in the hope that, as this story continues, it will extend beyond trauma—and those from our community will help us to do this.

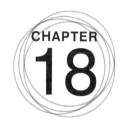

CHAPTER
18

Conclusions

Doing Whatever It Takes to Leave a Better System

LEARNING OBJECTIVES

- To conclude the book
- To share what happened to the kids

ICONS USED IN THIS CHAPTER

Essential Point

Case Discussion

Congratulations! You've made it through with us. We assume if you are still here, that you remain undaunted by the central TST commitment: to do *whatever it takes* to help a traumatized child. If you are still here, your eyes have not yet been averted from the reality of the drowning child who is in the river before us. You join with us as we wade into the water together to do everything possible to help the child reach safety.

As we described in the first chapter, we aimed to write a book to honor the courage of those who would join us in this difficult work. Accordingly, we made a pledge to you at the beginning, which—we hope—you feel we have kept. We repeat that pledge here:

- We write about the reality you face as you help with the reality your children face.

- We simplify this reality only to help us focus on what is most important. We do everything we can to *not* oversimplify.

- We offer practical solutions that will work in the world in which most people practice. In order for these solutions to work, clinical care must be embedded in the right type of organizational and systems-level approach and to be financially viable within these organizations and systems. We address these areas methodically, practically, and clearly.

- We aim to provide an approach that offers value to whoever uses it, based on what is most important to them. The user may be a provider, an administrator, a parent, or a child. The only evidence base that matters to us is the accumulating evidence that our approach yields this type of value.

- We write to honor the courage of those who choose to do whatever it takes and to help with *your* very real needs as you take this difficult road.

Although the work requires a lot of courage, and it is hard to get it right, we know that small things can sometimes make an enormous difference in peoples' lives. TST is about finding those small things that, if changed, can change lives and provide the tools for providers and their agencies to go "all in" to achieve those small but (truly) pivotal changes. We conclude by telling you what happened to some of the children described in this book. Of course, the vignettes that describe each child are composites to protect the privacy of individual children and families but, at this point, we've been involved in the care of a great number of children by a great number of providers and agencies. We are confident that the postscripts we describe are fully achievable because we have seen these achievements happen a great many times.

Remember Gerald?

 Gerald is now 15. His dad is still in jail, but Gerald is able to talk about him without becoming upset. In fact, in his beyond trauma sessions Gerald talked a lot about how he wanted to be a father someday and that he was going to "do it differently." Gerald's mother continues to struggle with depression, but is actively seeking treatment and has begun to talk about how her own traumatic reactions from the domestic violence she experienced sometimes make it hard to parent Gerald and his brother in the way that she wants to. Gerald's older brother was arrested and placed in Division of Youth Services (DYS) custody, and at Mom's request, the TST team has been working with DYS providers to create a discharge plan that will help him get trauma treatment services. And Gerald?

Gerald just completed a successful year in a specialized classroom. He passed all of his courses, and did particularly well in his student leadership class. His concentration has improved, and within the structured classroom, he is able to focus relatively well. He no longer expresses any suicidal ideation and, in fact, does not seem to experience any symptoms of depression. He has not had a survival-in-the-moment state in a very long time. Although he still sometimes "thinks about what happened" in the past, he says that it no longer "takes over."

Remember Denise?

 Denise's TST treatment team felt strongly that unless some of the key environmental stressors were removed, Denise was going to continue to have trouble. In fact, they felt that arguably one of the most important things they could do to help Denise would be to get her a bedroom door. Through services advocacy and writing letters clearly noting the link between the substandard housing and Denise's health problem, the recalcitrant landlord finally had a door installed. Meanwhile, the treatment team provided Denise's mom with a lot of education around trauma, domestic violence, and how the ongoing abusive relationship with her boyfriend might be contributing to problems for everyone in the family. Things got worse before they got better, and Denise's mom threatened to "pick my boyfriend over my daughter if I have to," but after working closely with the home-based TST team during safety-focused treatment, she admitted that she was staying with her boyfriend because she was afraid to leave. With the help of the team she broke off the relationship and filed a restraining order. And Denise? At home, Denise began to feel markedly safer and her nightmares stopped. Some men she sees around town still remind her of her abuser, but she says "I just make myself look at the guy again and say to myself: 'He can't hurt me, that's not the same guy.'" She is now finishing her GED and applying to a local community college.

Remember Robert?

 When Robert first started TST the primary environmental threat—his stepfather—was already out of the picture. But Robert was having such trouble regulating survival-in-the-moment states that almost anything seemed to trigger him, including typical playground teasing. Robert, his mom, and his TST team spent a lot of time and energy working on emotion regulation skills. Psychopharmacology helped to dampen Robert's arousal, but he still became dysregulated at school. He moved to a more structured classroom, where he was able to successfully complete the year without any suspensions. He is starting now in a mainstream classroom, and his mother reports that, with the exception of gym class (which gets a little rambunctious), he hasn't had any problems. She told the TST team that she had already been to the school to talk about having him moved to a smaller gym class. In her words, "I know he can do it! He just needs the right setting until *he* knows he can do it."

And then there's Tanisha . . .

Tanisha completed beyond trauma treatment just as she was completing fifth grade and planning her transition to middle school. Her verbal rages and physical aggression had long since ceased, her self-loathing and sense of isolation and sadness had diminished, and she was able to tolerate and put in perspective comments from peers that had, at an earlier time, been her undoing. Ms. Williams was advocating within the child welfare system to become permanent legal guardian for Tanisha, and the pieces were lining up for this to happen. "I can do it right this time," Ms. Williams had confided in Tanisha's therapist at one point. "I can do for Tanisha what I never knew how to do for her mother." At her fifth-grade graduation, Tanisha's teachers asked if she would give the class address. Tanisha worked diligently on a piece of writing. On the day of graduation she stood on stage, hands slightly trembling as she held her speech and looked out over the audience and into Ms. Williams's face. "Today we end the world we know," she started, "and tomorrow we are sixth graders. But who we are, and the people who love us, will still be with us."

No child's journey through TST looks quite the same. These are the stories of a few of the children who have benefited from TST. We hope that you'll have your own stories—because more than any outcome study, more than any balanced budget sheet, more than any symptom reduction score, it's these stories that tell us that what we're doing is working. It's these kids, and their successes, that keep us going. It's these kids who helped us develop TST. We've seen their courage, and this has given us the courage to help them. As the TST community grows—and the numbers of children who are helped expands—and the courage expended by these children, families, providers, and agencies becomes increasingly evident—the change becomes formidable and irreversible. And then we, *all* of us, will have left a better system.

Appendices

TST Organizational Planning Form

Leadership Team	Name of Organization/Program	Ways to Reach

1. Organizational Priority Problems: *What are the problems my organization **most** needs to address?*

Priority Problem #1:	
Priority Problem #2:	
Priority Problem #3:	

2. Organizational Solutions: *How does the proposed TST program help to address those problems?*

Solution #1:	
Solution #2:	
Solution #3:	

(continued)

3. Partners: *Which programs will participate in our TST program? What are their specific roles (e.g., home-based, psychopharmacology, legal advocacy, psychotherapy)?*

Program (and Agency Name)	Specific Role in TST Program	Program Leader

4. Population: *Who is our TST program designed to help? What are the criteria for admission?*

5. Operations: *How will our planned TST program operate?*

Scale *How many teams will provide TST and how many children will each team treat?*	**Startup:** **Full Scale:**
Intake *How will children and families be referred to our program? How will intakes be conducted?*	
Case Assignment and Monitoring *How will decisions be made about case assignments and the designation of a primary provider for each case? How will cases be supervised?*	

(continued)

TST Team *Who will be the members of the team? Who will lead the team?*	
Program Oversight *How will the leadership team be managed? What level of authority does the team have for decision making within our organization?*	

6. Training and Staff Development: *How will we build our expertise?*

Staff Engagement *How will we introduce this organizational change process to our staff? What are the likely impediments to change?*	
TST Training Plan *What is the plan to train staff to provide TST?*	
Professional Development *What other training/development needs does our staff have related to TST?*	
Secondary Traumatic Stress *What is our plan to address the emotional impact of the work for our staff?*	

7. Finances: *What resources are needed to provide TST and sustain our program?*

Training and Consultation *What is the cost for training and consultation? Where will these resources come from?*	

(continued)

Services *What is the additional cost to our organization for services provided within TST? Where will these resources come from?*	
Additional Costs *What additional costs do we anticipate for providing TST? Where will these resources come from?*	

8. Evaluation: *How will we evaluate our program?*

Success Indicators *What indicators of success will we track for each of our identified organizational priority problems?*	
Method *How will we track each of the identified success indicators?*	
Quality Improvement *How will we use the information related to changes in identified success indicators to improve the quality of our program?*	

Additional Notes:

_____

_____

_____

_____

_____

_____

_____

_____

_____

_____

TST Assessment Form

Child's name: _____ **Date of birth:** _____ **Record number:** ____

Instructions:

The purpose of this *TST Assessment Form* is to record the information that you have gathered about the child and family that you will use to establish an effective *TST Treatment Plan*. As detailed in Chapters 9 and 10 of the TST book, the treatment plan is based on your answers to five questions. The information you will use to answer each of these five questions should be recorded in the corresponding section of this form. Detailed instructions for completing this form are found in Chapter 9 of the TST book. The five sections—and their corresponding question/assessment information—are shown below:

Section 1: What problem(s) will be the focus of the child's treatment?

The information we need:

a. Moment-by-Moment Assessments of episodes of problematic emotion and/or behavior

b. Exposure to traumatic events

c. Other problems that may need to be addressed in treatment, including:
   i. Comorbid psychiatric or developmental disorders
   ii. Enduring trauma-related cognitions
   iii. Current social problems that impact the child's health and development

Section 2: Why are these problems important and to whom are they important?

The information we need:

a. The functional impact of the identified problems

b. The level of concern about these problems from the child, the family, and others

c. The identification of what is most important/concerning to the child, the family, and others

Section 3: What interventions will be used to address the child's problems?

The information we need:

a. The child's vulnerability to shift to survival state

b. The environment's capacity to help and protect the child

Section 4: What strengths will be used to address the child's problems?

The information we need:

a. The child's strengths

b. The family's strengths

c. The strengths in the social environment

Section 5: What will interfere with addressing the child's problems?

The information we need:

a. The child and family's understanding of trauma and mental health intervention

b. The practical barriers to engage in treatment

(continued)

SECTION 1: WHAT PROBLEM(S) WILL BE THE FOCUS
OF THE CHILD'S TREATMENT?

a. Moment-by-Moment Assessment of episodes of problematic emotion and/or behavior

Please identify the episodes of problematic emotion and/or behavior that will be evaluated during the assessment period. Record the date that each episode was evaluated with a Moment-by-Moment Assessment (blank Moment-by-Moment Assessment Sheets are found in Appendix 3). At least three episodes should be recorded during the assessment process.

Date of Episode	Brief description of episode	Date Moment-by-Moment Assessment Sheet complete

b. Exposure to traumatic events

Please check any event(s) the child may have experienced and record any relevant detail such as age and duration of event.

☐ Sexual abuse	☐ Injury or illness	☐ Lack basic needs
☐ Physical abuse	☐ Disaster	☐ Homelessness
☐ Violence exposure	☐ Terrorism	☐ Removal from family
☐ Witness violence	☐ War and/or displacement	☐ Caregiver mental illness/ substance abuse
	☐ Loss of close family member or friend	☐ Other (specify)

(continued)

c. Other problems that may need to be addressed in treatment

Please provide information on any other problem(s) that may need to be addressed in treatment

    i. Comorbid psychiatric and/or developmental problems (e.g., depression, ADHD, autism, mental retardation). Please make sure the symptoms of the problem you identify are clearly distinct from survival-in-the-moment episodes:

    ii. Enduring trauma-related cognitions (e.g., feelings of worthlessness, hopelessness, shame, guilt):

    iii. Current social problems (e.g., caregiver mental illness/substance abuse, parental divorce/separations):

SECTION 2: WHY ARE THESE PROBLEMS IMPORTANT AND TO WHOM ARE THEY IMPORTANT?

a. The functional impact of the identified problems

What has been the impact of the episodes of problematic emotional/behavioral expression on the child's functioning? What has been the impact of any other identified problem on the child's functioning? Has the problem interfered with learning and school, or with family and peer relations? How big a problem is this?

(continued)

b. The level of concern about the identified problems from the child, the family, and others

Who is concerned about the identified problems? Is the child concerned? Are family members concerned? Who else is concerned? Does the level of concern correspond to the level of functional impact for the child?

c. The identification of what is most important/concerning to the child, the family, and others

What is most important/concerning to the child and to family members? What are their sources of pain? What are their goals and priorities?

 i. Child's main goals, concerns, sources of pain:

 ii. Caregiver's/family member's main goals, concerns, sources of pain:

(continued)

SECTION 3: WHAT INTERVENTIONS WILL BE USED
TO ADDRESS THESE PROBLEMS?

Within TST, interventions are selected based on the phase of treatment that is appropriate for the child's problems. The information used to determine the TST treatment phase (detailed in Chapter 10 on treatment planning), concerns the degree to which the child is vulnerable to switch to survival states and the degree to which the social environment is able to help and protect the child. Please use the table below to record your ratings, *using the definitions provided.*

Child's Vulnerability to Switch into Survival States	Definitions
☐ **No Survival States**	1. Does not display episodes of survival-in-the-moment (shifts in *awareness, affect, and action*) when a threat is perceived in the present environment. 2. If the child displays shifts in awareness, affect, and action when a threat is perceived, neither the episode itself, nor the anticipation of such episodes, results in any problem with the child's functioning.
☐ **Survival States**	1. Displays episodes of survival-in-the-moment (shifts in *awareness, affect, and action*) when threat is perceived in the present environment. 2. The shift in *action* during such episodes does not include potentially dangerous behaviors (e.g., self-destructive, aggressive, substance-abusing, risky eating, or sexual behaviors). 3. Such episodes, or their anticipation, result in problems with the child's functioning.
☐ **Dangerous Survival States**	1. Displays episodes of survival-in-the-moment (shifts in *awareness, affect, and action*) when threat is perceived in the present environment. 2. The shift in *action* during such episodes includes potentially dangerous behaviors (e.g., self-destructive, aggressive, substance-abusing, risky eating, or sexual behaviors). 3. Such episodes, or their anticipation, result in problems with the child's functioning.
Justification of Rating:	

(continued)

The Social Environment's Capacity to Help and Protect the Child	Definitions
☐ **Helpful and Protective**	1. The child's immediate caregivers are sufficiently available and apply sufficient competence to *help* with the child's vulnerability to switching into survival states and to *protect* the child from perceived and actual threats; *or* 2. Other adults in the child's life are sufficiently available and apply sufficient competence to *help* and *protect* the child; *or* 3. The appropriate child service system is sufficiently available and applies sufficient competence to *help* and *protect* the child.
☐ **Insufficiently Helpful and Protective**	1. The child's immediate caregivers are insufficiently available and/or apply insufficient competence to *help* with the child's vulnerability to switching into survival states or to *protect* the child from perceived threats; *and* 2. Other adults in the child's life are insufficiently available and/or apply insufficient competence to *help* or *protect* the child; *and* 3. The appropriate child service system is insufficiently available and/or applies insufficient competence to *help* or *protect* the child.
☐ **Harmful**	1. The child's immediate caregivers are insufficiently available and/or apply insufficient competence to *protect* the child from actual threats; *and* 2. Other adults in the child's life are insufficiently available and/or apply insufficient competence to *protect* the child from actual threats; *and* 3. The appropriate child service system is insufficiently available and/or applies insufficient competence to *protect* the child from actual threats.
Justification of Rating:	

(continued)

SECTION 4: WHAT STRENGTHS CAN BE USED
TO ADDRESS THE CHILD'S PROBLEMS?

Please record information about the strengths that might be available to help address the child's problems. Record enough detail about the strength so that decisions can be made for its possible use in the child's treatment.

a. **Child strengths** (e.g., intellectual, social–emotional skills, talents):

b. **Caregiver strengths** (e.g., parenting skills, motivation and dedication, organizational strengths, flexibility, emotional attunement, openness to help):

c. **Social–environmental strengths** (e.g., strengths and resources among friends, neighbors and neighborhood, culture, religion, school, or service system):

SECTION 5: WHAT CAN INTERFERE WITH ADDRESSING
THE CHILD'S PROBLEMS?

Please record information about the factors that can interfere with the child and family's engagement in treatment.

a. **The child and family's understanding about trauma and mental health intervention**

b. **The practical barriers in the way of treatment engagement, such as transportation, scheduling, child care, language, parent limitations, treatment concerns**

Additional Notes:

TST Moment-by-Moment Assessment Sheet

Child's name: _____ **Record number:** ___ **Date:** _____

Step 1: Finding what flipped the switch

Instructions: What flipped the switch, such that the *episode of problematic emotion and/or behavior,* happened? <u>First</u>: Consider the period of time just before the *episode*. What was the child doing (**A**ction)? What was he or she feeling (**A**ffect)? Where/what was the child's focus of attention/thought (**A**wareness)? <u>Second</u>: Consider the period of time during the *episode*: What of the **three A's** changed during the *episode*? <u>Third</u>: Consider the present environment throughout this process. Record any feature of the *present environment* that you think may have been related to the *episode* (whatever it is). Any of these features may turn out to be responsible for flipping the switch. If assessment revealed sufficient detail about the **four R's**, you can skip the "During the Episode" box and complete Step 2.

Before the Episode *(possible "usual state"/regulating)*	**During the Episode** *(possible "survival-in-the-moment")*
Action:	Action:
Affect:	Affect:
Awareness:	Awareness:

Features of the Present Environment *(possible "switch"/"cat hair")*

(continued)

Step 2: Understanding what happened when the switch was flipped*

Instructions: Once you have understood what flipped the switch, you may be able to see important details about the *episode* in question. If the *episode* represents *survival-in-the-moment,* the child will have switched from a *usual state* (**R**egulating) to the three *Survival-in-the-Moment* states of **R**evving, **R**eexperiencing, and **R**econstituting. Each of these states will be characterized by changes in the **three A's**. Consider the *episode* assessed in Step 1: Record information in your *present environment* during these respective states. See Chapter 9, Section 1, of the TST book for details about conducting this assessment.

Revving	Reexperiencing	Reconstituting
Action:	Action:	Action:
Affect:	Affect:	Affect:
Awareness:	Awareness:	Awareness:
Present Environment:	Present Environment:	Present Environment:

Was the episode you have assessed an expression of survival-in-the-moment?	How confident are you in your answer to this question?
☐ Yes ☐ No	☐ Very confident ☐ Confident enough ☐ Not so confident ☐ Not at all confident

*In the first few Moment-by-Moment Assessments of a child's episodes, you may not be able to see these details. The more you get to know a child—through these Moment-by-Moment Assessments—the more you will be able to see how a child's **three A's** change across the **four R's**. Seeing these details is very important for planning an effective treatment.

Sample Completed TST Assessment Form

Child's name: _Tanisha_   **Date of birth:** _7/29/02_   **Record number:** _909_

Instructions:

The purpose of this *TST Assessment Form* is to record the information that you have gathered about the child and family that you will use to establish an effective *TST Treatment Plan*. As detailed in Chapters 9 and 10 of the TST book, the treatment plan is based on your answers to five questions. The information you will use to answer each of these five questions should be recorded in the corresponding section of this form. Detailed instructions for completing this form are found in Chapter 9 of the TST book. The five sections—and their corresponding question/assessment information—are shown below:

Section 1: What problem(s) will be the focus of the child's treatment?

The information we need:

a. Moment-by-Moment Assessments of episodes of problematic emotion and/or behavior

b. Exposure to traumatic events

c. Other problems that may need to be addressed in treatment, including:
   i. Comorbid psychiatric or developmental problems
   ii. Enduring trauma-related cognitions
   iii. Current social problems that impact the child's health and development

Section 2: Why are these problems important and to whom are they important?

The information we need:

a. The functional impact of the identified problems

b. The level of concern about these problems from the child, the family, and others

c. The identification of what is most important/concerning to the child, the family, and others

Section 3: What interventions can be used to address the child's problems?

The information we need:

a. The child's vulnerability to shift to survival state

b. The environment's capacity to help and protect the child

Section 4: What strengths will be used to address the child's problems?

The information we need:

a. The child's strengths

b. The caregiver's strengths

c. The social-environmental strengths

Section 5: What will interfere with addressing the child's problems?

The information we need:

a. The child and family's understanding of trauma and mental health intervention

b. The practical barriers to engage in treatment

(continued)

SECTION 1: WHAT PROBLEM(S) WILL BE THE FOCUS
OF THE CHILD'S TREATMENT?

a. Moment-by-Moment Assessment of episodes of problematic emotion and/or behavior

Please identify the episodes of problematic emotion and/or behavior that will be evaluated during the assessment period. Record the date that each episode was evaluated with a Moment-by-Moment Assessment (blank Moment-by-Moment Assessment Sheets are found in Appendix 2). At least three episodes should be recorded during the assessment process.

Date of Episode	Brief description of episode	Date Moment-by-Moment Assessment Sheet complete
9/9/14	Mom's unannounced visit. Whispered GM cannot love her as much as Mom does. Assaulted GM.	9/12/14
9/18/14	Family friends visited. Assaulted GM after being told to play with other girl.	9/19/14
10/1/14	Pushed and kicked girl on playground.	10/1/14

b. Exposure to traumatic events

Please check any event(s) the child may have experienced and record any relevant detail such as age and duration of event.

☐ Sexual abuse	☐ Injury or illness	☒ Lack basic needs
☐ Physical abuse	☐ Disaster	☐ Homelessness
☐ Violence exposure	☐ Terrorism	☒ Removal from family
☒ Witness violence	☐ War and/or displacement	☒ Caregiver mental illness/ substance abuse
	☐ Loss of close family member or friend	☒ Other (specify) *Emotional abuse*

Between birth and age 6, Tanisha lived with her mother and father, where she was exposed to neglect, inconsistent parenting, and being put into the middle of her parents' fights. Her mother often asked her to take sides between her and her father, and told her she must take her mother's side if she loves her. Tanisha also witnessed frequent domestic violence between her parents. Neighbors called the police several times, and the last time the police arrested her father for severely injuring her mother. Child Protection was called, and removed Tanisha, placing her into foster care. Over the next 5 years, Tanisha had three different foster care placements, before being placed with her grandmother, Ms. Williams. This is the fourth home she has had since being removed from her home at age 6.

(continued)

c. Other problems that may need to be addressed in treatment

Please provide information on any other problem(s) that may need to be addressed in treatment.

    i. Comorbid psychiatric and/or developmental problems (e.g., depression, ADHD, autism, mental retardation). Please make sure the symptoms of the problem you identify are clearly distinct from survival-in-the-moment episodes:

Past diagnosis of depression, but will determine whether depressive symptoms are part of survival state, or not.

    ii. Enduring trauma-related cognitions (e.g., feelings of worthlessness, hopelessness, shame, guilt):

Tanisha often feels she is "bad," and when something negative happens, she blames herself and becomes hopeless, and assumes she will be rejected and given up on. When she gets in trouble at school, she is quick to assume she will be expelled. When she has a conflict with her grandmother, she becomes very afraid that she will have to leave the home.

    iii. Current social problems (e.g., caregiver mental illness/substance abuse, parental divorce/separations):

Grandmother is quite stressed and has her own health problems. She will need a lot of support and possibly referral to her own treatment.

SECTION 2: WHY ARE THESE PROBLEMS IMPORTANT AND TO WHOM ARE THEY IMPORTANT?

a. The functional impact of the identified problems

What has been the impact of the episodes of problematic emotional/behavioral expression on the child's functioning? What has been the impact of any other identified problem on the child's functioning? Has the problem interfered with learning and school, or with family and peer relations? How big a problem is this?

Tanisha has had three failed foster placements. Each foster family said they cared about her, but was unable to handle her explosive outbursts. She has also been suspended from school multiple times due to her aggressive behavior. She has had a hard time keeping friendships, both due to her aggression and to having moved multiple times.

(continued)

b. The level of concern about the identified problems from the child, the family, and others

Who is concerned about the identified problems? Is the child concerned? Are family members concerned? Who else is concerned? Does the level of concern correspond to the level of functional impact for the child?

Tanisha is very worried about maintaining her placement. She is extremely concerned that she will have to leave her grandmother's home, as she has never had a stable placement that lasted for long. She is aware that her lack of control over her behavior causes problems for her grandmother, and she is terrified that she will be rejected yet again.

Ms. Williams is also very concerned. She loves her granddaughter, and wants her to remain in her home, but is very worried that she won't be able to manage her outbursts. The team is also very concerned, and wants this placement to work out.

c. The identification of what is most important/concerning to the child, the family, and others

What is most important/concerning to the child and to family members? What are their sources of pain? What are their goals and priorities?

i. Child's main goals, concerns, sources of pain:

Tanisha wants to be a teacher. She hates that she gets aggressive and "kicked out of school." Tanisha says, "How can I be a teacher when I can't stay in school? I hate myself when I lose my temper in school." She also wants desperately to stay in her grandmother's home.

ii. Caregiver's/family member's main goals, concerns, sources of pain:

Ms. Williams feels guilty about her daughter's severe drug abuse and mental health problems. She wants to be a better mother for Tanisha than she was for her daughter. She wants this placement to work out.

SECTION 3: WHAT INTERVENTIONS WILL BE USED TO ADDRESS THESE PROBLEMS?

Within TST, interventions are selected based on the phase of treatment that is appropriate for the child's problems. The information used to determine the TST treatment phase (detailed in Chapter 10 on treatment planning), concerns the degree to which the child is vulnerable to switch to survival states and the degree to which the social environment is able to help and protect the child. Please use the table below to record your ratings, *using the definitions provided.*

(continued)

Child's Vulnerability to Switch into Survival States	Definitions
☐ **No Survival States**	1. Does not display episodes of survival-in-the-moment (shifts in *awareness, affect, and action*) when a threat is perceived in the present environment. 2. If the child displays shifts in awareness, affect, and action when a threat is perceived, neither the episode itself, nor the anticipation of such episodes, results in any problem with the child's functioning.
☐ **Survival States**	1. Displays episodes of survival-in-the-moment (shifts in *awareness, affect, and action*) when threat is perceived in the present environment. 2. The shift in *action* during such episodes does not include potentially dangerous behaviors (e.g., self-destructive, aggressive, substance-abusing, risky eating, or sexual behaviors). 3. Such episodes, or their anticipation, result in problems with the child's functioning.
☒ **Dangerous Survival States**	1. Displays episodes of survival-in-the-moment (shifts in *awareness, affect, and action*) when threat is perceived in the present environment. 2. The shift in *action* during such episodes includes potentially dangerous behaviors (e.g., self-destructive, aggressive, substance-abusing, risky eating, or sexual behaviors). 3. Such episodes, or their anticipation, result in problems with the child's functioning.

Justification of Rating:

Tanisha has had three recent episodes of extreme physical aggression.

The Social Environment's Capacity to Help and Protect the Child	Definitions
☐ **Helpful and Protective**	1. The child's immediate caregivers are sufficiently available and apply sufficient competence to *help* with the child's vulnerability to switching into survival states and to *protect* the child from perceived and actual threats; *or* 2. Other adults in the child's life are sufficiently available and apply sufficient competence to *help* and *protect* the child; *or* 3. The appropriate child service system is sufficiently available and applies sufficient competence to *help* and *protect* the child.

(continued)

☒ **Insufficiently Helpful and Protective**	1. The child's immediate caregivers are insufficiently available and/or apply insufficient competence to *help* with the child's vulnerability to switching into survival states or to *protect* the child from perceived threats; *and* 2. Other adults in the child's life are insufficiently available and/or apply insufficient competence to *help* or *protect* the child; *and* 3. The appropriate child service system is insufficiently available and/or applies insufficient competence to *help* or *protect* the child.
☐ **Harmful**	1. The child's immediate caregivers are insufficiently available and/or apply insufficient competence to *protect* the child from actual threats; *and* 2. Other adults in the child's life are insufficiently available and/or apply insufficient competence to *protect* the child from actual threats; *and* 3. The appropriate child service system is insufficiently available and/or applies insufficient competence to *protect* the child from actual threats.

Justification of Rating:

Tanisha's mother recently came to the home unannounced, and Ms. Williams, despite agreeing with her caseworker that the visits must be supervised, has allowed her daughter into the home to see Tanisha. Ms. Williams needs help to set firmer limits and to learn to better meet Tanisha's needs.

SECTION 4: WHAT STRENGTHS CAN BE USED TO ADDRESS THE CHILD'S PROBLEMS?

Please record information about the strengths that might be available to help address the child's problems. Record enough detail about the strength so that decisions can be made for its possible use in the child's treatment.

a. **Child strengths** (e.g., intellectual, social–emotional skills, talents):

Tanisha loves creative writing and reading. She is a talented artist and likes to illustrate her own stories. She has clear ambitions to teach and help others. She is very bright and quick to understand what others say and to take in new information. She is proud of herself when she does well, like when she won a trophy in the writing competition at the community center. She feels very calm when she reads and writes, and she successfully uses these strengths to manage emotion.

(continued)

b. **Caregiver strengths** (e.g., parenting skills, motivation and dedication, organizational strengths, flexibility, emotional attunement, openness to help):

Ms. Williams is very motivated to learn and help. She is very warm and loving toward Tanisha and well connected to her community.

c. **Social–environmental strengths** (e.g., strengths and resources among friends, neighbors and neighborhood, culture, religion, school, or service system):

Tanisha has her own room and plenty of books to read. She has a library card and frequently spends time in the library near her home. There is a community center one block from her apartment that has a good arts program that Tanisha really enjoys.

SECTION 5: WHAT CAN INTERFERE WITH ADDRESSING THE CHILD'S PROBLEMS?

Please record information about the factors that can interfere with the child and family's engagement in treatment.

a. The child and family's understanding of trauma and mental health intervention

Tanisha has not had the experience of treatment being helpful to her, and is thus hesitant to engage in the process. She will need much support and psychoeducation about the process.

Ms. Williams has had negative experiences with attempts to get treatment for her daughter, but is motivated to "do what it takes" for Tanisha. Neither Tanisha nor Ms. Williams has much understanding of trauma or how TST, or treatment in general, can work.

b. The practical barriers in the way of treatment engagement, such as transportation, scheduling, child care, language, parent limitations, treatment concerns

Ms. Williams has very limited funds, and does not live close to the agency. The agency gives her money for public transportation, but the only bus route takes a very long time. Ms. Williams prefers meetings in the morning.

Additional Notes:

There are many strengths in this system, but also real risks. The team needs to work quickly to engage Tanisha and Ms. Williams, to leverage these strengths, and to establish a treatment plan that will maximize the likelihood of stabilizing the system in order to maintain this placement.

Sample Completed TST Moment-by-Moment Assessment Sheet

Child's name: _Tanisha_   **Record number:** _909_   **Date:** _9/12/14_

Step 1: Finding what flipped the switch

<u>Instructions</u>: What flipped the switch, such that the *episode of problematic emotion and/or behavior*, happened? <u>First</u>: Consider the period of time just before the *episode*. What was the child doing (**A**ction)? What was he or she feeling (**A**ffect)? Where/what was the child's focus of attention/thought (**A**wareness)? <u>Second</u>: Consider the period of time during the *episode*: What of the **three A's** changed during the *episode*? <u>Third</u>: Consider the present environment throughout this process. Record any feature of the *present environment* that you think may have been related to the *episode* (whatever it is). Any of these features may turn out to be responsible for flipping the switch. If assessment revealed sufficient detail about the **four R's**, you can skip the "During the Episode" box and complete Step 2.

Before the Episode *(possible "usual state"/regulating)*	**During the Episode** *(possible "survival-in-the-moment")*
Action: *Reading book in her bedroom on her bed.*	Action: *"Tore up the house," throwing things, yelling, broke a glass, broke a chair.*
Affect: *Calm. Feeling good. Very excited by adventure story.*	Affect: *Rage*
Awareness: *Focused on adventure story. Her imagination was engaged in the book.*	Awareness: *Focused on mother saying something "that was so unfair . . . why does she say this to me . . . she knows I hate when she does that."*

Features of the Present Environment   *(possible "switch"/"cat hair")*
Tanisha's mother came over unannounced, Ms. Williams let her in, and the mother told Tanisha she must choose her over grandmother.

(continued)

Step 2: Understanding what happened when the switch was flipped*

Instructions: Once you have understood what flipped the switch, you may be able to see important details about the *episode* in question. If the *episode* represents *survival-in-the-moment*, the child will have switched from a *usual state* (**R**egulating) to the three *Survival-in-the-Moment* states of **R**evving, **R**eexperiencing, and **R**econstituting. Each of these states will be characterized by changes in the **three A's**. Consider the *episode* assessed in Step 1: Record information in your *present environment* during these respective states. See Chapter 9, Section 1, of the TST book for details about conducting this assessment.

Revving	Reexperiencing	Reconstituting
Action: *Sat still. Listening to mother talk. Legs shaking.*	Action: *Yelling at Ms. Williams, throwing things, breaking glass and furniture, accidentally cuts her hand.*	Action: *Rocking on the floor. Crying. Begging Ms. Williams to forgive her.*
Affect: *Anxious. Worried about what mother would say. Getting angry.*	Affect: *Enraged*	Affect: *Anxious. Ashamed.*
Awareness: *Focused on mother's words. "I wish she'd stop talking."*	Awareness: *Thinking about what mother whispered to her.*	Awareness: *Focused on damage she had caused and worried that her grandmother would be fed up with her.*
Present Environment: *Mother arrives unannounced. Mother tells Tanisha she must hug her and tell her she loves her, and whispers that she must not love her grandmother because she is not her mother.*	Present Environment: *Just after mother left, Ms. Williams entered Tanisha's room wanting to know what the mother said and urged her to tell her.*	Present Environment: *In living room, begging Ms. Williams's forgiveness as Ms. Williams tries to reassure her.*

Was the episode you have assessed an expression of survival-in-the-moment?	How confident are you in your answer to this question?
☒ Yes ☐ No	☒ Very confident ☐ Confident enough ☐ Not so confident ☐ Not at all confident

*In the first few Moment-by-Moment Assessments of a child's episodes, you may not be able to see these details. The more you get to know a child—through these Moment-by-Moment Assessments—the more you will be able to see how a child's **three A's** change across the **four R's**. Seeing these details is very important for planning an effective treatment.

Sample Completed TST Moment-by-Moment Assessment Sheet

Child's name: _Tanisha_   **Record number:** _909_   **Date:** _9/19/14_

Step 1: Finding what flipped the switch

<u>Instructions</u>: What flipped the switch, such that the *episode of problematic emotion and/or behavior,* happened? <u>First</u>: Consider the period of time just before the *episode*. What was the child doing (**A**ction)? What was he or she feeling (**A**ffect)? Where/what was the child's focus of attention/thought (**A**wareness)? <u>Second</u>: Consider the period of time during the *episode*: What of the **three A's** changed during the *episode*? <u>Third</u>: Consider the present environment throughout this process. Record any feature of the *present environment* that you think may have been related to the *episode* (whatever it is). Any of these features may turn out to be responsible for flipping the switch. If assessment revealed sufficient detail about the **four R's**, you can skip the "During the Episode" box and complete Step 2.

Before the Episode *(possible "usual state"/regulating)*	**During the Episode** *(possible "survival-in-the-moment")*
Action: *Reading her new creative fiction kids' magazine.*	Action: *Ran at Ms. Williams. Tried to punch and kick her.*
Affect: *Calm, relaxed*	Affect: *Rage*
Awareness: *Reading magazine, funny story.*	Awareness: *Remembers thinking "I hate her." Only fragmented memory for punching and kicking her.*

Features of the Present Environment   *(possible "switch"/"cat hair")*
Ms. Williams told Tanisha to play with visiting children. Told her that Tanisha embarrasses her when she resists.

(continued)

Step 2: Understanding what happened when the switch was flipped*

<u>Instructions</u>: Once you have understood what flipped the switch, you may be able to see important details about the *episode* in question. If the *episode* represents *survival-in-the-moment,* the child will have switched from a *usual state* (**R**egulating) to the three *Survival-in-the-Moment* states of **R**evving, **R**eexperiencing, and **R**econstituting. Each of these states will be characterized by changes in the **three A's**. Consider the *episode* assessed in Step 1: Record information in your *present environment* during these respective states. See Chapter 9, Section 1, of the TST book for details about conducting this assessment.

Revving	Reexperiencing	Reconstituting
Action: *Puts magazine down. Looks away from Ms. Williams toward wall.*	Action: *Threw book at Ms. Williams. Ran toward her and tried to punch and kick her.*	Action: *Sitting still in bed. Crying and urging Ms. Williams to forgive her.*
Affect: *"Getting angry"*	Affect: *Rage*	Affect: *Frightened and ashamed*
Awareness: *"I wish she'd stop talking and leave me alone."*	Awareness: *"I remember hating her, but I can't remember much else after that."*	Awareness: *Worried that Ms. Williams will "be fed up and kick me out."*
Present Environment: *Friends of the family (not well known to Tanisha) visiting for the afternoon. Ms. Williams came to room and asked Tanisha to stop what she was doing to play with the other children.*	Present Environment: *Ms. Williams stayed in room and continued to urge Tanisha to stop reading her magazine and to play with the children. Ms. Williams began raising her voice to Tanisha, saying that Tanisha was embarrassing her.*	Present Environment: *On bed. Mrs. Williams trying to help her calm down and reassure her.*

Was the episode you have assessed an expression of survival-in-the-moment?	How confident are you in your answer to this question?
☒ Yes ☐ No	☒ Very confident ☐ Confident enough ☐ Not so confident ☐ Not at all confident

*In the first few Moment-by-Moment Assessments of a child's episodes, you may not be able to see these details. The more you get to know a child—through these Moment-by-Moment Assessments—the more you will be able to see how a child's **three A's** change across the **four R's**. Seeing these details is very important for planning an effective treatment.

Sample Completed TST Moment-by-Moment Assessment Sheet

Child's name: _Tanisha_   **Record number:** _909_   **Date:** _10/1/14_

Step 1: Finding what flipped the switch

<u>Instructions</u>: What flipped the switch, such that the *episode of problematic emotion and/or behavior*, happened? <u>First</u>: Consider the period of time just before the *episode*. What was the child doing (**A**ction)? What was he or she feeling (**A**ffect)? Where/what was the child's focus of attention/thought (**A**wareness)? <u>Second</u>: Consider the period of time during the *episode*: What of the **three A's** changed during the *episode*? <u>Third</u>: Consider the present environment throughout this process. Record any feature of the *present environment* that you think may have been related to the *episode* (whatever it is). Any of these features may turn out to be responsible for flipping the switch. If assessment revealed sufficient detail about the **four R's**, you can skip the "During the Episode" box and complete Step 2.

Before the Episode *(possible "usual state"/regulating)*	During the Episode *(possible "survival-in-the-moment")*
Action: *Tanisha and her friends are gossiping, and laughing, having fun.*	Action: *Pushed friend to ground and kicked her.*
Affect: *Calm, happy, laughing*	Affect: *Enraged*
Awareness: *Sitting on park bench with friends. Focused on conversation. Wants to say things that will make her friends laugh.*	Awareness: *Thinking, "How dare she tell me who to like" and "She's such a bitch."*

Features of the Present Environment
(possible "switch"/"cat hair")

One of Tanisha's friends took her aside to talk about another one of Tanisha's close friends. She asked Tanisha if she is her best friend, and if she likes her more. She tells her not to be friends with the other girl.

(continued)

From Glenn N. Saxe, B. Heidi Ellis, and Adam D. Brown. Copyright 2016 by The Guilford Press. Permission to photocopy this material is granted to purchasers of this book for personal use only (see copyright page for details). Purchasers can download and print a larger version of this material (see the box at the end of the table of contents).

Step 2: Understanding what happened when the switch was flipped*

Instructions: Once you have understood what flipped the switch, you may be able to see important details about the *episode* in question. If the *episode* represents *survival-in-the-moment,* the child will have switched from a *usual state* (**R**egulating) to the three *Survival-in-the-Moment* states of **R**evving, **R**eexperiencing, and **R**econstituting. Each of these states will be characterized by changes in the **three A's**. Consider the *episode* assessed in Step 1: Record information in your *present environment* during these respective states. See Chapter 9, Section 1, of the TST book for details about conducting this assessment.

Revving	Reexperiencing	Reconstituting
Action: *Listening quietly to what her friend was saying about the other friend.*	Action: *Pushed girl to ground and kicked her.*	Action: *Sitting on bench with best friend. Crying.*
Affect: *Getting angry*	Affect: *Rage*	Affect: *Embarrassed. Anxious.*
Awareness: *Thinking: "How can she say this? She's talking about my close friend."*	Awareness: *Thinking: "Who are you to tell me who to like?" Doesn't remember pushing and kicking.*	Awareness: *Worried no one will like her or be her friend.*
Present Environment: *Private conversation with friend who is asking her about another girl.*	Present Environment: *On park bench. Tanisha was attacking friend, crowd gathered, adults broke up the fight.*	Present Environment: *Sitting on bench with best friend. Friend trying to reassure her.*

Was the episode you have assessed an expression of survival-in-the-moment?	How confident are you in your answer to this question?
☒ Yes ☐ No	☒ Very confident ☐ Confident enough ☐ Not so confident ☐ Not at all confident

*In the first few Moment-by-Moment Assessments of a child's episodes, you may not be able to see these details. The more you get to know a child—through these Moment-by-Moment Assessments—the more you will be able to see how a child's **three A's** change across the **four R's**. Seeing these details is very important for planning an effective treatment.

TST Treatment Plan

Child's name: _____ **Date of birth:** _____ **Record number:** _____

Instructions:

This *TST Treatment Plan* is based on answers to five treatment-planning questions. Use the information that you have recorded in the child's *TST Assessment Form* to answer these five questions. The TST Treatment Plan—like the TST Assessment Form—has five sections: Each section corresponds to one of the five questions. Detailed instructions for completing this form are found in Chapter 10 of the TST book. The five questions and the decisions you need to make to answer them are shown below:

Section 1: What problem(s) will be the focus of the child's treatment?

The decisions we need to make:

a. The child's TST priority problem(s) and their relation to the child's trauma history
b. Other problem(s) that will be addressed in treatment, including:
    i. Comorbid psychiatric and developmental disorders
    ii. Enduring trauma-related cognitions
    iii. Social problems that impact the child's health and development

Section 2: Why are these problem(s) important and to whom are they important?

The decisions we need to make:

a. The order of priority of the TST priority problem(s) and any other identified problem(s)
b. The strategy to engage the child and family to address the identified problem(s)
c. The strategy to engage others to address the identified problem(s)

Section 3: What interventions will be used to address the child's problem(s)?

The decisions we need to make:

a. The phase of treatment to initiate
b. The statement about how the treatment will be directed to address the identified problem(s)
c. The role and expectations of each member of the team in implementing the treatment
d. The role and expectations of the child and the family members in implementing treatment

Section 4: What strengths will be used to address the child's problem(s)?

The decisions we need to make:

a. The child's strengths that will be used in the treatment
b. The family members' strengths that will be used in the treatment
c. The strengths in the social environment that will be used in treatment

Section 5: What will interfere with addressing the child's problem(s)?

The decisions we need to make:

a. The approach to address the psychoeducational needs of the child and family
b. The approach to surmount practical barriers

(continued)

SECTION 1: WHAT PROBLEM(S) SHOULD BE THE FOCUS
OF THE CHILD'S TREATMENT?

a. The Child's TST Priority Problem(s) and their relation to the child's trauma history

Use the information from the TST Priority Problem Worksheets to record at least one TST priority problem in the section below:

Priority Problem 1

When _____ is exposed to _____ ,
     Child's name   Description of perceived threat

She/he responds by _____ .
                        Description of Survival State

This pattern can be understood through past experience(s) of:

_____
Description of past trauma to inform Survival State

Priority Problem 2

When _____ is exposed to _____ ,
     Child's name   Description of perceived threat

She/he responds by _____ .
                        Description of Survival State

This pattern can be understood through past experience(s) of:

_____
Description of past trauma to inform Survival State

Priority Problem 3

When _____ is exposed to _____ ,
     Child's name   Description of perceived threat

She/he responds by _____ .
                        Description of Survival State

This pattern can be understood through past experience(s) of:

_____
Description of past trauma to inform Survival State

(continued)

b. Other problem(s) that will be addressed in treatment

Record any other problem (e.g., comorbid psychiatric or developmental disorder, enduring trauma-related cognition, social problem) that will be addressed in treatment. Make sure to select only problems from Section 1.b of the TST Assessment Form (Appendix 2) that you think are important enough to address (remember TST Principle 5: *Put scarce resources where they will work*). If no other problem will be addressed in treatment, leave this section blank.

SECTION 2: WHY ARE THE CHILD'S PROBLEM(S) IMPORTANT AND TO WHOM ARE THEY IMPORTANT?

a. The order of priority of the TST priority problem(s) and any other identified problem(s)

Identify the problems that are of highest priority (based on the functional impact of each identified problem recorded in Section 2.a of the TST Assessment Form). Describe the possible impact to the child and family if the identified problem(s) are not effectively addressed.

b. The strategy to engage the child and family to address the identified problem(s)

Describe your strategy to engage the child and relevant family members (based on both the degree they are concerned about the identified problems, and what you have identified is most important to them (recorded in Section 2 of the TST Assessment Form). How may the identified problems(s) impact what is most important to the child and family (including their goals and pain sources)?

(continued)

The child:

Family members:

c. The strategy to engage others concerned about the child's problem(s)

Describe your strategy to engage any other parties (e.g., teachers, neighbors, grandparents, coaches) whom you believe are concerned about the child.

(continued)

SECTION 3: WHAT INTERVENTIONS WILL BE USED
TO ADDRESS THE CHILD'S PROBLEM(S)?

a. The phase of treatment to initiate

Use the information recorded in Section 3.a of the TST Assessment Form to identify the phase that will be initiated in treatment.

TST Treatment Planning Grid		The Environment's Help and Protection		
		Helpful and Protective	**Insufficiently Helpful and Protective**	**Harmful**
The Child's Survival States	**No Survival States**	Beyond trauma	Beyond trauma	Safety-focused
	Survival States	Regulation-focused	Regulation-focused	Safety-focused
	Dangerous Survival States	Regulation-focused	Safety-focused	Safety-focused

☐ Safety-Focused   ☐ Regulation-Focused   ☐ Beyond Trauma

b. The overall strategy to address the identified TST priority problems and other identified problem(s)

Succinctly describe your overall strategy to address the child's identified problem(s) within the phase in which he or she will begin treatment. How will you reduce environmental stimuli that provoke survival-in-the-moment responses? How will you enhance the child's ability to regulate emotion/behavior to the stimuli you have identified?

(continued)

c. The roles and expectations of each member of the team in implementing TST treatment

Describe the role/expectation of each team member in the child's treatment.

Team Member	Contact information	Intervention Modality* *skill-based, home-based, pharmacology, etc.	Role/Expectation

(continued)

d. The role/expectations of the child and family members in implementing TST treatment

Describe the role/expectation of the child and relevant family members in the child's treatment.

Child/Family	Contact information	Role/Expectation

SECTION 4: WHAT STRENGTHS WILL BE USED
TO ADDRESS THE CHILD'S PROBLEM(S)?

a. How will the child's strengths be used in treatment?

Describe your plan for integrating the child's strengths into their treatment.

b. How will family members' strengths be used in treatment?

Describe your plan for integrating family members' strengths into treatment.

c. How will the strengths of the social environment be used in treatment?

Describe your plan for integrating the strengths of the social environment into treatment.

(continued)

SECTION 5: WHAT WILL INTERFERE WITH ADDRESSING THE CHILD'S PROBLEM(S)?

a. The approach to address the psychoeducational needs of the child and family.

b. The approach to surmount the practical barriers in the way of treatment engagement.

TST Priority Problem Worksheet

Shift to Survival State

Episode 1

Episode 2

Episode 3

Past Trauma Environment

Pattern of Survival-in-the-Moment

Pattern of Perceived Threat

Perceived Threat in Present Environment

Episode 1

Episode 2

Episode 3

TST Priority Problem Statement

When _____ is exposed to _____
       Child's name   Description of perceived threat

She/he responds by _____
                    Description of Survival State

This pattern can be understood through past experience(s) of:

_____
Description of past trauma to inform Survival State

Sample Completed TST Treatment Plan

Child's name: _Tanisha_   **Date of birth:** _7/29/02_   **Record number:** _909_

Instructions:

This *TST Treatment Plan* is based on answers to five treatment-planning questions. Use the information that you have recorded in the child's *TST Assessment Form* to answer these five questions. The TST Treatment Plan—like the TST Assessment Form—has five sections: Each section corresponds to one of the five questions. Detailed instructions for completing this form are found in Chapter 10 of the TST book. The five questions and the decisions you need to make to answer them are shown below:

Section 1: What problem(s) will be the focus of the child's treatment?

The decisions we need to make:

a. The child's TST priority problem(s) and their relation to the child's trauma history
b. Other problem(s) that will be addressed in treatment, including:
   i. Comorbid psychiatric and developmental disorders
   ii. Enduring trauma-related cognitions
   iii. Social problems that impact the child's health and development

Section 2: Why are these problem(s) important and to whom are they important?

The decisions we need to make:

a. The order of priority of the TST priority problem(s) and any other identified problem(s)
b. The strategy to engage the child and family to address the identified problem(s)
c. The strategy to engage others to address the identified problem(s)

Section 3: What interventions will be used to address the child's problem(s)?

The decisions we need to make:

a. The phase of treatment to initiate
b. The statement about how the treatment will be directed to address the identified problem(s)
c. The role and expectations of each member of the team in implementing the treatment
d. The role and expectations of the child and the family members in implementing treatment

Section 4: What strengths will be used to address the child's problem(s)?

The decisions we need to make:

a. The child's strengths that will be used in the treatment
b. The family members' strengths that will be used in the treatment
c. The strengths in the social environment that will be used in treatment

Section 5: What will interfere with addressing the child's problem(s)?

The decisions we need to make:

a. The approach to address the psychoeducational needs of the child and family
b. The approach to surmount practical barriers

(continued)

SECTION 1: WHAT PROBLEM(S) SHOULD BE THE FOCUS OF THE CHILD'S TREATMENT?

a. The Child's TST Priority Problem(s) and their relation to the child's trauma history

Use the information from the TST Priority Problem Worksheets to record at least one TST priority problem in the section below:

Priority Problem 1

> When _Tanisha_ is exposed to _a situation when she feels her loyalty and love are being questioned_ ,
>
> Child's name   Description of perceived threat
>
> She/he responds by _becoming enraged, then aggressive and dissociative_ .
>
> Description of Survival State
>
> This pattern can be understood through past experience(s) of:
>
> _severe neglect, witnessing domestic violence, inconsistent parenting, and coercive statements about love and loyalty_
>
> Description of past trauma to inform Survival State

Priority Problem 2

> When _____ is exposed to _____ ,
>
> Child's name   Description of perceived threat
>
> She/he responds by _____ .
>
> Description of Survival State
>
> This pattern can be understood through past experience(s) of:
>
> _____
>
> Description of past trauma to inform Survival State

Priority Problem 3

> When _____ is exposed to _____ ,
>
> Child's name   Description of perceived threat
>
> She/he responds by _____ .
>
> Description of Survival State
>
> This pattern can be understood through past experience(s) of:
>
> _____
>
> Description of past trauma to inform Survival State

(continued)

b. Other problem(s) that will be addressed in treatment

Record any other problem (e.g., comorbid psychiatric or developmental disorder, enduring trauma-related cognition, social problem) that will be addressed in treatment. Make sure to select only problems from Section 1.b of the TST Assessment Form (Appendix 2) that you think are important enough to address (remember TST Principle 5: *Put scarce resources where they will work*). If no other problem will be addressed in treatment, leave this section blank.

As noted in the TST assessment, Tanisha often feels she is "bad," and when something negative happens, she blames herself, and becomes hopeless, and assumes she will be rejected and given up on. For example, she often says things such as "I'm a bad kid, what's the point, nothing good is going to happen for me." When she gets in trouble at school, she is quick to assume she will be expelled. When she has a conflict with her grandmother, she becomes very afraid that she will have to leave the home. We need to be cautious of how these negative cognitions may be easily triggered and may contribute to hopelessness, and to survival-in-the-moment states. One of the goals of treatment will be to help Tanisha become aware of these pervasive and automatic thoughts, in order to learn to break the patterns that lead to survival in the moment states.

SECTION 2: WHY ARE THE CHILD'S PROBLEM(S) IMPORTANT AND TO WHOM ARE THEY IMPORTANT?

a. The order of priority of the TST priority problem(s) and any other identified problem(s)

Identify the problems that are of highest priority (based on the functional impact of each identified problem recorded in Section 2.a of the TST Assessment Form). Describe the possible impact to the child and family if the identified problem(s) are not effectively addressed.

Tanisha's priority problem is this: When Tanisha is exposed to a situation in which she feels her loyalty and love are being questioned, she becomes enraged, aggressive, and dissociative, which can be understood by her history of extreme neglect, witnessing domestic violence, inconsistent parenting, and coercive statements about love and loyalty. This problem is a priority because it poses a very real threat to Tanisha's stated goal of becoming a teacher, as well as to the stability of her placement in her grandmother's home. If the current pattern of triggered survival-in-the-moment episodes continues, Tanisha may end up being expelled from school, hospitalized, placed in a new foster home or in residential treatment. The team's priority is to put measures in place to attempt to make sure these outcomes do not occur. If successful, Tanisha will begin to function better both at school and at home.

b. The strategy to engage the child and family to address the identified problem(s)

Describe your strategy to engage the child and relevant family members (based on both the degree they are concerned about the identified problems, and what you have identified is most important to them [recorded in Section 2 of the TST Assessment Form]). How may the identified problem(s) impact what is most important to the child and family (including their goals and pain sources)?

(continued)

428

The child:

Tanisha wants to become a teacher because she wants to "help kids have the best chance in life." This goal relates to her own life experience. She derives great pleasure out of reading and writing and wants to help "kids who go through tough times feel good when they read and write." The team will keep Tanisha's goal of becoming a teacher front-and-center and will continue to help Tanisha see that her efforts to gain more control over her behavior through engaging in the treatment will increase the likelihood of her being successful at becoming a teacher. She questions her ability to achieve this goal, however, whenever she is triggered, and her negative beliefs and inability to manage her impulses overcome her ability to maintain control. Tanisha's triggered pattern of survival-in-the-moment states is jeopardizing her performance in school and even ability to stay in her current school. If this pattern continues, it will clearly interfere with her goal of becoming a teacher. When Tanisha states "How can I be a teacher when I can't stay in school? I hate myself when I lose my temper in school," she is becoming aware of the connection between her behavior and her ability to achieve her goal. The team will continue to help Tanisha develop this awareness to help her come up with strategies to overcome this pattern so that she can achieve her goal.

Family members:

Ms. Williams wants to be a "better mother" to Tanisha than "the mother I was to my daughter." To Ms. Williams this means that she was not present enough, not loving enough, and too permissive about her daughter's behavior. When Ms. Williams sees Tanisha lose control over her behavior, it reminds her about how her daughter would lose control, and then Ms. Williams feels that her caregiving is ineffective and harmful. Ms. Williams feels that her daughter is "not able to function in society" and is "completely irresponsible" (she also wishes that this were not true, and this wishful thinking motivates her permission of her daughter's visits). She very much sees the opportunity to parent Tanisha as a way of "repenting" for the damage she believes she has caused. Whenever Tanisha has a survival-in-the-moment state, particularly at home, it confirms her belief that she is a failure as a mother. Although Ms. Williams had not made the direct connection, it was very easy for her to see it once it was identified. The team, through building a trusting, therapeutic relationship with Ms. Williams, will help her to see that her inability to limit her daughter's visits, and thereby protect Tanisha, continues to lead to Tanisha's survival-in-the-moment states, which then undermine Ms. Williams's belief in herself as a good mother.

c. The strategy to engage others concerned about the child's problem(s)

Describe your strategy to engage any other parties (e.g., teachers, neighbors, grandparents, coaches) whom you believe are concerned about the child.

It will be very important to engage key staff at Tanisha's school as members of the treatment team. Success in school is important to Tanisha, as it is an essential component of helping her to achieve her goal of becoming a teacher. Her behavior problems in school, however, lead to suspensions, which interfere with her academics and trigger her negative beliefs about herself. If the school can become active members of the TST team, they can help to identify situations in which she is likely to be triggered there, and can help to put proactive plans in place, such as identifying a supportive person she can go to when she feels upset. The school, if effectively engaged, could also create opportunities for Tanisha to tutor younger children in reading and writing, which would capitalize on her strengths and help her counter her negative beliefs by giving her opportunities that make her feel successful. It will also be important, if possible, to attempt to engage Tanisha's mother in the treatment. Ideally, the team would attempt to determine the mother's priorities and sources of pain, in order to enlist her as a key member of Tanisha's treatment team.

(continued)

SECTION 3: WHAT INTERVENTIONS WILL BE USED TO ADDRESS THE CHILD'S PROBLEM(S)?

a. The phase of treatment to initiate

Use the information recorded in Section 3.a of the TST Assessment Form to identify the phase that will be initiated in treatment.

TST Treatment Planning Grid		The Environment's Help and Protection		
		Helpful and Protective	**Insufficiently Helpful and Protective**	**Harmful**
The Child's Survival States	**No Survival States**	Beyond trauma	Beyond trauma	Safety-focused
	Survival States	Regulation-focused	Regulation-focused	Safety-focused
	Dangerous Survival States	Regulation-focused	Safety-focused	Safety-focused

☑ Safety-Focused   ☐ Regulation-Focused   ☐ Beyond Trauma

b. The overall strategy to address the identified TST priority problems and other identified problem(s)

Succinctly describe your overall strategy to address the child's identified problem(s) within the phase in which he or she will begin treatment. How will you reduce environmental stimuli that provoke survival-in-the-moment responses? How will you enhance the child's ability to regulate emotion/behavior to the stimuli you have identified?

Tanisha shifts to survival states when she is in a situation that makes her feel as though she must choose one person over another or in which she feels as though she may lose someone she cares about, or may lose her sense of self. When this happens she becomes aggressive, usually toward someone she is close to, such as her grandmother or her friends. She is thus at great risk to lose her friends, her school, and her placement with her grandmother. The team must create a trusting relationship with both Tanisha and Ms. Williams, through which to help them both understand Tanisha's behavior in the context of her traumatic history. Once they both understand trauma and survival-in-the-moment, they may become more open to working with us, and more likely to engage in the treatment process. We will do this by helping them each to see how Tanisha's survival-in-the-moment states are triggered by situations in which she feels her love and loyalty are being challenged. We will also help each to see how these patterns interfere with Tanisha's goal of becoming a teacher, and with Ms. Williams's goal of being the best possible parent to Tanisha that she can be. We will offer to meet with both Tanisha and with Ms. Williams on a weekly basis to provide psychoeducation, support, and practical help. We will also attempt to engage with the school to help them better plan for Tanisha's emotional needs. Our relationship with social services and the caseworker will be critical to make sure the case plan is well enforced.

(continued)

c. The roles and expectations of each member of the team in implementing TST treatment

Describe the role/expectation of each team member in the child's treatment.

Team Member	Contact information	Intervention Modality* *skill-based, home-based, pharmacology, etc.	Role/Expectation
Clarissa Holmes (home-based therapist)		Home-based care	Tanisha is starting in safety-focused treatment. Ms. Holmes will conduct two visits per week, primarily in the home to make sure visits with mother are reduced and that the types of loyalty binds that lead to dysregulation are minimized. There will need to be meetings at the school to help teachers and guidance counselor understand Tanisha's vulnerabilities and to address them. Certainly a lot of coordination with Mr. Martinez (caseworker) is indicated.
Carlos Martinez (caseworker)		Caseworker from Agency for Children's Welfare	Mr. Martinez well understands the importance of supporting Ms. Williams to stop all visits with Tanisha's mother. He will support this need in the case plan and work with Ms. Williams to reinforce it.
Dr. Sam Edwards (psychiatrist)		Psychopharmacology	Dr. Edwards will provide a medication follow-up visit. When Tanisha saw Dr. Edwards for an evaluation during her assessment, we thought medications might be helpful for Tanisha's aggression (but were not absolutely necessary). Based on Ms. Williams and Tanisha's preferences, we thought it made sense to try other ways of helping first. We believe it makes sense to have a reassessment in 1 month.
Dr. Susan Jennings (treatment supervisor)		Home- & community-based stabilization Fidelity monitoring and oversight	Provide help to advocate with the school to get a meeting to review Tanisha's educational plan. Review fidelity to the model, and help make sure the team is on track with TST interventions.

(continued)

431

d. The role/expectations of the child and family members in implementing TST treatment

Describe the role/expectation of the child and relevant family members in the child's treatment.

Child/Family	Contact information	Role/Expectation
Tanisha and Ms. Williams		Both will participate fully with all home-based sessions, school observation visit, and reassessment visit with Dr. Edwards.
Ms. Williams		Ms. Williams will limit all visits with Tanisha's mother and will comply with Department of Social Services requirements.
		Ms. Williams will work with Dr. Holmes to set up school education plan meeting.

SECTION 4: WHAT STRENGTHS WILL BE USED TO ADDRESS THE CHILD'S PROBLEM(S)?

a. How will the child's strengths be used in treatment?

Describe your plan for integrating the child's strengths into their treatment.

The team will advocate with the school to encourage Tanisha's talent for writing and love of reading by suggesting that the school provide her with extra opportunities to engage in writing and reading, and perhaps allowing for her to tutor younger students.

The team can also work with Ms. Williams to build in time where the two of them, together, do things they both enjoy. The more Tanisha feels successful and acknowledged for what she does well, the more she will feel accepted and appreciated, and the more likely she is to stay regulated in difficult moments.

b. How will family members' strengths be used in treatment?

Describe your plan for integrating family members' strengths into treatment.

The team will praise and reinforce Ms. Williams's love for and devotion to Tanisha, and support her in every way possible to be the best parent she can be.

c. How will the strengths of the social environment be used in treatment?

Describe your plan for integrating the strengths of the social environment into treatment.

The team will work with Ms. Williams to encourage Tanisha's love of art by enrolling her in art classes at the community center, in addition to the creative writing class, and will arrange for Ms. Williams to get her there. The team will also look for opportunities for Tanisha to tutor or otherwise help other children.

(continued)

SECTION 5: WHAT WILL INTERFERE WITH ADDRESSING THE CHILD'S PROBLEM(S)?

a. The approach to address the psychoeducational needs of the child and family.

The team, during meetings with Tanisha and Ms. Williams, will use the TST psychoeducational materials to help them both better understand how trauma impacts emotions and behavior, how factors in the environment can trigger problematic reactions, and how TST can help address these patterns.

b. The approach to surmount the practical barriers in the way of treatment engagement.

There is a practical barrier about transportation to our clinic for treatment. Fortunately, Tanisha will start in safety-focused treatment so the work will largely be home-based initially. This will give us time to help with the scheduling of clinic-based treatment and possibly to access a transportation stipend to help for when Tanisha is ready for regulation-focused treatment.

The team will advocate with the school to get a Committee on Special Education meeting for Tanisha to better address her emotional and academic needs.

The team will continue to advocate with the Agency for Children's Welfare to have the visits with Tanisha's mother stopped, as defined in the service plan.

Sample Completed TST Priority Problem Worksheet

Perceived Threat in Present Environment

Episode 1

Mother arrived unannounced. Asked for hug. Whispered that grandmother can't love her because she is not her mother.

Episode 2

Grandmother asked her to spend time with other kids when she wanted to do something else.

Episode 3

Girl told her not to be friends with other girl. Asked if she was "best friend."

Past Trauma Environment

History of neglect and witnessing family violence. Multiple foster home placements. Coercive communication about love and loyalty.

Shift to Survival State

Episode 1

Became enraged. Ran at grandmother. Tried to punch and kick her.

Episode 2

Became enraged, yelled at grandmother. Broke furniture. Threw glass.

Episode 3

Became enraged and knocked girl to ground, kicking her.

Pattern of Perceived Threat

Put in loyalty conflict by others where she must choose between people.

Pattern of Survival-in-the-Moment

Becomes enraged related to loyalty bind and responds with aggressive behavior and some dissociation.

TST Priority Problem Statement

When ___Tanisha___ is exposed to ___loyalty binds/choosing between people___ .
   Child's name   Description of perceived threat

She/he responds by ___becoming enraged, aggressive, and dissociative___ .
                          Description of Survival State

This pattern can be understood through past experience(s) of:

___neglect, witness to violence, coercive communication re: loyalty___ .
         Description of past trauma to inform Survival State

Treatment Agreement Letter

☑ Draft (team's ideas)   ☐ Final (by discussion and agreement with family)

Child name _____   **Date of birth** _____   **Record number** _____

Dear _____,

We've asked you a lot of questions so that we may best know how to help you. We have developed some ideas about how we can work with you to give you the help that you need. This form provides our ideas about working with you. It indicates what we think should be the goals of treatment, based on our understanding of what is most important to you. It also indicates what we intend to do to help and what we think you can do to help. We want to make sure we've *got it right*, so please look at the information in this form very carefully. We are glad to discuss any of it with you and to change anything if you think we have missed important information. Once we agree on how we will work together, this form will be the guide for our work.

Sincerely,

_____, _____

_____, _____

1. **Our work will be about helping you achieve what is most important to you. We understand what is most important to you is:**

2. **We believe you have several strengths that will really help you to achieve what is most important to you. These strengths are:**

(continued)

3. **We have identified a number of problems that we believe should be the focus of the treatment. These problems are:**

4. **These problems make what is most important to you worse. The way these problems can make what is most important to you worse is:**

5. **Here is what we will do to help:**

6. **Here is what you will do to help:**

(continued)

7. If our treatment helps, you will know it in the following way:

8. If our treatment does not help, you will know it in the following way:

9. Here is everyone's agreement:

Name	What I will do	How to reach me	Signature

Sample Completed Treatment Agreement Letter

☑ Draft (team's ideas)　　　☐ Final (by discussion and agreement with family)

Child name _Tanisha_　　　**Date of birth** _7/29/02_　　　**Record number** _909_

Dear _Tanisha and Ms. Sally Williams_　　　　　,

We've asked you a lot of questions so that we may best know how to help you. We have developed some ideas about how we can work with you to give you the help that you need. This form provides our ideas about working with you. It indicates what we think should be the goals of treatment, based on our understanding of what is most important to you. It also indicates what we intend to do to help and what we think you can do to help. We want to make sure we've *got it right*, so please look at the information in this form very carefully. We are glad to discuss any of it with you and to change anything if you think we have missed important information. Once we agree on how we will work together, this form will be the guide for our work.

Sincerely,

Ms. Clarissa Holmes (home-based therapist) , _Mr. Carlos Martinez (ACW caseworker)_

Dr. Sam Edwards (psychiatrist)　　　　, _Dr. Susan Jennings (treatment supervisor)_

1. **Our work will be about helping you achieve what is most important to you. We understand what is most important to you is:**

   Tanisha: You told us you want to become a teacher because you want to "help kids have the best chance in life." You told us that you love to read and write and that you want to help "kids who go through tough times feel good when they read and write."

   Ms. Williams: You told us that you want to be a "better mother" to Tanisha than "the mother I was to my daughter."

2. **We believe you have several strengths that will really help you to achieve what is most important to you. These strengths are:**

   Tanisha: We see that you are talented at art, you love to read and write, you are a good friend, and you want to help other people.

   Ms. Williams: We see that you are very loving, caring, and supportive of Tanisha, and that you are willing to accept help and work with the TST team.

(continued)

3. **We have identified a number of problems that we believe should be the focus of the treatment. These problems are:**

The main problem we see is that when Tanisha feels she is put in a position in which she has to choose between people she cares about, she gets very angry and then can do things to hurt other people. Sometimes, she doesn't even remember what she has done in such a situation. We've seen this happen most recently when her mother came to visit unannounced, when those family friends visited, and when that girl at school asked her to say who is her best friend.

4. **These problems make what is most important to you worse. The way these problems can make what is most important to you worse is:**

Tanisha: These problems may interfere with your being able to finish school so that you can achieve your goal of becoming a teacher. Your record of aggression in school may also interfere with this goal.

Ms. Williams: These problems may make it hard for you to achieve your goal of protecting and supporting Tanisha.

5. **Here is what we will do to help:**

- Ms. Holmes will provide two visits a week. These will mainly occur at home, but sometimes will occur at school. We'll work on Tanisha's sensitivity to having to choose between people and will help support the two of you so you can best communicate with each other. We'll also arrange at least one school visit to observe Tanisha in school and with peers. This visit will include meetings with relevant teachers and the school psychologist to make recommendations of what will help.
- We will provide a medication follow-up visit with Dr. Edwards. When Tanisha saw Dr. Edwards for an evaluation during the assessment, we thought medications might be helpful for Tanisha's aggression (but were not absolutely necessary). Based on Ms. Williams's and Tanisha's preferences, we thought it made sense to try other ways of helping first. We believe it makes sense to have a reassessment within the next week or so.
- Mr. Martinez is a part of our team and he will work with Ms. Williams to provide support with her daughter and will certainly support the child welfare case plan.
- Dr. Edwards will advocate with the school to get a meeting to review Tanisha's educational plan.

6. **Here is what you will do to help:**

- Participate fully with all home-based sessions.
- Participate (Tanisha) in school observation visit.
- Participate in reassessment visit with Dr. Edwards.
- Ms. Williams will limit all visits with Tanisha's mother and will comply with the Agency for Child Welfare case plan.
- Ms. Williams will work with Dr. Holmes to set up school education plan meeting.

(continued)

7. If our treatment helps, you will know it in the following way:

Tanisha's behavior will be in much better control. She will feel better about her ability to be in control and will worry less about how her behavior may interfere with the possibility of becoming a teacher.

Ms. Williams will observe that Tanisha is much better able to control her behavior and will feel better about herself as a good parent. She will feel less sad and hopeless about the care she provides for Tanisha and will worry less about Tanisha's future.

8. If our treatment does not help, you will know it in the following way:

Tanisha will continue to have difficulty controlling her behavior at school and at home. She may be hospitalized again and may be asked to leave her school. Tanisha will feel very bad about herself that she can't control her behavior and will continue to worry about whether she will ever become a teacher.

Ms. Williams will continue to observe Tanisha's out-of-control behavior and continue to feel that she is a "bad" parent. She will continue to worry about Tanisha's future. It may become too difficult for Tanisha to remain in Ms. Williams's home.

9. Here is everyone's agreement:

Name	What I will do	How to reach me	Signature
Tanisha	Participate in visits at home and school visit. Participate in appointment with Dr. Edwards.		*Tanisha*
Ms. Williams	Participate in visits at home and appointment with Dr. Edwards. NO VISITS FROM DAUGHTER ALLOWED. Work toward school meeting with Ms. Holmes and with child welfare plan.		*Ms. Williams*
Mr. Carlos Martinez (ACW)	Work with Ms. Williams to support her with stress of managing her daughter. Make sure visits do not occur, as required within our service plan.		*Mr. Martinez*
Dr. Clarissa Holmes	Provide visits to home twice weekly to help Tanisha and Ms. Williams, particularly with communications between them and exposure to loyalty binds. Work with school on these issues, as well.		*Dr. Holmes*
Dr. Sam Edwards	Provide a reassessment of Tanisha's need for medication. Provide my best recommendation to Tanisha and Ms. Williams based on the results of my reassessment.		*Dr. Edwards*

Safety-Focused Guide

Helping to establish and maintain safety

Child's name _____ **Clinician's name** _____ **Date** _____

Anchoring Safety-Focused Treatment

1. *How will the child's overall treatment strategy be used in safety-focused treatment?*

_____

_____

_____

_____

_____

Implementing Safety-Focused Treatment

SECTION 1: ESTABLISHING SAFETY

Caring for Caregivers: As you go about the process of establishing safety, make sure to have a completed "Planning for Emergencies" from the HELPers Guide. Introduce "Handling the Difficult Moments" as a way of supporting caregivers who have difficulty managing their own emotions.

A safe-enough environment is defined by:

i. Caregivers who will *protect* their child from actual threats, and

ii. Caregivers who will *help* their child regulate dangerous survival states and *protect* their child from stimuli that provoke those dangerous survival states.

Step 1: Appraise whether the current environment is safe enough.

A. The Safe-Enough Environment Standard

What—at minimum—needs to be in place for the environment to be considered safe enough for the child?

_____

_____

_____

_____

_____

(continued)

B. The Current Evidence

What is the evidence that caregivers are currently providing a safe-enough environment (as defined above)?

_____

_____

_____

_____

_____

_____

What supports do caregivers rely on to provide the current level of safety (e.g., family, friends, service system interventions/supports)? How reliable are these supports?

_____

_____

_____

_____

_____

_____

C. The Realistic Appraisal

What do you conclude from the evidence about safety in the child's environment?

☐ At or above the safe-enough standard

☐ Below the safe-enough standard

Step 2: Develop the plan to establish a safe-enough environment.

You have decided that the child's environment falls below the safe-enough standard. This means, by definition, that there is risk for the child, or someone else, to be hurt in that environment. You need to work with all concerned to establish safety by bringing the environment to the defined safe-enough standard.

What is your plan to do this?

_____

_____

_____

_____

_____

_____

(continued)

442

What will be expected from anyone you need to implement the plan (e.g., caregivers, neighbors, providers in service system, TST team members)?

_____

_____

_____

_____

_____

_____

Step 3: Determine the risk to establishing safety in the current environment (with the safety plan).

A. Safety Plan Time Limit

Please rate the maximal time that you believe the safety plan should be attempted in the effort to bring the environment to the safe-enough standard, before you will conclude that it is too unsafe for the child to continue to stay in that environment: _____ days.

B. Safety Plan Confidence Level

Consider the strengths and limitations of all those caregivers/providers who are needed to successfully implement the safety plan. Based on this consideration, please rate your level of confidence that the safety plan will result in achieving the safe-enough standard within the defined time limit*: _____

1. *Very confident*: I am very confident that the safety plan will be implemented so successfully that it will result in the environment reaching the safe-enough standard within the defined time limit.

2. *Somewhat confident*: I am somewhat confident that the safety plan will be implemented so successfully that it will result in the environment reaching the safe-enough standard within the defined time limit.

3. *Hardly confident*: I am hardly confident that the safety plan will be implemented so successfully that it will result in the environment reaching the safe-enough standard, within the defined time limit.

4. *Not at all confident*: I am not at all confident that the safety plan will be implemented so successfully that it will result in the environment reaching the safe-enough standard within the defined time limit.

*Note: The rating for your level of confidence should consider the following factors for each caregiver/provider who is needed to implement the safety plan.

- His or her understanding of what is expected.
- His or her motivation to do what is expected.
- His or her ability to do what is expected.
- His or her track record of following through on other expectations.
- His or her track record of taking responsibility for problems he or she has caused related to safety in the environment.

(continued)

Justification of Confidence Rating:

Please provide the justification of your confidence rating, using the factors listed above:

_____

_____

_____

_____

_____

Confidence Level	Level of Risk to Establish Safety in the Current Environment
1	Manageable Risk The risk is manageable. Stick with the plan but monitor the keeping of agreements and the safety information carefully.
2	Marginally Manageable Risk You may not need to intervene immediately, but the situation poses a level of risk that is marginally manageable. If you are not able to devote a high level of vigilance to monitoring safety over the period of the safety plan time limit, you should bring the child to a safe-enough environment.
3	Unmanageable Risk The risk is unmanageable. You should bring the child to a safe-enough environment. In unusual circumstances the child could stay in the current environment for a very brief period of time while awaiting placement (within 1 day), as long as safety can be monitored very carefully within this time frame.
4	Critical Risk The child must be brought to a safe-enough environment immediately.

Step 4: Reach the decision on whether to keep the child within the current environment, based on the risk.

Consider the level of risk entailed by implementing the safety plan while the child remains in the current environment. Record your decision about the management of this risk.

☐ The risk is manageable enough. The child will stay in his or her current environment. We will work with all relevant parties to establish the Safety Plan written in section B. We will establish a safe enough environment within _____ days or we will bring the child to a safe-enough environment. Here is where we will bring the child if the Safety Plan is not effective within the Safety Plan Time Limit:

_____

_____

_____

(continued)

☐ The risk is not manageable enough. The child will be brought to a safe-enough environment. That environment is:

_____

_____

_____

Step 5: Reach the decision on whether (and under what conditions) to return the child to the environment, based on the risk (for children who have been placed in a new environment).

If the child is placed in a new environment because a safe-enough standard has not been reached, the TST team has two roles: (1) work with those in the child's previous environment to bring it to the safe-enough standard while the child is in placement (or to determine that a return to that environment is too risky), and (2) work with those in the child's new environment to make sure it is safe enough, given the child's vulnerabilities. In this section, we focus on the first role. In the maintaining safety section, we focus on the second. Only complete this section if the child is placed in a new environment.

Safety in the previous environment

What—at minimum—needs to be in place for the child's previous environment to be considered safe enough for the child to return to it?

_____

_____

_____

_____

_____

How can you work to support caregivers in putting these things in place?

_____

_____

_____

_____

Can these things be accomplished before the child is planning to return? If not, how will you communicate these concerns and to whom?

_____

_____

_____

_____

_____

(continued)

SECTION 2: MAINTAINING SAFETY

Caring for Caregivers: During this phase of maintaining safety, continue working with caregivers using the HELPers Guide. Continue working on "Handling the Difficult Moments" and introduce "Learning Parenting Skills." As always, keep the "Planning for Emergencies" section updated and on hand.

Activity 1: Clean out the cat hair.

What stressors, or cat hair, make it difficult for the child to stay regulated?

_____

_____

_____

What needs to be done to address this? Make a plan for each stressor, considering whether you need to help the child tolerate it (through introducing emotional regulation skills), reduce/eliminate it (possibly using advocacy tools), or both.

Stressor 1: _____

Plan: _____

Stressor 2: _____

Plan: _____

Stressor 3: _____

Plan: _____

Activity 2: Support emotional regulation.

A. Emotional Regulation Skill Introduction

Identify easy-to-implement strategies from Appendix 11. Monitor how they work for the child.

Emotional regulation skill	Notes about utility	Keep, modify, discard

(continued)

446

B. Psychopharmacology Plan

Consider a referral for psychopharmacology. Make notes here about any medications, dosage changes, or communications with a psychopharmacologist. Make sure the psychopharmacologist is aware of your assessment of, and interventions within, the social environment.

_____
_____
_____
_____
_____
_____
_____
_____
_____

C. Supporting the Child's Basic Health Needs

Review the categories below and make a plan to support the child's basic health needs where necessary:

Basic health needs	Concerns noted	Plan for intervention
Sleep: Is the child getting enough? Is it uninterrupted?		
Nutrition: Are the child's nutritional needs being met? Are unhealthy foods, including caffeine, appropriately limited?		
Health: Does the child have health problems that are not being attended to? Is the child getting sufficient physical activity in the day?		

(continued)

Activity 3: Advocate for needed services.

A. Define the problem that needs the intervention/service.

_____

_____

B. Identify the intervention/service the child needs for the defined problem.

_____

_____

C. Propose how the intervention/service should be used to address the defined problem, including:

The potential impact of the intervention/service on the child's functioning

_____

The potential impact on the child's functioning should the child not receive it

_____

The maximal time frame the child could wait to receive it, without significant impact on the child's functioning

_____

D. Engage the relevant organizations/providers who are responsible for delivering the intervention/service.

E. Evaluate the quality of this engagement, the implementation of the needed intervention/service, and the results of this implementation.

F. Adjust the plan based on these results.

HELPers Guide

Child's name _____ **Parent's name** _____ **Date** _____

All children and families go through difficult times. If you are reading this HELPers Guide, your family is going through one right now. This guide will give you some ways to help your family make it through this difficult time. This guide will help you with the following four areas:

1. **H**andling the difficult moments.
2. **E**njoying your child.
3. **L**earning parenting skills.
4. **P**lanning for emergencies.

Before we get started, here are a few things to know:

You are not alone! There is a team of people here to help you, your family, and your child make it through this difficult time. Here's who they are and how to contact them:

Name	Agency/role	Best way to contact

Also, you may have other people who are close to your child and who are also HELPers. The HELPers Guide can help them too. They are:

Name	Agency/role	Best way to contact

Finally, you are the most important person in your child's life. We are here to help you help your child.

(continued)

1. HANDLING THE DIFFICULT MOMENTS

When a child gets very upset, he or she can behave in ways that can be very difficult to be around. Sometimes a child says things or does things that are hurtful or scary. Sometimes it takes a lot of energy and patience to be around a child who gets easily upset.

- When a child gets upset, it is easy for a parent to get upset.
- When a parent gets upset, it is hard to do the things that you need to do to calm your child.

Staying calm when your child is upset can be hard, but there are things you can do that generally make it easier to stay calm (sort of like exercising gets you in shape for sports competition) and also some things you can do in the moment. Here are ways to "get in shape" for parenting in the difficult moments:

1. **Take a break!**

    It can be challenging taking care of a child who is having a lot of difficult emotions; making sure you can take a break will help you keep up the energy and patience you need to do your best job. Make a plan to give yourself some time away from your child:

2. **Take care of yourself.**

    Being a parent of a child who is having difficult emotions is like being a marathon runner; you need to take care of your body so you are in shape to go the distance. You need to get enough sleep, eat healthy foods, and avoid drugs and alcohol. Make a plan for how you can take care of yourself:

3. **Seek support.**

    Difficult times are when we need friends and supportive family the most, but sometimes we are so caught up in managing everything that we don't make time to get this support. Make a plan for seeing friends or supportive family members:

(continued)

Here is a **survive-the-moment** plan to help you when your child is in the midst of having a difficult time:

1. Is my child in danger (i.e., at risk to harm self or others, at risk to be harmed)?

   Yes → Go to the emergency plan at the back of this guide.

   No → Keep going.

2. Am I upset (e.g., angry, frightened, worried I might lose control)?

   Yes → Walk away and take 10 deep breaths, think a calming thought, or tense and release muscles in different parts of your body. Ask yourself again, "Am I calm?" Keep taking space and deep breaths or use other coping skills until you are calm.

   No → Keep going.

3. Offer help to your child.

   Make a plan with your child's therapist for how to help your child when he or she is upset and write it here. Keep track of what works best:

   ```
   
   
   
   
   
   
   
   ```

2. ENESTILL... JOYING YOUR CHILD

2. <u>E</u>NJOYING YOUR CHILD

Sometimes when a child is having difficulty, it is easy to forget the good times. But having good times is very, *very* important. Good times are what give everyone the strength and courage and love to make it through the difficult times.

Make a "good times" album here and in your head. Recall a time when you and your child had a good time together:

```




```

Make a mental picture of this good time, like a snapshot that you keep in your head. Try to pull this out a few times a day. If you can think of other good times, write them down. Try to stop every now and then and go through this "album" of good times.

(continued)

1. **Make a "good times" date.**

    Think of something your child particularly loves to do and that you could do with your child. Make a plan to do this together.

2. **Make a "good kid" slogan.**

    Go through the "My Kid" Adjectives list on page 455 and circle all that apply to your child. Pick your three favorites and make a statement:

    My child is _____, _____, and _____.

    Write this statement on cards and put it in a few places you will see during the day, such as in your wallet or on the refrigerator.

3. LEARNING PARENTING SKILLS

Living with a child who has challenging behavior can be difficult. Here are three basic principles of parenting that will help to make things go more smoothly in the home. Your child's therapist can help you come up with specific plans around how to do these things.

1. **Focus on the positive!**

    Children do more of whatever is noticed—good or bad! Usually bad behavior is easier to notice, but it is very important to notice when your child is doing something good as well. The more you notice and comment on your child when he or she is doing something good, the more your child will do that thing! Practice these two parenting strategies:

    a. Say something out loud when you notice your child doing something good. You can just observe the behavior, such as saying "I notice that you put your shoes away," or you can praise the behavior by saying, for example, "Great job! You put your shoes away, and it looks so nice to walk in the front door!" Set a goal for yourself about noticing good behavior and apply it every day.
    b. Use a reward system to create good habits. Sometimes when a child is not in the habit of doing something, providing an incentive to develop the habit helps. Incentives do not have to be big or expensive; sometimes a sticker, a later bedtime, or a special activity with you as a reward is enough!

    Pick a daily habit that you wish your child had, and that right now involves a lot of nagging from you, like doing homework, cleaning their room, or brushing their teeth. Work with your child's therapist to develop a reward plan to encourage the habit.

(continued)

2. Set clear, firm limits.

Children do best when they know what is expected of them, and when these expectations stay the same from day to day. Think about some areas that you and your child typically struggle around, like how much TV is permissible or how late the child can stay up.

Make a plan with your child's therapist for what you think the limits should be on these things, how you want to communicate them to your child, and how you will help your child respect those limits.

3. Have a plan for what to do if your child does something he or she shouldn't do.

All children do things that they shouldn't do sometimes. Parents need a plan for how to help their children learn not to do those things. Some parents take away privileges for a short period of time, some parents give children a "time-out" away from activity, some parents use "logical and natural" consequences (e.g., not replacing a toy the child breaks). The important point is that whatever you do does not shame or hurt your child. Work with your child's therapist to come up with a plan for what to do when your child does something he or she shouldn't:

These three skills will help make family life go more smoothly. Sometimes, however, children who have been through very stressful experiences have strong emotions in response to stressors or triggers. These are called "survival-in-the-moment states." At these times, some of the parenting strategies that *normally* work may not work. It is important to have a plan for these moments too. Go back to page 2 of this guide and review your survive-the-moment plan.

4. PLANNING FOR EMERGENCIES

When unexpected things happen, it can sometimes be hard to know what to do. When someone in your family is not safe, it is important to act right away. When something upsetting happens but no one is in danger, sometimes waiting to get advice or help is OK. *Knowing the difference between these two situations, and knowing what to do when unexpected things happen, can make everything run more smoothly.*

Work with your child's therapist to come up with examples of behaviors that are emergency life-threatening behaviors (e.g., child is in danger of hurting self or others; someone else is hurting child), emergency non-life-threatening behaviors (e.g., nonsuicidal self-harm behaviors such as cutting, substance use), and nonemergency dysregulated behaviors (e.g., temper tantrums,

(continued)

dissociative states with no risk of harm). Work with therapist to identify whom you should call or contact depending on the type of behavior (e.g., 911, people identified on front of guide) and what you can do to help keep your child safe (e.g., move to a safe environment).

	Emergency: Life-Threatening Behaviors	Emergency: Non-Life-Threatening Behaviors	Nonemergency: Dysregulated Behaviors
Describe behavior			
Whom can you call?			
What can you do?			

"My Kid" Adjectives

1. Enthusiastic		20. Sociable
2. Excited		21. Lively
3. Energetic		22. Upbeat
4. Passionate		23. Vivacious
5. Persistent		24. Fiery
6. Determined		25. Fearless
7. Diligent		26. Courageous
8. Tenacious		27. Curious
9. Ambitious		28. Smart
10. Focused		29. Bright
11. Bold		30. Inventive
12. Eager		31. Clever
13. Motivated		32. Spunky
14. Assertive		33. Entertaining
15. Self-assured		34. Spirited
16. Independent		35. Free-spirited
17. Confident		36. Unique
18. Outspoken		37. Sensitive
19. Outgoing		

Regulation-Focused Guide (RFG)

Helping to build children's emotional regulation skills

Child's name _____ **Clinician's name** _____ **Date** _____

Anchoring Regulation-Focused Treatment

1. *How will the child's overall treatment strategy be used in regulation-focused treatment?*

_____

_____

_____

_____

2. *What agreements about stabilizing the social environment need to be kept to enable regulation-focused treatment? How will you monitor these agreements?*

What is the agreement, and with whom is it made?	Why is it necessary?	Plan to monitor agreements

(continued)

Implementing Regulation-Focused Treatment

BUILDING AWARENESS

Activity 1: Clarify the problem.

Write the version of the TST priority problem used in the treatment agreement letter for the child.

_____

_____

_____

_____

Are you and the child still on same page about this problem? If no, write a revised problem here.

_____

_____

_____

_____

Activity 2: Explore the problem in different situations.

A. Select at least three Moment-by-Moment Assessment Sheets you have gathered about the TST priority problem.

B. Review each with the child (and caregiver, if appropriate).

C. Describe how the priority problem clarified in the previous section manifests in each of the situations assessed in the Moment-by-Moment Assessments.

_____

_____

_____

_____

D. Help the child (and caregiver, if appropriate) see the patterns of threat signals and survival states.

E. Make sure there is a good-enough shared understanding of the patterns to proceed to the next activity.

Activity 3: Understand how the problem happens (MEG—Step 1).

A. Introduce the MEG and describe how it works.

B. Use the information from different Moment-by-Moment Assessments to help the child see commonalities of their three A's and four R's in response to similar threat stimuli.

C. Help the child (and caregiver, if appropriate) complete Step 1 of the MEG.

Note: It may take several sessions to complete Step 1 of the MEG.

(continued)

Activity 4: Identify the earliest detectable warning signal (EDWS).

A. Ask the child to think about each episode at the time the revving state happened.

B. Ask if the child could remember the first thing he or she noticed that something was different—perhaps a feeling in the body, or a sight, sound, or smell.

C. Encourage the child to describe whatever comes to his or her mind, even if he or she thinks it is not relevant or important.

Write it down:

_____

_____

_____

_____

APPLYING AWARENESS

Activity 1: Identify the tools to use.

A. Go to the Strengths sections of the TST Assessment Form and TST Treatment Plan. What strengths might you use to help the child manage emotion? List them in the following table, and describe when you think they should be used (i.e., during regulating, revving, reexperiencing, or reconstituting).

B. Go to the regulation-focused exercises in Appendix 11. Select the exercises that you think will be particularly helpful for the child. List the exercises in the following table and describe when you think they should be used (i.e., during regulating, revving, reexperiencing, or reconstituting).

Child's strength to manage emotion		Regulation-focused exercise	
What is it?	When and how should it be used?	What is it?	When and how should it be used?

(continued)

C. Review your list of "tools" with the child and caregiver. Get their feedback and ideas. Identify if there are any new tools or approaches they might suggest.

D. Refine your "toolbox" based on that discussion.

Activity 2: Decide when to apply each tool (MEG—Step 2).

A. Introduce Step 2 of the MEG and describe how it works.

B. Help the child (and caregiver, if appropriate) complete Step 2 of the MEG, based on the "tools" identified in Step 1.

Note: It may take several sessions to complete Step 2 of the MEG.

Activity 3: Get ready to regulate.

A. Review Step 2 of the MEG with the child (and caregiver) and discuss how this may be implemented in different situations.

B. Consider role playing with the child (and caregiver) to test whether the activities specified in the MEG are practical enough.

C. Rehearse what the child and caregiver have agreed to do in Step 2 of the MEG to make sure they are as prepared as possible.

D. Direct attention to the regulation-focused exercises selected for use. Practice these exercises with the child and, when relevant, with the caregiver. Build these skills so they will be strong enough when needed.

E. Give child (and caregiver) homework to practice.

Note: Activity 3 will take at least three sessions.

Activity 4: Get it better.

A. Review the child's (and caregiver's) experience implementing the MEG.

Was there exposure to a threat stimulus at any point after the previous session and this one? What happened? Was Step 2 of the MEG implemented, as planned? Did it work as planned? Document these occasions in the table below.

Date	What threat stimulus was encountered?	What skill/approach was implemented from MEG—Step 2?	What was the result?

(continued)

B. Appraise whether the emotional regulation plan detailed in Step 2 of the MEG is working as expected.

If not, why not? _____

_____

C. Revise the MEG based on your appraisal.

D. Review the revised MEG with child (and caregiver).

SPREADING AWARENESS

Activity 1: List who is needed and the plan to engage them.

Complete the table below about everyone needed to implement the MEG, and the plan to engage them.

Name	What he or she needs to do	How we will engage him or her to do it

(continued)

Activity 2: Engage and enable others who can help.

Use the following table to document your efforts to engage and enable the people you need, and the results of your efforts.

Date	Person/ organization contacted	Nature of contact (e.g., phone call, meeting)	Results

Activity 3: Monitor whether it worked.

A. Review occasions when another person was expected to help the child, as specified in MEG—Step 2. Record results in the following table.

Date	What was expected of the other person?	What did he or she do?	Did it help?

B. Revise MEG—Step 2, based on the information of what other people did to help and the results.

(continued)

OTHER COMPONENTS OF REGULATION-FOCUSED TREATMENT

Psychopharmacology

If the child is in pharmacological treatment, make sure you understand what is occurring in that treatment so that you can best appraise the emotional reactions of the child, as some reactions may be related to medications and their effects.

Make sure your plans to build emotional regulation skills are well understood by the psychopharmacologist.

If the child is not treated with psychotropic agents and is not making expected progress regulating emotion, consider psychopharmacology evaluation.

Caring for Caregivers

Are the caregiver's emotional needs addressed sufficiently to participate in regulation-focused treatment? If not, update the TST Treatment Plan to address these needs, including referral to mental health providers.

Are the caregiver's practical needs addressed sufficiently to participate in regulation-focused treatment? If not, update the TST Treatment Plan to address these needs.

APPENDIX 10
Managing Emotions Guide (MEG)

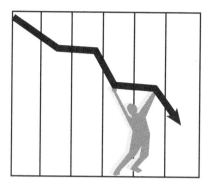

The MEG is a tool that helps children and families understand the ways they react when reminded of traumatic or really stressful events, or when they experience "triggers," and to help them use healthier strategies to handle strong emotions or behavior that is hard to control. The MEG will be used by you, your parents, your therapist, and the rest of the treatment team to break down events, piece by piece, and figure out what led to problems. As you can see from the Moment-by-Moment Assessment Forms and the Priority Problem Form, it is possible for you to go from being in a "regulated state" (where you feel calm and are in control) to getting extremely "dysregulated" (where you start getting upset and stop being in control of how you feel and how you act). The goal of the exercises you will learn in treatment is to practice being able to think more clearly in future situations, recognize triggers, and choose healthier ways to react when you are upset.

With your permission, copies of this guide can be given not only to your family, but also to anyone in your life who might be able to help you stay in control, whether it is a grandparent, social worker, teacher, or school counselor. Sometimes it is hard to realize that things going on around you can make you lose control. For that reason, your parents or caregivers can help you understand and manage strong emotions or intense reactions you might have when you get upset.

This first step of the MEG is to understand changes in your ability to be in charge of your emotions during times of stress or when you are triggered or reminded of bad things that happened in the past. The second step is to find things you can do when you get upset so that you can stay more in charge of your feelings and reactions.

(continued)

Managing Emotions Guide

BY:

FOR: (List everyone who should get a copy. Possibilities include YOU, therapist, parent, teacher, psychiatrist, home-based clinicians, and anyone else who you think knows you well and can help you when things get tough!)

MY PRIORITY PROBLEM I AM WORKING ON:

(continued)

STEP 1: UNDERSTAND YOUR EMOTIONS (<u>B</u>UILDING AWARENESS).

Usual State	Survival-in-the-Moment States		
Environment—Past	Environment—Past	Environment—Past	Environment—Past
Environment—Present	Environment—Present	Environment—Present	Environment—Present
Action Affect Regu-lating Awareness	Action Affect Revving Awareness	Action Affect Reexper Awareness	Action Affect Reconst Awareness
Regulating Being in control	**Revving** Getting upset	**Reexperiencing** Losing contol	**Reconstituting** Getting it back together again

Environment—Present: What was going on around you? What triggered your upset feelings?

Awareness: What are you thinking? What are you paying attention to? Are you spaced out?

Affect: What do you feel? What does your face show? What does your body feel like?

Action: What are you doing? What are you saying? What do you feel like doing?

(continued)

STEP 2: MANAGE YOUR EMOTIONS (<u>A</u>PPLYING AWARENESS).

Regulating Being in control	Revving Getting upset	Reexperiencing Losing contol	Reconstituting Getting it back together again
Things you can do to continue to feel good and in control	*Things you can do when you start to become upset*	*Things you can do to stay safe and keep yourself from losing control*	*Things you can do to calm down and fix any problems that happened when you lost control*
Things you can do			
Things an adult or friend can help you with			

Regulation-Focused Exercises

Tips and Tools for Building Emotion Regulation Skills

Once the MEG has been used to check in about the past week and to guide the first half of the session, the focus then shifts to introducing or practicing specific skills. The activities or skills can be tailored to the child's developmental level, personal interests, and needs. There are two primary types of skills that need to be built:

1. Emotion coping skills
2. Emotion identification skills

The next two sections detail the goals of each of these skill areas and provide examples of activities that encourage skill development.

1. EMOTION COPING SKILLS

Not all of the activities listed here are going to work with every child. Make sure you think about the child's developmental level and natural interests when selecting an activity. For instance, visualization techniques may be too quiet, demanding of the imagination, or difficult to focus on for some (particularly younger) children. If this is the case, try making the exercises shorter and more concrete. Some clients may not be comfortable closing their eyes. Younger clients may be able to engage in drawings that follow themes similar to the visualizations suggested below.

Relaxation

Relaxation skills are critical to help the child calm down, counteract physiological arousal, take a mental and behavioral "pause," and create an opportunity to shift an escalating trajectory. Learning to relax can also help a child gain a greater awareness of changes in his or her body, and to become more attuned to when his or her body is reacting to a stressor. Relaxation skills can encompass body movement, breathing, and visualization.

Relaxation Toolbox: Body Movement, Breathing, and Visualization Activities

Activity: Mirror

Skills: Body awareness, sense of control over body, mindfulness, physiological calming

Stand facing the client. Tell the child that you are each looking into a magical mirror, where each person is the other's reflection. Start by having the child make slow movements and mirror his or her body movements with your own body. After a few minutes, switch, so that the child follows yours. Then change again, with neither person identified as the lead—this time either person can make movements, and you both take turns without verbally telling the other when

(continued)

you are changing. Try making different emotional expressions and moving very slowly. Rules: No touching the mirror (the other person), use slow-motion movements, and make no sound.

Activity: Hand drawing

Skills: Body awareness, visualization

Place a blank piece of paper in front of both you and your client. Explain that you are each going to draw a picture of your own hands, and that you have to place your hand on the table in such a way that you can't see the paper while you draw. You may need to tape the paper down so that it doesn't move. Encourage your client to draw lots of details on the hand, like fingernails and knuckle wrinkles. When both of you have finished, look at the drawings you made. This is an important activity to participate in with your client, because usually the drawings are very silly looking. Rules: No peeking at the paper and keep your eyes on the hand you are drawing the entire time.

Activity: Strike a pose

Skills: Body awareness, sense of body control

Take turns having you or the client strike a pose. The other person has to mimic that pose. The initiator then has to comment on three things he or she notices about the pose (e.g., all your weight is on your left foot, it's hard to balance, and the world looks upside down!) before you can shift out and have the other person strike a pose. Try finding some poses that are more inward-focused (e.g., hugging your knees or placing your arms tight across your chest) and some positions that are very open (e.g., arms flung up and out or stretched toward the sky on tiptoes). Talk about the different feelings you have in each of the poses. Rules: The position has to be physically possible for both therapist and client!

Activity: Statue

Skills: Body awareness, collaboration, trust

Explain to the child that one of you is a great artist who is going to make a statue out of some magical putty. The putty is magical because it will move where you want it to move—without being touched! All the sculptor has to do is describe to the putty what to do. Unfortunately, the putty doesn't understand things unless the words are very specific; for instance, it won't respond to "Sit down"—you have to say "Bend the left knee, lower your bottom toward the floor, put the left foot on the floor. . . ." Take turns being the "sculptor" and the "putty" and talk each other into sculpture positions. The sculptor needs to tell the putty as specifically as possible how to move (e.g., "Take your left arm and move it up—now take your thumb and make it stick up, curl your other fingers into a fist"). The putty needs to listen carefully and respond very literally to the commands. Rules: No touching or inappropriate positions.

Activity: Being a noodle

Skills: Body awareness, muscle relaxation, visualization

Ask the child if he or she has ever seen a spaghetti noodle before and after it's been cooked. Talk about how stiff and rigid it is before, and how floppy and flexible it becomes. Then have the child act like an uncooked noodle (guide him or her verbally to tighten different muscles, stand stiff, and be as tight and rigid as possible). Talk the child through the cooking process, relaxing him or her as you go: "OK, the noodle is being put in a big pot of hot water. It's in there, and OH! It's starting to get sort of soft in the middle! It's bending a little bit at the middle . . . now up top

(continued)

468

it's getting a little floppy, relax your neck a little bit . . . now the arms are beginning to wiggle around a little bit . . . uh-oh, the legs are getting so soft I'm not sure they'll be able to hold the noodle straight anymore!" Continue in this fashion until the child is totally relaxed. Then let the child take a turn cooking you.

Activity: Connect to the universe

Skills: Body awareness, body control, sense of groundedness

Start by talking about how, thanks to gravity, it is virtually impossible not to be connected to the Earth. Explain that today we're going to see just *how* connected we can get. Start by observing how many different points of the body are touching the Earth just then (e.g., two feet on the ground, one bottom on the chair, an arm on the armrest makes four points). Then ask the child if he or she can make zero points touch the ground (e.g., by jumping). Ask the child to place one point down (e.g., one foot, one bottom). Keep increasing the number of points, until the child can't put any more points down. Talk about how different it feels when you have one point versus eight (or whatever limit was reached).

Activity: Walking and breathing (adapted from Linehan, 1993)

Skills: Control over body, physiological calming, breathing awareness

Begin by walking slowly around the room in pace with your client. Have the child count how many steps he or she is taking with each breath. After about five steps, ask the child to slow his or her breathing to three steps per breath. Continue gradually increasing the number of breaths per step until the breaths are long and slow, but not to the point of being forced.

Activity: Deep breathing

Skills: Physiological calming, breathing awareness, control over body

Have your client sit in a comfortable position or lie on the floor on his or her back. Have the child breathe normally, and verbally draw attention to the way the stomach and chest moves as he or she breathes. Start by commenting "Breathe in . . . breathe out" in time with the child's natural breathing pace. Gradually slow them down so that the child is pausing a moment at the top of the breath before slowly exhaling. Do this for about 10 breaths. For young children, place a stuffed animal on their abdomen and have them watch it move up and down with their breathing.

Addendum: Particularly for the child who finds deep breathing boring, it can be helpful to include a before and after "pulse test." Have the child find the pulse while he or she is breathing normally, and count the beats for 10 seconds. Multiply this number by 6 to get the pulse rate. Then complete the deep breathing and retake the pulse. Compare the numbers and see if the child was able to bring his or her heart rate down.

Activity: Favorite room

Skills: Distraction, self-soothing, mindfulness

Help your client visualize a room that feels safe and comfortable. Ask questions about what furniture and toys the child would put in the room. Who would he or she let come to visit in this room? What kinds of games would people play, or what would they talk about in the room? Are there windows? What is the view from the window? Are there pictures on the wall? What is in the pictures? Is there music playing? Make the child the queen or king of the room and be in control of the imaginary space.

(continued)

Activity: Four Seasons Mountain Meditation

Skills: Self-soothing, mindfulness, focus

Have the client sit comfortably, preferably in a cross-legged position (like a mountain). Ask him or her to think of a mountain, a beautiful mountain, real or imagined. Provide the child with a series of elaborations, such as "There is a stream that falls over some rocks on the mountain. What does the stream sound like? Imagine an animal drinking from the stream. What kind of animal do you see?" Include trees, the sky, and the ground. Ask about details that appeal to different senses, like temperature, bird, or wind sounds, or the feel of the ground under the feet. After the child has a sufficiently elaborate mountain in mind, say that fall is coming, and have the child imagine changes. Then bring in a winter storm and snowfall, and have the child imagine again how things change. Do this yet again for spring and summer, ending on an image that is full of life.

Affect Management

Another key area of coping skills, affect management, provides children with tools to calm themselves when they are upset. These skills are focused on in-the-moment activities that help to calm a child and prevent him or her from acting impulsively. Affect management skills include refocusing and self-coaching.

Affect Management Toolbox: Refocusing and Self-Coaching

Activity: My list of things I do

Skills: Refocusing

Work with parent and child to generate a list of things the child likes to do. Try to get them to really stretch beyond the usual (e.g., "I like to draw and watch TV"), and come up with an exhaustive list. Does the child like to skip down the hall? Sit on the top stair and watch the light coming in the window? Eat apples with the skin peeled off? Wash hands in hot water? Take a bubble bath? Try to come up with sensory activities. Have the child decorate the list or turn it into a poster, so that it can go up at home in a visible place. When the child is feeling upset, have him or her pick something off the list and do it, whether he or she feels like it or not. If the child is scientifically minded, you can have the child create a rating column next to the activities so he or she can rate how well they worked (or create a rating of how distressed the child is on a 1–10 scale before he or she tries it, and then after).

Activity: Affirmations (adapted from James, 1989)

Skills: Inserting a wedge of cognition, refocusing, positive self-talk

Collaborate with the child to find an affirmation, slogan, word, or phrase that he or she can repeat to self or visualize when having a hard time. For instance: "I am lovable"; "I am here to learn, and I don't have to get it right the first time—just try"; "I know people who believe in me." When a booster message has been selected, you can reinforce it by making banners, using puffy-paint on a T-shirt, or making a poster. Have the child practice saying it aloud as well as silently. When the child begins to get upset, encourage him or her to visualize the poster, or repeat the slogan in his or her mind 10 times.

(continued)

Activity: Imaginary school bus

Skills: Internalizing positive self-image, idea generation

Work with the child to generate a list of people who are supportive of the child, or who the child thinks would support him or her (e.g., superheroes or celebrity figures). Feel free to put yourself on the list, teachers, or anyone else the child might not think of who you suspect could be a supportive person. Then ask the child to visualize getting on a school bus and seeing each of those people in a seat. Help the child visualize this scene in a way that is easiest for him or her—by drawing a picture of the bus, putting names of people in seats (who would sit next to whom?), or closing his or her eyes and having you describe all the people in the bus. Have the child imagine which seat he or she would pick—near whom would the child sit? Have the child imagine that all the people on the bus want the child to sit next to them. If the child is having a specific problem (e.g., teasing from friends at school), ask the child to imagine the whole bus of people generating ideas of what he or she could do. What would Mom say? What would Katie Perry say?

Activity: Coach the therapist

Skills: Idea generation, self-talk

Talk with the child about a sports coach (the child may have one he or she admires, or you can talk about a hypothetical team coach). Talk about how a coach's job is to encourage and support team members, as well as to challenge them to do their best. Have the child imagine how a coach stands at the side of the basketball court, calling out encouragement and suggestions. Now suggest that the child be the coach, and you be the player. Pick a recent incident when the child was having a little trouble regulating emotions (e.g., having trouble staying in his or her seat at school). Do a role play, with you acting like the child (and verbalizing out loud your thoughts and reactions). Ask the child to play the coach and to stand on the sideline, yelling support and encouragement and providing suggestions and tips. If the child is having trouble playing the coaching role, switch roles and you be the coach, then switch back so the child has practice verbalizing the coaching. Suggest that the child can visualize his or her coach when next in school. You can refer back to this image later, asking questions like "What would the coach say?" when the child comes in with a new problem.

Activity: Bigger than a breadbox, or emotion continuum

Skills: Emotion identification, self-confidence, emotion regulation

This exercise works best when the child has had trouble regulating emotions in the past week and comes in with a specific incident to talk about (e.g., got in a fight at school when someone teased him or her). Ask the child to pick up a handful of rocks (or crayons, jelly beans, paper clips, or whatever small object you have on hand in large quantity) and make a pile to show how angry the child felt during that time. Then ask the child to think of another time he or she was angry, but a little less angry (place a smaller pile of rocks in front of the child). Ask how he or she coped with that time. Keep going down in size, until the child finally reaches a point where he or she tells a story about a time he or she was angry but successfully coped with it. Compare the two piles of rocks—one that represents how much anger the child felt when he or she successfully regulated him- or herself, and one that represents how much anger was felt when he or she was dysregulated. Point out that the child really *does* know how to regulate, and the trick will be gradually working on coping with more and more rocks (angry feelings) in successful ways.

(continued)

2. EMOTION IDENTIFICATION SKILLS

Being able to experience, identify, and express emotions forms the foundation for successful emotional regulation. These abilities are also essential for cognitive processing. Part of the goal of the regulation-focused phase is to make sure the child has the skills to experience, identify, and express feelings. If the child has trouble identifying his or her feelings when you go through the Regulation-Focused Guide, that's a good clue that you need to spend some time on these skills. You can do emotion identification skills interchangeably with emotion coping skills during the second half of the session; both types of activities reinforce the other.

We've divided emotion identification skills into two sections: (1) Observing and naming skills focus on helping the child become aware of his or her emotions and put words to the feeling. (2) Expressing feelings, on the other hand, focuses on ways of allowing that feeling to be shared with another person, or even fully experienced by oneself. For children who experience numbing or avoidance of feelings, these skills may form the central portion of the regulation-focused treatment work.

Observing and Naming Feelings

Observing and naming feelings are critical underlying skills for all emotion regulation work. In the course of using the MEG, children will become more familiar with observing their internal and external responses and putting words to those emotions. The process of playing and talking in session will frequently give rise to opportunities to explore how the child is feeling in the moment. Pausing in your activities to discuss physiological changes, action urges, and emotions provides the child with immediate feedback and practice in labeling feelings in the moment.

The therapist's own emotional responses provide another opportunity for modeling the process of observing and naming feelings. Particularly if a child appears to be attempting to elicit a certain emotion (e.g., anger) from you, it can be helpful to pause and identify for the child the fact that you are feeling that emotion, as well as how you plan to handle it. Using your own responses in session allows you to model that emotions are knowable and controllable, and that the child's actions have an effect on the environment.

In-session process work can be augmented by skill-building activities that help the child develop a vocabulary for, and understanding of, a wide range of emotions.

Expressing Feelings

Skills for expressing feelings can be divided into two groups: skills that allow a child to experience feelings (e.g., expressing them to self), and skills that help a child communicate these feelings with others. Expression of feelings skills can involve art, dance, music, writing, or any medium that resonates with that particular child. For some children who are especially numb to feelings, or who actively avoid anything that leads to certain physical sensations, activities that elicit different emotions and give them the chance to safely experience the physical sensations associated with feelings may be necessary.

Activities that help children experience emotions are most important for those children who avoid experiencing emotions, avoid situations that might lead to such emotions, or are numb to some or all emotions. They may not be appropriate for children who have difficulty controlling their anger. Skills involving communicating with others may also help increase children's social skills: How do you express your anger to someone through words, rather than fists? How can you communicate to someone else the different feelings you have about something?

(continued)

Emotion Identification Toolbox: Observing, Naming, and Expressing (ONE)

Activity: Emotion portfolio

Skills: Emotion identification, self-awareness, emotion vocabulary

Part 1: Emotion faces. On a piece of paper, trace or draw a large circle. Ask the child to name an emotion and draw a corresponding face. Have the child write the name of the emotion at the top. Do this for as many emotions as the child can think of (or until you have a range of basic emotions), each on a different sheet of paper. If there are any critical emotions missing (e.g., anger, fear), prompt the child by thinking about scenarios in which that feeling is likely to occur. If the child is having difficulty thinking of what the facial expression looks like for a particular emotion, take turns trying to act out that feeling and showing it on your face. You can also take this time to talk about how different people show emotions in different ways.

Part 2: "I feel [name of emotion] when. . . ." On the bottom of each emotion face page, write "I feel [name of emotion] when. . . ." Help the child brainstorm different activities or events that make him or her feel a certain way, and write these on the bottom of the face page. Some items may show up on more than one emotion face page. Point this out, and talk about how you can have more than one feeling about the same thing.

Part 3: Emotion words. On the back of each emotion face page, brainstorm a list of related emotion words. By taking turns with the child thinking of other related emotions, you can introduce the child to words that he or she may not know. Spend some time thinking together about how the different words might provide different information (e.g., *glad* vs. *joyful* vs. *content*), and making up scenarios where you (or a puppet, or a friend) might feel the different ways.

The emotion portfolio can be worked on and developed over time. New experiences or words can be added to the face sheets as you go. Ultimately, the different emotion face sheets can be collected and made into a book.

The emotion portfolio can also be adapted for different ages. Older children, for instance, may choose to do more abstract representations of feelings within the circle on the page. Younger children may need to have the face predrawn, and then they can participate by trying to guess the feeling depicted.

Activity: Emotional drama

Skills: Emotion identification, emotion vocabulary

Write a variety of emotion words on different slips of paper and put them in a hat. Hand a copy of "The Boring Script" (at the end of this appendix) to both you and the child. (The boring script can be the one provided in this book, something you have made up beforehand, or something that you write together. The idea is to have a script of a brief, neutral dialogue that the two of you can enact.) Read through the script together once, with each of you taking a role. Now have each of you draw an emotion from the hat, without showing the other. Reread the script, but this time each person enacts his or her role as if experiencing the emotion drawn from the hat. Try to guess each other's emotion, and give feedback about why you guessed that emotion.

Continue drawing slips with emotions named on them and reenacting the script until all of the slips have been drawn and the emotions enacted.

(continued)

Activity: The feelings interview (adapted from James, 1989)

Skills: Emotion identification, physiological awareness, normalizing

Provide the child with a set of about 10 sheets of paper that have the following format:

WHAT PEOPLE'S BODIES DO WHEN THEY ARE MAD			
Reaction	Yes	No	What Helps?
SHAKING			
GET HOT			
CRY			
FEEL SICK TO STOMACH			
GET TIGHT/TENSE			
OTHER			

Together, fill out the left column (the list of possible reactions to when someone is mad). Then ask the child to interview 10 people in the next week about times when they were mad and if they have ever had their body react a certain way (e.g., shaking). Also have the child ask what each person does to feel better. When the child brings the forms back, discuss how bodies respond to anger. You can do a similar activity for different feelings.

Activity: Basket of feelings (from James, 1989)

Skills: Identify feelings, understand mixed emotions, communicate feelings

Have the child come up with a list of feelings and write each one in large letters (or draw a face showing it) on a different piece of paper. Spread the paper out in front of you. Then show the child a basket with a bunch of things in it—a bunch of crayons, lots of little stones, jelly bellies, whatever comes in many little pieces. Model for the child bringing up a time when you had a strong feeling (e.g., when you had to give a talk in front of a bunch of people). Then for each feeling you had during that experience, place a handful of the objects—a big handful if you had a lot of those feelings, a little handful if you had a little. You might have lots of jelly beans on nervous and scared, and a few on excited, and one or two on confident. Then have the child do the same thing, either with his or her own emotional experience or a specific event that you are helping the child talk about. This activity can be done over and over during the course of treatment, to talk about how feelings change. It can also be used to help communicate to parents how a child feels about something.

Activity: Color your life (adapted from James, 1989)

Skills: Communicating emotions, identifying feelings

Have the child make a list of feelings, each in a different color. Then draw a large circle on a piece of paper, tell the child that the circle represents him or her right now, and have the child fill the circle in with colors that represent the different feelings. Then do this for other events in the child's life or for other people and how the child perceives his or her feelings about these different experiences/areas. You can have family members, and yourself, do this as well and compare the different perspectives on how people felt with the child.

(continued)

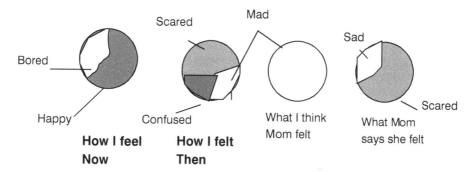

An alternative is to have the child color a timeline of his or her life, going from left (birth) to right (present). Then go back and have the child explain what events are represented by the different changes in color.

Activity: Name that feeling/name that tune

Skills: Identifying feelings, experiencing emotions

Bring in a selection of music (the child can as well). Take turns playing the music and being the "feeling actor." The feeling actor needs to decide what feeling a particular piece of music evokes, and then act it out (with facial expressions and body language). The other person needs to guess the feeling. Talk about whether listening to different types of music actually makes you feel different.

Activity: Stop everything and feel!

Skills: Identifying feelings, generating coping strategies

Write a story together, alternating lines or having the child dictate it (if the child can generate it on his or her own). Periodically ring a bell (or clap, bang a drum, etc.). Whenever the bell rings, the story stops and you answer the following questions: How is the character feeling? How can you tell the character feels that way? What can the character do next to let people know he or she feels that way? Does the character want to keep feeling this way? If not, what could the character do to change her feelings? When you've had a sufficient discussion about the character's feelings, ring the bell and let the story continue. The character does not have to take the advice you might have come up with during the discussion (e.g., does not have to express feelings to someone, or change the way he or she feels).

Activities: The last straw, sit and spin, and hearts up (adapted from Barlow, Allen, & Choate, 2005)

Skills: Experiencing emotions

Each of these activities is for children who avoid different physical sensations because they associate them with feeling upset. "The last straw" is for children who avoid feeling lightheaded or hyperventilate, "sit and spin" is for children who avoid feeling dizzy, and "hearts up!" is for children who avoid having their heart beat fast.

If a child is very avoidant of emotions, explain that you want to help the child get used to feeling different sensations in his or her body and learning that it's OK, nothing really bad happens. Talk about how everyone has different feelings all the time—like an itch, for instance—that are pretty normal. But if you get too focused on that feeling, or too scared that that feeling "means something" or is the beginning of something bigger and worse, then simply having that little itch

(continued)

475

can throw off your whole day. For some kids that "itch" might be their heart speeding up a little, or their head feeling a little light, or getting a little dizzy on the tire swing. Talk about how these are normal daily feelings that come and go, and that if a child is really avoiding one of them, or scared by one, it's good to get used to having it and not being afraid. Ultimately, you want the child to understand that the feeling itself isn't a problem and that sometimes that feeling is very manageable. The following activities can help a child experience whichever feeling he or she is avoiding in a safe, controlled way.

Sit and Spin. Have the child sit in an office chair that can spin. Ask the child to list any sensations noticed in the body, and any thoughts in their mind. "Can you feel your heart beat? Do you notice the speed of your breath?" Then tell the child that you are going to spin him or her around very fast in the chair, and you want the child to pay attention to see if there are any changes to the feelings, sensations, and thoughts just identified. Spin the chair long enough for the child's physiology to react, usually between 30 seconds and 2 minutes. Then stop the chair and ask the child the same questions you asked prior to spinning. "What has changed? Does the feeling in your body remind you of an emotion? Have you felt that way before? Have you ever done something to avoid feeling that way?" Help the child track how the feelings keep changing over time, gradually becoming less intense. Talk about "riding the wave" of emotion, and how there is a moment of peak intensity that is typically followed be a drop off. Once the child has "ridden the wave" back down, try another exercise to start another wave. If the child is reticent to do this, remind the child that this is different from other emotional experiences because here the child is literally in the "driver's seat" choosing to start the wave.

The Last Straw. Have on hand two drinking straws. Tell the child that you are both going to breathe through the straw for a while. First have the child note all the physical sensations, thoughts, and feelings he or she can identify. Do this again after breathing through the straw long enough to feel your own internal sensations change. Did the internal sensations remind the child of a feeling he or she has had before? Did the child notice his or her emotions change, or that emotions appeared? Talk about "riding the wave," as described in the exercise above. Now try a coffee straw. . . .

Hearts Up! For this exercise, follow the basic outline described above (having the child note his or her physical sensations, thoughts, feelings, etc.). Then pick a cardiovascular exercise—say, running in place, or running up the stairwell. As described above, have the child note changes in his or her feelings, changes in emotions, and talk about "riding the wave."

Activity: Feelings . . . are they really worth it?

Skills: Experiencing emotions

If some children are very resistant to the idea of experiencing emotions, you may need to start by helping them (and sometimes their parents) understand the value of emotions. Here are several situations you can pose to children. In each case, see if they can think of any important things that come out of having that emotion or physical sensation.

1. "The burner on the stove is hot, and you put your hand on it. What if you couldn't feel any pain? What might happen then? What does pain lead you to do?"
2. "You have a test at school at the end of the week and you haven't read the chapter yet. What if you don't feel anxious at all—what might you do? What might you do differently if you did feel anxious? How might reading the chapter change what you feel? How might reading the chapter change how you do on the test?"
3. "You borrow a friend's new shirt and get a big stain on it. What are some emotions you might

(continued)

feel? What might those feelings motivate you to do? Let's say you didn't have *any* feelings. Would that change what you did? Let's say you returned the shirt to the friend with the stain (even though you have enough money to buy the friend a new one, or even though you could have tried spot remover on it). How might that action affect your friend and your friendship?"

Then ask the child to think of other examples that show how emotions can be helpful: "Can you think of times when you had emotions that were helpful, or when having a certain emotion would have helped?"

Activity: Picture this (adapted from Barlow et al., 2005)

Skills: Experiencing emotions

Have a selection of photographs or magazine pictures on hand that evoke different emotions. Look at them with the child, and ask some questions to get him or her thinking about the image. "What is happening in the picture? What might the people in the picture be feeling? What are you feeling as you look at the picture?" If the child identifies a feeling, spend some time helping him or her describe that feeling and any associated thoughts or fears the child might be having related to that feeling. After the feeling has been explored, move to the next picture. At the end, reflect back on how those feelings were transient, how they could be changed, and how the child was able to tolerate all of those different feelings without anything bad happening. Pay attention to whether the child is trying to avoid experiencing emotions during this time, for example, by looking away from the pictures or trying to distract him- or herself. The child may need some encouragement to go ahead and really *feel*—you can remind the child about how sometimes feelings end up being helpful.

Activity: Avoiding avoidance (adapted from Barlow et al., 2005)

Skills: Experiencing emotions

This activity is designed for children who are avoiding some essential part of life in an effort to avoid becoming distressed. First identify the activity or setting that is being avoided, and talk about why that is an essential part of life. Examples include going to school (essential for learning, making friends, and achieving independence), riding in a car (essential for getting around), being in public (essential for being a part of one's community, doing other things one needs to do). Once you've picked an "avoided" activity to work on, help the child construct a list of ways you could start chipping away at doing that activity. For instance, if a child is avoiding getting in the car because he or she was in a car accident, the list might include:

1. Look at a picture of a car.
2. Look at a car.
3. Watch someone else drive around in a car.
4. Sit in the car with it turned off, then on.
5. Ride in the car for a short distance.
6. Ride in the car for a long distance. With the child, put the list in order from easiest to hardest. Working from the list, have the child start with the easiest activity and report on his or her emotions and physical sensations while engaged in the task: "How are you feeling? What are you thinking?" The key to this exercise is that the child has to stick with it until any wave of emotion has subsided. You may need to do the activity several times (show several pictures, or the same picture again and again) until the child's emotions get less intense, and the emotions dissipate faster. Then move to the second step on the list. Moving through the whole list may take several sessions.

(continued)

THE BORING SCRIPT

Following is a very boring script for use in the emotional drama exercise.

Setting: A donut shop.

CUSTOMER: Hello, I'd like to have a coffee, with milk, and a donut.

SALES CLERK: We're out of coffee.

CUSTOMER: Oh. Out of coffee? I'll just have tea then.

SALES CLERK: We're out of tea.

CUSTOMER: Oh. Well, could I just have the milk then?

SALES CLERK: Nope, no milk either.

CUSTOMER: What? No milk?

SALES CLERK: No milk. None at all.

CUSTOMER: Well, I guess I will just have the frosted donut.

SALES CLERK: We're out of donuts.

CUSTOMER: You are out of donuts?

SALES CLERK: Yup. Out.

CUSTOMER: Well, OK, I guess I'll have to go somewhere else. Is there anywhere else I can go around here for a cup of coffee and some donuts?

SALES CLERK: Out the door and to the left. Third door down.

CUSTOMER: Thanks. Goodbye.

SALES CLERK: Have a nice day.

(We *told* you it was boring . . .)

Beyond Trauma Guide

Helping Children Move into a Safe and Healthy Future

Child's name _____ **Clinician's name** _____ **Date** _____

ANCHORING BEYOND TRAUMA TREATMENT

1. *How will the child's overall treatment strategy be used in regulation-focused treatment?*

_____

_____

_____

_____

2. *What agreements about stabilizing the social environment need to be kept in order to enable beyond trauma treatment? How will you monitor these agreements?*

What is the agreement, and with whom has it been made?	Why is it necessary?	Plan to monitor agreements

3. *What regulation-focused skills have been the most useful for the child, and could be called on again?*

_____

_____

_____

_____

(continued)

IMPLEMENTING BEYOND TRAUMA TREATMENT

Step 1: Strengthening Cognitive Skills

A. Review the CAL related to any stressful events or situations from the last week. If the child did not complete a CAL for that event or situation, fill one out together.

B. Using the CAL, identify potentially unhelpful cognitions and the child's level of awareness: What thinking traps did the child fall into? Is the child able to challenge them? Can the child identify positive thoughts and more helpful cognitions?

Step 2: Telling Your Story: The Trauma Narrative

Note: This section of the intervention is begun ONLY when the child's cognitive restructuring skills are strong.

A. Are the child's cognitive skills sufficiently mastered that he or she is able to easily complete the CAL and demonstrates consistent success in applying skills to real-world situations? If not, remain focused on cognitive skill building in session. If yes, continue.

B. Identify whether "Trauma Narrative: Specific Event" or "Trauma Narrative: Chronic Trauma" is indicated (see the final section in this appendix, "Trauma Narrative Type," for these two categories of possible narratives).

C. Identify the child's strengths in communication, the preferred medium for the child's narrative construction, and the most appropriate approach for the narrative construction (e.g., collage, poetry, cartoons).

D. Work in session to develop the trauma narrative.

E. Once the narrative is complete, move to cognitive processing of it.

F. See "Step 5: Nurturing Parent–Child Relationships," on page 483.

Step 3: Reevaluating Needs

A. Conduct a reassessment of the child's social-emotional needs. This should be done at the beginning of beyond trauma treatment and in any further assessment or intervention throughout treatment to make sure these needs are being addressed.

Consider the following chart:

Area	Not a concern	Needs further assessment	Needs intervention
Attention disorder			
Executive function problems (e.g., problems in organization, planning)			
Oppositional disorder/conduct problems			
Developmental disorders			
Cognitive limitations			
Learning disorders			
Social skills			

(continued)

Area	Not a concern	Needs further assessment	Needs intervention
Psychotic processes			
Substance abuse			
Other (specify)			
Other (specify)			

B. For all areas identified as in need of further assessment, create a plan for either further evaluation by the TST team or for referral to outside provider for specialized evaluation:

_____
_____
_____
_____
_____
_____

C. For all areas identified as in need of intervention, create a plan for either additional treatment foci under the TST team or for referral to outside provider for specialized intervention:

_____
_____
_____
_____
_____
_____

Step 4: Orienting to the Future

A. Are the trauma narrative and associated cognitive processing components completed? If not, return to the narrative and determine if (a) additional traumatic events need detailing, or (b) additional detail and processing need to be added to the current narrative. If yes, continue.

B. The self as worthy of healthy, intimate relationships.

How does the child see him- or herself?

_____
_____
_____
_____
_____

(continued)

Identify any unhelpful or inaccurate elements of the child's self-image.

_____

_____

_____

_____

C. Help the child complete a CAL for the above. Focus on the "thinking" and "feeling" aspects of the CAL, rather than the "situation" or "what I did" sections.

D. Working toward life goals.

What progress has been made toward the child's achieving his or her goals?

_____

_____

_____

_____

What more needs to be done for the child to achieve his or her goals?

_____

_____

_____

_____

What is the plan to continue facilitating the achievement of these goals for the future?

_____

_____

_____

_____

Are there any new goals that the child wants to set now?

_____

_____

_____

_____

What is the plan to meet these new goals?

_____

_____

_____

_____

(continued)

Step 5: Nurturing Parent–Child Relationships

A. Assess caregivers' understanding and perspective of the trauma. If any of the following concerns are noted, make a plan for addressing them (e.g., individual sessions with provider, referral to outside provider):

Area of concern	Yes	No	If yes, plan for addressing:
Does parent blame child?			
Does parent become emotionally overwhelmed and distraught when discussing the trauma?			
Does parent believe child's story?			
Does parent believe that talking about the trauma is unhelpful or unnecessary?			
Does parent demonstrate any unhelpful or inaccurate thoughts about the trauma?			
Any other concerns?			

B. Once the caregiver demonstrates the necessary skills for supporting the child, hold joint sessions for child to share trauma narrative with him or her.

Step 6: Going Forward

A. One of the most critical aspects of this step is to *go forward* without treatment. Set aside time to talk about it—even though it may be difficult. Recall the three basic steps of termination:

Anticipate the goodbye early.

Acknowledge the meaning of the work.

Acknowledge the meaning of the relationship.

Date planned for termination:	Date in advance of this when discussion of termination to begin:	Strategies for discussing termination and timeline:

(continued)

B. In addition, recall that as a child leaves the work with *you*, he or she is also continuing his or her engagement with the world beyond. Take some time to talk with the child about what needs to be in place to continue supporting the child toward his or her life goals:

People and places that support child in life goals:	Already in place?	Barriers to keeping or putting in place?	Plan to overcome barrriers

TRAUMA NARRATIVE TYPE

Trauma Narrative: Specific Event

Chapter 1: All about Me The therapist should introduce the book with nonthreatening questions. Following are suggested topics to ask about: Things the child likes about him- or herself Things he or she is good at Favorite food Favorite color Favorite TV show Person he or she is closest to His or her best friend	**Goals of Chapter 1:** Introduce the book, help the child become comfortable writing about him- or herself through easy, familiar topics. **Notes:**
Chapter 2: My Family Who are the people in the child's family? Who does the child live with? What does his or her home look like? Who are the people who take care of him or her? Who does the child get along with the best? What does he or she like about his or her family? What doesn't he or she like?	**Goals of Chapter 2:** Introduce key players and discussion of both positive and negative aspects of a child's life. Depending on the child's situation, this chapter may already delve into difficult territory. In this case, adding questions about supportive people outside the family will be important. **Notes:**

(continued)

Chapter 3: Something Bad Happened to Me **For first two sessions:** Facts about the traumatic event (who, what, when, where, why) Does child remember sights, sounds, smells? Does child remember what he or she said or did? Who else was involved? What did he or she say and do? **Next two sessions:** What was the child thinking and feeling during the traumatic event? What did the child's body feel like? Are there parts of the event that he or she can't remember? What does the child say other people were thinking and feeling during the event? What was the worst part? What does child wish would have happened instead?	**Goals of Chapter 3:** The goal of Chapter 3 is to help the child recall and begin to verbalize what happened during the traumatic event. The therapist should plan to spend at least four sessions working on this chapter with the child. **Notes:**
Chapter 4: Things Changed After the Bad Thing Happened The therapist should help the child describe things that may have changed immediately after the traumatic event as well as over time (e.g., removal of perpetrator from home, mother became depressed, moved to a new location).	**Goals of Chapter 4:** This chapter can help a child explore the many different ways that the trauma may have affected his or her life—for better or for worse. On the positive side, there may be people who stepped up to help, or changes that led to greater safety. It's also possible that the traumatic event led to grieving, problems at school, or new difficulties at home. In writing this chapter, it may become evident that the child should write another book focusing on other traumatic events. **Notes:**
Chapter 5: Some Things Stayed the Same After the Bad Thing Happened The therapist should help the child describe things that have remained consistent since the traumatic event. These can be both positive and negative (e.g., child still does well in school, child still enjoys playing basketball, child still argues with siblings).	**Goals of Chapter 5:** This chapter is useful in helping the child feel reassured that, amidst all of the changes that may have taken place since the trauma, he or she can count on a number of things to remain the same. **Notes:**

(continued)

Chapter 6: People Who Care about Me The therapist should help the child list as many people as possible that he or she can rely on (the therapist should remember to add him- or herself to the list if the child forgets). The list can include family, friends, teachers, guidance counselors, clergy, as well as religious/spiritual figures. **Chapter 7: What I Can Do to Protect Myself in the Future** The therapist should help the child generate a list of possible safety measures that he or she could take in the event that something like this were to happen again. It is obviously important to strike a balance between providing the child with a sense of an internal locus of control while not inadvertently sending a message that the child is to blame for what happened. **Chapter 8: Skills I Have Learned to Use When My Bad Thoughts Get in the Way** The therapist should help the child describe coping skills that he or she has learned in therapy, including thought stopping, using positive self-statements, engaging in enjoyable activities, and talking to a trusted adult/friend.	**Goals of Chapters 6–8:** The next set of chapters serves to help the child identify supports and strengths in his or her life—both what other people bring to the child, as well as what the child has learned him- or herself. The goal of these chapters is to help the child feel empowered, as well as to review the skills covered in earlier therapy sessions. **Notes:**
Chapter 9: What I Learned from the Bad Thing The therapist should help the child reflect on any positive life lessons that may have resulted from the traumatic event. If the child has trouble, the therapist can ask what he or she would say to someone who just experienced the same traumatic event. What advice or wisdom would he or she give to the person? **Chapter 10: My Future Is Bright** The therapist should have the child describe what he or she hopes to do in the future (e.g., career goals, family aspirations, travel). The therapist should help the child generate steps that he or she can take, beginning right now, to reach his or her goals.	**Goals of Chapters 9–10:** The final chapters are meant to empower the child and help him or her recognize that the traumatic event does not have to define the child's identity or future self. As the child is working on his or her book, it will be important to share the child's progress with the caregiver. This is done to ensure that the caregiver is kept up to date with the child's trauma processing, to provide an opportunity for gradual exposure with the caregiver alone, and to assess the caregiver's thoughts and feelings with regard to the trauma. **Notes:**

(continued)

Trauma Narrative: Chronic Trauma

Chapter 1: All about Me Same as above version. **Chapter 2: My Family** Same as above, with additional questions if the child is having trouble defining *family*: "There's no one definition for what a family is, so there's no right or wrong answers here. What do you think *family* means? What is the job of a family? Does anyone do that for you? Do you think families stay the same, or do they change? Can you think of families that look different from one another, but are both still families? What makes each of them a family?"	**Goals of Chapters 1 and 2:** Same as above. Note that for children who have experienced many changes in who they live with, it may be hard to define *family*; some sample questions to help the child decide who should go in this chapter are provided. **Notes:**
Illustration 1: My Timeline The therapist can help the child draw a timeline with all of the important events of his or her life. It can help to start with a blank page with "My Birth" on the far left side of the page and "Today" on the far right side of the page. Explain how a timeline works, and ask the child to put important events along it. You may need to help younger children sequence things as they go. The child can decide what is important. After the child has filled in all that he or she can think of, ask some probe questions. Has the child always lived with the same caregivers or in the same city? If not, make sure these changes get noted. Has the child lost anyone important to him or her? Did anything upsetting happen? Did anything really good happen? By this time, the therapist usually knows if there are certain events that were important parts of the child's history and can ask appropriate probes to help the child acknowledge and sequence these things.	**Goals of Timeline:** The goal of this exercise is both to help the child begin the process of putting order to his or her life events, as well as for you to learn which life events are most salient to the child. If a child seems to be avoiding some important events (e.g., there is no mention of when child was taken from parents and placed in foster care), it will be important to introduce this event and help the child acknowledge and place it on the timeline. **Notes:**
Chapter 3: When I Was a Baby In this chapter the therapist helps the child to assemble facts known from infancy and early childhood. This section will largely rely on what the child has heard from others, and may also include questions that are unanswered. Some areas to ask about include: Facts about the child's birth—who took care of the child, where he or she lived	**Goals of Chapters 3–5:** In this set of chapters, the therapist helps the child begin to verbally sequence events and to make his or her life story into a narrative. Children who have had very inconsistent caregiving may have more questions than answers.

(continued)

Who were important people in the child's life when he or she was a baby?

What has the child been told about their infancy and early childhood? What was the child told they were like as a baby?

- What has the child been told about what his or her mom and dad were like back then?
- What does the child know about other caregivers he or she had during that time?

Facts about important events that took place during the child's infancy and early childhood

The therapist can also ask the child what he or she wishes he or she knew knew about his or her life as a baby, or what he or she imagines things would have been like (see the following examples): "What sorts of things do you think would have been scary to you when you were a baby? What sorts of things do you think you would have liked to do when you were a baby? What made you special as a baby?

Have the child write down questions he or she wants to know the answer to.

Chapter 4: When I First Went to School

In this chapter, the therapist helps the child put together a narrative about their school years. They should include facts about going to school (age, where he or she was living, name of school, who he or she lived with then). The therapist can help the child reflect on what he or she was like in school, what he or she enjoyed or disliked about school. Then move to questions that may be more difficult, such as:

What kinds of things were scary to you back then?

What was it like to come home after school? What kinds of stuff did you do at home? Who else lived with you in your home? What kinds of stuff did they do?

What are some important things that happened when you were just starting school?

Who were the important people in your life back then? (Look back at the list of important people from when the child was a baby—were those people still important?)

Chapter 5: My Life Today

Here the therapist helps the child organize a narrative about his or her current life, building from the past. This should include facts about the child's life today (How old is he or she? Where does he or she live? Who does he or she live with? Where does he or she go to school?).

The time frame you pick to help the child build the chapters should be changed depending on how the child remembers events—for instance, instead of "When I Started School," you might choose to call the chapter "When I moved to Grandma's House." Regardless of the timelines, an important thread to follow through the child's life is important people—who is still there, who has left.

Notes:

(continued)

488

How is his or her life different now than when he or she had just started school? How is it different from when he or she was a baby? How is his or her family different? How is his or her home different? How is he or she different? The therapist should also strive to help the child identify strands of continuity. What aspects of his or her life or self have remained the same over time?	
Chapter 6: Best and Worst, Hopes and Fears In this chapter the therapist helps the child articulate which life events punctuated his or her life in the most important ways. The therapist can use some of the following questions to guide the conversation: Looking back over the last chapter and your timeline, what were the best times? What made them the best? What were the worst times? What made them the worst? Looking ahead, what do you hope will happen in your life? What would you like to see happen tomorrow? Next year? Five years from now? When you are a grown-up? What about worries—do you have any fears or worries about what will happen in the future? What do you worry about for tomorrow? Next year? Five years from now? When you are a grown-up?	**Goals of Chapter 6:** This chapter asks the child to reflect back on the life events he or she has ordered and identify the most difficult times—and the best times. The second half of the chapter—hopes and fears—orients the child toward the future. **Notes:**
Illustration 2: My Support Tree In this section, the therapist helps the child draw something called a *support tree* (or the child draws it on his or her own). The support tree is like a family tree, only in this tree all the different kinds of people who are supportive toward the child are listed: family the child lives with, family the child doesn't live with, friends, and mentors. Go through each category with the child and help him or her think of who is supportive, and then have the child list each person on the tree. During this time, the therapist can also ask about people who used to be important but are not on the support tree. **Chapter 7: People Who Care about Me** The therapist can help the child write about the people on the support tree. Who helps with what kinds of problems? Who does the child trust and talk to?	**Goal of illustration 2 and Chapter 7:** The goal of these sections is to help the child identify supports in their life. **Notes:**

(continued)

Chapter 8: What I Have Learned from the Tough Times	Goals of Chapters 8 and 9:
The therapist should help the child describe coping skills that he or she has learned in therapy, including thought stopping, using positive self-statements, engaging in enjoyable activities, and talking to a trusted adult/friend. The therapist should help the child think of what he or she would tell someone else who was having a tough time. **Chapter 9: My Future Is Bright** The therapist should have the child describe what he or she hopes to do in the future (e.g., career goals, family aspirations, travel). The therapist should help the child generate steps that he or she can take, beginning right now, to reach his or her goals.	Chapter 8 helps the child to be the expert on him- or herself and the life experiences described, and to reflect on what he or she has learned. Chapter 9 orients the child to the future; you can even add a future timeline, so that the child can imagine events that he or she hopes will happen in the future.

Cognitive Awareness Log (CAL)

Meet detective CAL! CAL can help you get through challenging situations. After you've had a stressful or difficult time with something, think through the situation with CAL. First, answer these questions:

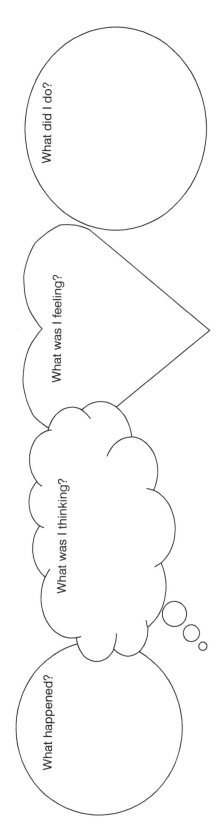

What happened?

What was I thinking?

What was I feeling?

What did I do?

Now help detective CAL think it through. Talk through your answers to his questions.

- What, exactly, happened in the situation? "Just the facts, ma'am."
- Have you ever been through a similar situation? What happened?
- Have you ever had a similar thought? What happened?
- Now consider the thought you have about this situation. What is the evidence for it being true? What is the evidence that things could be different?
- What is an alternative, more calming thought that could be true about this situation?

(continued)

Cognitive Awareness Log *(page 2 of 3)*

CAL to the Rescue!

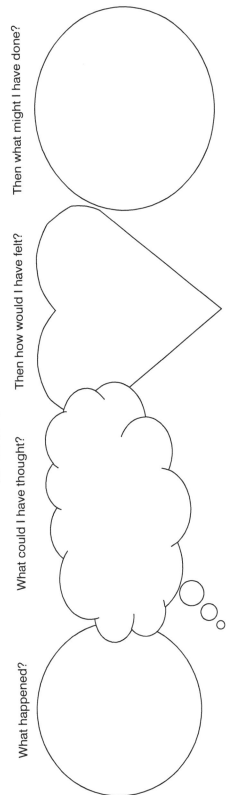

What happened?

What could I have thought?

Then how would I have felt?

Then what might I have done?

Remember that how you *think* about things changes how you *feel.* Sometimes there are more accurate, helpful thoughts that are true about a situation. Catching unhelpful thoughts and replacing them with helpful thoughts can make everything go more smoothly.

The next time you find yourself having a worrisome, angry, or unhelpful thought, ask yourself "What would CAL say?"

(continued)

Thought Stopping with CAL

Sometimes people have unwanted thoughts that pop into their head—upsetting images, memories, or thoughts about terrible things that happened in the past. If these thoughts get in the way of your being able to do what you need to do, thought stopping could help. Thought-stopping strategies are ways of immediately distracting yourself from the unwanted thoughts. You and your therapist can come up with some different strategies to try.

When this kind of thing happens . . .

and I have unwanted thoughts like this . . .

then I will put a STOP to that thought by doing this:

How did it work?

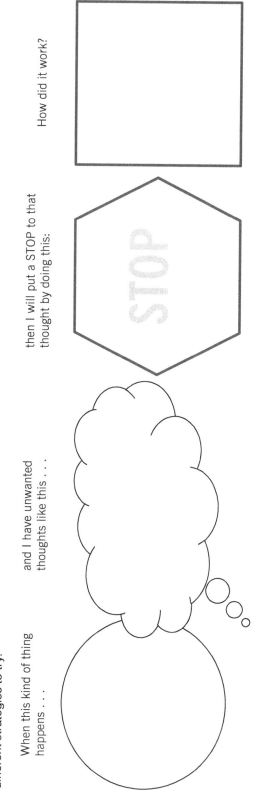

References

Albano, A. M., & DiBartolo, P. M. (2007). *Cognitive-behavioral therapy for social phobia in adolescents: Stand up, speak out therapist guide.* Oxford, UK: Oxford University Press.

American Heritage Dictionary (4th ed.). (2000). Boston: Houghton Mifflin.

Barlow, D. H., Allen, L., & Choate, M. L. (2005). *The unified protocol for treatment of the emotional disorders.* Unpublished manual, Boston University.

Beck, A. T., Rush, A. J., Shaw, B. F., & Emery, G. (1979). *Cognitive therapy of depression.* New York: Guilford Press.

Bowlby, J. (1979). On knowing what you are not supposed to know and feeling what you are not supposed to feel. *Canadian Journal of Psychiatry, 24*(5), 403–408.

Bronfenbrenner, U. (1979). *The ecology of human development.* Cambridge, MA: Harvard University Press.

Bronfenbrenner, U., & Ceci, S. J. (1994). Nature–nurture reconceptualized in developmental perspective: A bioecological model. *Psychological Review, 101*(4), 568–586.

Chemtob, C. M., Griffing, S., Tullberg, E., Roberts, E., & Ellis, P. (2010). Screening for trauma exposure and posttraumatic stress disorder and depression symptoms among mothers receiving child welfare preventive services. *Child Welfare, 90*(6), 109–127.

Chess, S., & Thomas, A. (1991). Temperament and the concept of goodness of fit. In J. Strelau & A. Angleitner (Eds.), *Explorations in temperament* (pp. 15–28). New York: Springer.

Cohen, J. A., Mannarino, A. P., & Deblinger, E. (2006). *Treating trauma and traumatic grief in children and adolescents.* New York: Guilford Press.

Cohen, J. A., Mannarino, A. P., & Deblinger, E. (2012). *Trauma-focused CBT for children and adolescents.* New York: Guilford Press.

Damasio, A. (1999). *The feeling of what happens: Body and emotion in the making of consciousness.* Fort Worth, TX: Harcourt College.

Darwin, C. R. (1859). *On the origin of species by means of natural selection, or the preservation of favoured races in the struggle for life.* London: John Murray.

Deblinger, E., & Heflin, A. H. (1996). *Treating sexually abused children and their nonoffending parents: A cognitive-behavioral approach*. Thousand Oaks, CA: Sage.

Donnelly, D. A., & Murray, E. J. (1991). Cognitive and emotional changes in written essays and therapy interviews. *Journal of Social and Clinical Psychology, 10*(3), 334–350.

Dweck, C. S. (2006). *Mindset: The new psychology of success*. New York: Random House.

Esterling, B., L'Abate, L., & Murray, E. J. (1999). Empirical foundations for writing in prevention and psychotherapy: Mental and physical health outcomes. *Clinical Psychology Review, 19*(1), 79–96.

Felitti, V. J., Anda, R. F., Nordenberg, D., Williamson, D. F., Spitz, A. M., Edwards, V., et al. (1998). Relationship of childhood abuse and household dysfunction to many of the leading causes of death in adults. The Adverse Childhood Experiences (ACE) Study. *American Journal of Preventative Medicine, 14*(4), 245–258.

Finkelhor, D., Turner, H., Ormrod, R., Hamby, S., & Kracke, K. (2009). *Children's exposure to violence: A comprehensive national survey*. Washington, DC: U.S. Department of Justice, Office of Justice Programs, Office of Juvenile Justice and Delinquency Prevention.

Frankl, V. E. (1962). *Man's search for meaning: An introduction to logotherapy*. Boston: Beacon Press.

Henggeler, S. W., Schoenwald, S. K., Borduin, C. M., Rowland, M. D., & Cunningham, P. B. (1998). *Multisystemic treatment of antisocial behavior in children and adolescents*. New York: Guilford Press.

Henggeler, S. W., Schoenwald, S. K., & Pickrel, S. G. (1995). Multisystemic therapy: Bridging the gap between university and community-based treatment. *Journal of Consulting and Clinical Psychology, 63*, 709–717.

Herman, J. (1997). *Trauma and recovery*. New York: Basic Books.

James, B. (1989). *Treating traumatized children: New insights and creative interventions*. New York: Free Press.

Karpman, S. (1968). Fairy tales and script drama analysis. *Transactional Analysis Bulletin, 7*(26), 39–43.

Kassner, B., & Kharasch, S. (1999). *Prevalence of violence exposure in adolescents who present to an emergency room*. Unpublished manuscript.

Kennedy, W. B. (1940). A review of legal realism. *Fordham Law Review, 9*(3).

Kurzweil, R. (2012). *How to create a mind: The secret of human thought revealed*. London: Penguin.

LeDoux, J. (1998). *The emotional brain: The mysterious underpinnings of emotional life*. New York: Simon & Schuster.

LeDoux, J. (2002). *Synaptic self: How our brains become who we are*. New York: Viking.

Linehan, M. M. (1993). *Cognitive-behavioral treatment of borderline personality disorder*. New York: Guilford Press.

March, J. S., Amaya-Jackson, L., Murray, M. C., & Schulte, A. (1998). Cognitive-behavioral psychotherapy for children and adolescents with posttraumatic stress disorder after a single-incident stressor. *Journal of the American Academy of Child and Adolescent Psychiatry, 37*, 585–593.

Ostroff, L. E., Cain, C. K., Bedont, J., Monfils, M. H., & LeDoux, J. E. (2010). Fear and safety learning differentially affect synapse size and dendritic translation in the lateral amygdala. *Proceedings of the National Academy of Sciences of the United States of America, 107*(20), 9418–9423.

Panksepp, J. (1998). *Affective neuroscience: The foundations of human and animal emotions*. New York: Oxford University Press.

Pennebaker, J. W., & Francis, M. E. (1996). Cognitive, emotional and language processes in disclosure. *Cognition and Emotion, 10*(6), 601–626.

Perry, B. D., Pollard, R. A., Blakley, T. L., Baker, W. L., & Vigilante, D. (1995). Childhood trauma, the neurobiology of adaptation, and "use-dependent" development of the brain: How "states" become "traits." *Infant Mental Health Journal, 16,* 271–291.

Perry, R., & Sullivan, R. M. (2014). Neurobiology of attachment to an abusive caregiver: Short-term benefits and long-term costs. *Developmental Psychobiology, 56*(8), 1626–1634.

Pynoos, R. S., & Nader, K. (1988). Psychological first aid and treatment approach to children exposed to community violence: Research implications. *Journal of Traumatic Stress, 1*(4), 445–473.

Saxe, G. N., Ellis, B. H., Fogler, J., & Navalta, C. P. (2011). Innovations in practice: Preliminary evidence for effective family engagement in treatment for child traumatic stress—trauma systems therapy approach to preventing dropout. *Child and Adolescent Mental Health, 17*(1), 58–61.

Saxe, G. N., Ellis, B. H., & Kaplow, J. B. (2006). *Collaborative treatment of traumatized children and teens: The trauma systems therapy approach.* New York: Guilford Press.

Saxe, G. N., Liebschutz, J. M., Edwardson, E., & Frankel, R. (2003). Bearing witness: The effect of caring for survivors of violence on health care providers. In J. M. Liebschutz, S. M. Frayne, & G. N. Saxe (Eds.), *Violence against women: Physician's guide to identification and management* (pp. 157–166). Philadelphia: American College of Physicians.

Saxe, G. N., Stoddard, F., Hall, E., Chawla, N., Lopez, C., Sheridan, R., et al. (2005). Pathways to PTSD, Part I: Children with burns. *American Journal of Psychiatry, 162*(7), 1299–1304.

Schiller, D., Levy, I., Niv, Y., LeDoux, J. E., & Phelps, E. A. (2008). From fear to safety and back: Reversal of fear in the human brain. *Journal of Neuroscience, 28*(45), 11517–11525.

Taylor, L., Zuckerman, B., Harik, V., & Groves, B. (1994). Exposure to violence among inner city children. *Journal of Developmental and Behavioral Pediatrics, 15,* 120.

Terr, L. (1990). *Too scared to cry: Psychic trauma in childhood.* New York: Basic Books.

U.S. Department of Health and Human Services. (1999). *Mental health: A report of the Surgeon General.* Rockville, MD: U.S. Department of Health and Human Services, Substance Abuse and Mental Health Services Administration, Center for Mental Health Services, National Institutes of Health, National Institute of Mental Health.

U.S. Department of Health and Human Services, Administration for Children and Families, Administration on Children, Youth, and Families, Children's Bureau. (2013). Child maltreatment 2012. Available from *www.acf.hhs.gov/programs/cb/research-data-technology/statistics-research/child-maltreatment.*

von Hippel, E. (2005). *Democratizing innovation.* Cambridge, MA: MIT Press.

Index

Page numbers followed by *f* indicate figure; *t* indicate table